WHAT
WHEN
WINE

A NO-EFFORT,
GOOD FOOD
DIET

FAST A LITTLE,
EAT A LOT

RAISE A GLASS!

WHAT
WHEN
WINE

Lose Weight and Feel Great
with Paleo-Style Meals,
Intermittent Fasting, and Wine

MELANIE AVALON

Foreword by Sarah Fragoso

THE COUNTRYMAN PRESS
A division of W. W. Norton & Company
Independent Publishers Since 1923

Foreword by Sarah Fragoso, international best-selling author of the Everyday Paleo cookbook collection

For information about permission to reproduce selections from this book, write to Permissions, The Countryman Press, 500 Fifth Avenue, New York, NY 10110

For information about special discounts for bulk purchases, please contact W. W. Norton Special Sales at specialsales@wwnorton.com or 800-233-4830

Manufacturing by Versa Press
Book design by Ellen Cipriano
Production manager: Devon Zahn

The Countryman Press
www.countrymanpress.com

A division of W. W. Norton & Company, Inc.
500 Fifth Avenue, New York, NY 10110
www.wwnorton.com

978-1-68268-203-6 (pbk.)

10 9 8 7 6 5 4 3 2 1

For my parents.
Thanks for providing the ingredients
so I could bake the proverbial (gluten-free) cake.
Love you more, most, so much!!

Contents

Melanie's FYI

Hi new friends!

I wrote this book to hopefully enhance your life, but let's be real: I don't actually know anything about you. I don't know whether you're just hoping to lose weight or whether you're looking to change your whole dietary lifestyle permanently. I don't know whether you have any genetic or medical conditions, allergies, or predispositions that perhaps make it a *not so good* idea for you to change your diet at the moment, practice fasting, drink wine, or do any of the other things I recommend in this book. Only you can know that. (And I'm *all about* finding what works for *you* personally!) So here are some very basic guidelines that I strongly encourage you to read as you consider implementing some or all of the steps that I discuss in this book:

IF YOU ARE DIABETIC, PREGNANT, OR NURSING: Please do not fast or drink alcohol unless you have been advised by a physician or other qualified health care provider that it is safe for you to do so. Consulting your doctor (more on that in a bit!) is particularly important if you suffer from any health condition or are experiencing any symptoms that may require treatment.

READING THIS BOOK: I know it's tempting to skip some stuff and read the chapters or sections that sound like they will have the biggest or most immediate impact on your life. And I freely confess that I may have gone off the deep end in describing so many studies (especially the ones on rats and mice). But I beg you to *read the whole book* before you act on any of my suggestions. First of all, this book describes multiple interacting lifestyle changes. Second, I sprinkle super vital pieces of information throughout the book. Some of this info may be *really key* for you, in terms of how you may react to these practices. Maybe that *one super important piece of info for you* is in one of the Q&A sections . . . or maybe it's in the "The Tipsy Elephants in the Room" chapter . . . or maybe it's on that *one random page you didn't read because you got distracted by life*. You just won't know unless you read everything, ya know?

MEDICAL CONSENSUS (OR LACK THEREOF): Not surprisingly, there are disagreements among doctors, nutritionists, and others about much of what I'm suggesting. Not everyone thinks intermittent fasting is a good idea, and for sure not everyone recommends drinking wine regularly, let alone daily! I've tried to point out where there are debates or contradictory studies, but unless I mention a study that contradicts the ones I discuss, I'm not aware of any.

CONSULTING YOUR DOCTOR: Please consult your doctor before you do anything—before you change your diet, before you start fasting, before you start (or increase) drinking, before you take any supplements, before you hit the gym like a warrior . . . anything!

CONSULTING YOUR DOCTOR (AGAIN): Consult your doctor if you have started to do any of the things I recommend and you begin to feel physically sick, tired, or mentally stressed out beyond just longing for your next meal (although that should totally stop happening once you adapt to intermittent fasting). The point of this book is to help you feel *good*, savvy?

WHAT TO EAT: Because everyone is different, I can give you guidelines about which foods have been shown to yield positive or harmful effects (oh hey, the whole "What?" section!), but I simply cannot tell you which exact foods are going to work best for *you*. I also can't know which foods you may be personally allergic or sensitive to. (So please keep that in mind when cooking any of the delicious recipes.) You have to figure all this out for yourself with self-experimentation. Which is sort of the theme of this book, and also where the fun begins! Yay for finding *your* perfect dietary protocol!

HOW MUCH TO EAT: For the same reasons, it's also pretty much impossible for me to recommend exactly *how much* of anything to eat, be it carbs, protein, fat, micronutrients, or total calorie intake. All I can do is encourage you to eat super nutritiously to satiety. If you'd like the official stance on the matter, check out the government's recommended dietary guidelines (health.gov/dietaryguidelines) and dietary reference intakes (ods.od.nih.gov/Health_Information/Dietary_Reference_Intakes.aspx).

HOW MUCH TO DRINK: Here in the United States, a "glass of wine" is usually five ounces. That said, different countries often use other standards, while the individual wines themselves can have different percentages of alcohol. So, when you read studies that involved people drinking "a glass" of wine, that "glass" may be smaller or larger than five ounces, and we likely don't even know how much alcohol the specific wine contained, to boot!

HOW MUCH TO EXERCISE: You should only exercise to the level of your own ability, even if you're just doing the few routines I suggest, like HIIT or wearing weights to the grocery store. If you've never exercised, then it could be a really bad idea to suddenly go crazy, especially if you're new to fasting as well. Plus, I'm *much* more a fan of getting your "exercise" from life, rather than potentially overexerting yourself at the gym anyway.

BRANDED PRODUCTS: Although I mention some branded products, including some that I take myself, I am not endorsing any particular brand *for you*. I can't say enough times that you have to try the things that appeal to you and see which ones make you feel best.

Okie dokie, so with all that cautionary stuff said, bring on #allthethings! You got this!

Melanie Avalon

FOREWORD

BY SARAH FRAGOSO

When I was first introduced to Melanie, we had an instant connection. Melanie has this fire—an innate awesome passion and drive to share her knowledge and experience of dieting. That she's kind and genuinely caring is instantly obvious and special! Plus, she's funny, and I'm a sucker for someone with a sense of humor.

I've been in the Paleo world for a really long time—some would even consider me to be the matriarch of the ancestral health movement (but please give me a few more years before you call me the grandmother . . .), and I've had the pleasure of seeing what used to be a fairly small circle of folks blogging and writing about Paleo turn into more websites, books, and "experts" then you can shake a stick at. The birth of my first book, *Everyday Paleo*, happened almost ten years ago, and it was the first Paleo cookbook and lifestyle guide to hit the market. There are now so many amazing resources out there; however, there's a lot of convoluted information as well, not just with Paleo but also with dieting advice in general. Melanie is one of the few who cuts through the cloudy, murky, crazy-laden diet world to give us some real useful tools to live by.

I'm not easily impressed when it comes to folks who are out there talking about Paleo; but Melanie—she's a gal who has done her homework, has lived this lifestyle, and has made it work for herself in an amazing way, and her passion is to share it with others in a fashion that just works!

Furthermore, she can back up what she's saying. I'm not a science gal by nature, but I personally want to know why I'm doing something as it pertains to my body, how it works, and when I'm supposed to do the thing I'm doing. Melanie covers all of these important bases in this book. *What* to eat (Paleo diet basics), *when* to eat (intermittent fasting)—and *wine*??? YES!! You see, Melanie is offering this thing called balance, BUT she's also giving you some serious scientific guidelines when it comes to the topic of intermittent fasting (IF) and, at the same time, she's also not giving you a one-size-fits-all perspective. Melanie offers reality and flexibility, without a bunch of dogma—which is rare in the health world. In this book, Melanie helps you figure out what works for YOU, not simply what works for HER, and she offers all this priceless info with a smart, sassy, fun approach.

Intermittent fasting can sound scary. It sounds like starvation and deprivation, but Melanie takes the fear out of this amazing lifestyle with easy-to-understand explanations of how it works. She also talks about whom this diet is good for, and whom it might not be good for, so once again: no more dogma, just science-backed information that's easy to read and apply to your life. IF is a natural go-to for many in the Paleo world, and some of us even end up doing it by accident! It's not about being miserable or counting calories but about living a natural lifestyle and making your health goals attainable in a busy, crazy, fast-paced world. Melanie even covers fitness in a functional, approachable manner, and as a strength and conditioning coach, it's so refreshing to hear someone suggest a sane approach to fitness rather than another author compelling the reader to "eat less and move more," which is an approach—in my not so humble opinion—that should have died with the dinosaurs . . .

Then there's the recipes and wine, because really, what's life worth living without a glass of wine here or there—and steak . . . with butter!? (Unless you're a plant-loving vegan—in which case, she's still totally got you covered!) I personally love food and consider myself a foodie. I love to cook, and I love to drink wine but I am not a savvy wine drinker. I simply pair red wine with red meat and white wine with fish or chicken. I haven't had the time or burning desire to learn a lot about wine and food pairing, so once again, here's Melanie to save the day! YAY! Now I can be a Paleo foodie and a wine snob (or at least pretend to be one) and that ups my game tremendously—being that my usual go-to bottle is whatever label looks cool (which, I know, I know, is so not cool.) Melanie also extensively covers the idea that drinking wine can be a healthy addition to life for many of us—so now I officially love her forever, and after you read this book I promise you will too!

What When Wine will show you how to kick-start your metabolism, rev up fat loss, and live a natural, healthy lifestyle without all the stress, hunger, and fuss typically associated with dieting. Your crazed, unhappy, hungry diet days will be a thing of the past. You'll end up with increased health, vitality, and a newfound zest for life. And steak. And butter. And WINE! Enjoy!

Introduction

A NEW WORLD

Sin and atonement color the Dieting World of Old: a place where we wear our past meals as scarlet letters and shudder at satiety's implications of *fat storage*. A world where we attempt to kill cravings with unfulfilling surrogate snacks, though they consistently leave us feeling suspiciously hungrier. When we do inevitably succumb to our cravings—processed temptations scientifically designed to lure our neurotransmitters—we wallow in shame and guilt. We consume decadent meals, only to hastily brush off such indulgences with Instagram filters, suppressing our anxiety with hashtags of #foodporn.

In fear of the creeping scale number, or of nebulous feelings of "bloatedness," we lash ourselves with fat-free salads and merciless cardio. "Take that, self!" we proclaim, hopeful that our willpower will wipe out past indiscretions. We remember *that one time* we successfully restricted for a week, and felt a surge of short-lived accomplishment.

If you're like me, or like the many others I know and could have known, a number of attempted protocols may line your diet resume, each carefully selected with dreams of a fitter figure. Yet despite the discipline they demanded, these promising diets yielded temporary and lackluster results. Like a hamster on a wheel, you may have made suspiciously little progress for your efforts.

Welcome to the paradigm shift.

Behind these proverbial doors awaits a New World, where dieting is a thing of the past. This new world is a place of timeless wisdom based on our biological constitutions, rather than of modern plastic promises that just swindle our money. A world where "hunger" is no longer an ominous wanting but rather a welcomed anticipation of enjoyable food to come. Where mealtime once again nurtures and fulfills, and you eat like a child, without fear, blissfully unaware of how many calories you may be consuming.

Soon you may welcome not only a lighter body but a changed composition, as uninvited deposits of fat, which once adamantly clung to love handles, sneak away in the night. You shall walk by temptations with ease, politely declining incandescently sprinkled cookies with a newfound sense of freedom. You might even indulge in luxurious meals, to the envy of onlookers, while your food scales and body scales collect dust in a corner. Beyond just feeling slimmer, you may experience newfound energy and alertness. Resistance to common ailments. Clearer skin and mind. *Resilience*.

A NEW MINDSET

I invite you to take a moment and evaluate your worldview. The natural state of your body is health, not disease. If your body stubbornly clings to excess weight, it is really grasping for life. Perhaps it's saving up energy reserves for future use, or instigating inflammation to fight dietary and environmental toxins. In any case, it is *not* trying to harm you. We simply don't harbor biological mechanisms geared for intentional self-harm.[1] There's a reason your body does what it does, and I'd wager it is *not* to make you feel fat, ugly, or out of control.

Common restrictive diets dispatch an SOS signal, indicating to our bodies that something is awry. These diets encourage a cellular mindset of jealous fat storage and ravenous appetite. With an absence of adequate nutrients, we spiral downward into a dreadful delirium of desire and discontent. It is my hope that you may switch from a restrictive mindset of punishing your body into weight loss to a mindset of love and abundance that naturally supports a healthy, lean state. Pushing and shoving is not allowed! Soon you shall see your body as friend, not enemy, as you love and savor your meals, which in turn nourish you.

Of course, reaching this state of appreciation may seem difficult at first, as it can feel so natural to mindlessly munch on treats at all hours, never realizing we lost our true appetite somewhere along the way . . .

ABOUT THIS BOOK

In this book, we'll explore the science of common eating patterns, and see why most weight-loss approaches simply don't work. We'll analyze how food affects the body on a foundational level, inviting health or disease depending on *your* personal constitution. We'll look at the reasoning behind the whole "Paleo" thing, and evaluate the scientific support for a historical approach to diet. We'll ascertain how to determine *your* perfect personal Paleo protocol.

We'll also see how eating in time windows—that is, "intermittent fasting" (IF)—can radically regulate metabolic health, generating not only weight loss but a multitude of health benefits. You'll learn how to adopt your own IF pattern that fits your fancy, and I'll address common fears and roadblocks, arming you with knowledge for those times your friends raise a proverbial (if not literal) eyebrow. For our metaphorical dessert, we'll see how alcohol can play a role in a healthy diet, and why you can (and perhaps should!) actually embrace wine as a not-so-guilty pleasure in your life.

Of course, why should you even listen to this Disney-loving blonde actress from Tennessee in the first place? Despite my mother's declarations of "You should be a doctor, Melanie!" I didn't attend medical school. My "official" medical credentials cap at a certification in holistic nutrition from the American Fitness Professionals and Associates, and I hold a double BA in film and theater from the University of Southern California. (Fight on!) That said, I *am* a science and literature geek who reads the conjoined form (scientific literature!) like a *Harry Potter* novel. As a guilty pastime, I binge-read medical journals, absorbing and analyzing all the information I can, laughing yet sighing at the bits of information the researchers often select to generate their persuasive abstracts and conclusions. (We all see what we want to see, now don't we?)

But perhaps most important, these are not approaches I've simply read about in school or looked at through a microscope, but protocols that I've *done*.

That I *do*. I actively and consistently self-experiment. This book is the result of living this lifestyle to find what *actually* works, not what *they* say works. Though I'm constantly trying new things, I've found the stuff worth doing tends to stick. And it's those sticky findings that revolutionized my world, and just may revolutionize yours as well!

Ultimately, I'm here as a resource for you in your journey. Let's be friends! If you have any questions whatsoever, please feel free to contact me—I'd love to hear how your journey goes! You can visit my blog, MelanieAvalon.com, for #allthethings, from free guides to more life ramblings to personal confessions (lots of those!). You can also check out *The Intermittent Fasting Podcast*, which I cohost with fellow intermittent fasting author Gin Stephens (*Delay, Don't Deny: Living an Intermittent Fasting Lifestyle*), if IF ends up rocking your world—which I just bet it might!

So if you're ready to bid a fine farewell to dieting, and say hello to a new you, take a fat-fueled walk with me! (And get ready for quite a few *Wizard of Oz* allusions en route.) You got this!

My Diet History

I first encountered the concept of "dieting" as an elementary school youngster—a time when primary concerns involved grades and sleepovers, and I was not yet tormented with woes of body image, scale numbers, and peer pressure. I was standing in the kitchen of our Sanibel Island summer condo when my aunt informed my mother that my older cousin Jeniffer was "on a diet." She said the words with a disapproving laugh, implying that the choice was simply silly. But as this was a cousin I admired, the idea of being *on a diet* sounded so *grown-up*. I didn't give it much thought beyond that, though it would remain silently etched in my mind.

THE ADOLESCENT YEARS

I soon would enter the "diet" universe—the cool thing to do in burgeoning adolescence. Accompanying middle school's trials and tribulations came a casual but nevertheless perpetual desire to lose weight. While never overweight by official BMI standards, I still eyed photoshopped celebrities with envy, and admired those friends I'd identified as maintaining *perfect* bodies. (Emily, I'm looking at you!) A vague sort of calorie counting and portion control defined my efforts to lose a pound or two. I distinctly remember seeing 110 pounds as ideal, 112 pounds as tolerable, and 113 pounds as wholly unacceptable. Because obviously that makes *so* much sense.

A far more sinister issue overshadowed my superfluous weight-loss desires:

My middle school years were plagued by acne. And I mean plagued. It was the bane of my existence. I flinched in the sunlight, wondering if those girls with flawless complexions appreciated their divine beauty. I loathed my so-called combination skin, dreaming of what it would be like to not panic over the state of one's foundation. I cried when a younger cousin told me my face looked like a volcano, and when a school friend made a "helpful" makeup suggestion to better cover my blemishes. I tried a myriad of topical treatments, and downed antibiotics prescribed for skin ailments. (I now wholeheartedly regret the latter—who knows what damage I did to my poor gut microbiome! More on all that to come.)

Sophomore year of high school, I began taking birth control and Accutane for acne. On the one hand, the drugs worked. Birth control made a dent, and Accutane essentially eradicated the condition. I was trying on dresses for the upcoming Valentine's Sadie Hawkins dance when I noticed something else had changed as well. Though I hadn't mustered up the courage to invite my crush Stewart to the dance, I figured I'd find the *perfect* pink dress to make him jealous. (Apparently I am now revealing my former crushes to the world? Yep. It happens.) In the Macy's dressing room under a pile of rejected gowns, I realized that somewhere along the line, I had jumped up two sizes. While my new size was not "overweight," it nevertheless marked very definite weight gain in a very small period of time, and without any discernible dietary change. I also noticed I was becoming more bloated in general, likely related to the hormone-adjusting pills I'd been popping.

So things got #real.

Calorie counting became the consistent tool in my arsenal, with appetite suppression as the goal. I figured if I could just find that *perfect* low-calorie meal to keep hunger at bay, I could survive until my *next* low-calorie meal to keep hunger at bay. I fostered an unsatisfying crush on microwaved Lean Cuisines. I secretly munched on SlimFast snack bars while studying Dante's Third Circle of Hell (Gluttony!) in honors English. (Shout-out to Coach Carruth!)

Motivation to lose weight intensified when I was accepted to the early-entrance program at USC in Los Angeles—a solid step in my entertainment-industry goals. This also meant I only had junior year of high school to get my act together and shed those lingering pounds. A year of calorie counting, hunger, and struggle later, I found myself at a weight acceptable for my rigid standards when I entered those Californian collegiate doors.

COLLEGE CRAZINESS

Freshman year at USC was a whirl of enthralling environments, new friends, and outstanding possibilities. It was also a time of food. So. Much. Food. Limitless buffets for every meal. Papers fueled by cakes and cookies. After all, there's no better motivation to write *just one more sentence* than making a pit stop at the local snack shop for a giant Coke Zero and a luscious blueberry muffin. Everyone knew the surefire way to draw a crowd to an extracurricular info session was by posting fliers proclaiming FREE PIZZA! Even finals week was marked by seven inspiring nights of food, from Diddy Riese cookies to tacos. Texting your friends, "Wanna get some food?" replaced grade school's "Want to sleep over on Friday?"

So it should come as no surprise that I gained the dreaded freshman fifteen (and then some!). Granted, I hadn't *actively* avoided it, figuring the constant storm of activity and biking to class on my pink beach cruiser would grant protection from any assaults in the weight department. And yet, as I nonchalantly stepped on the bathroom scale that spring break, I saw, to my chagrin, that I weighed 20 pounds more than when I'd left my home in Memphis.

So things, once again, got #real.

I resolved to lose the weight. I would and I could! Thankfully, sophomore year signified the transition from dormitory/dining-hall life to apartment/grocery-shopping life. It was much easier to make wise meal decisions when I was actively deciding what to purchase, compared to grazing at tempting unlimited buffets. Calorie counting returned with a vengeance, and daily life soon revolved around meals. I would wake up and eat breakfast (yum!), then busy myself with other matters until lunch. After lunch (yum!), I would busy myself until dinner. After dinner (yum!), the lovely cushion of sleep would suppress appetite until breakfast, in the whole *I want to keep eating more food, but I guess I can just go to bed and then eat more food in the morning* type way. Typical meals during this period involved carefully measured medleys of lettuce, chicken, and almonds, with low-fat, low-calorie salad dressings; or whole-grain quesadillas, featuring low-fat cheese and sugar-free teriyaki sauce. (I shudder just typing this.) I'd also visit the Lyon Center gym like an exercise Barbie lioness. I'm ashamed to confess I was one of "those girls" who wore a full face of makeup to work out, trying to make it look "natural." On rare occasions, I'd forgo the cosmetics and cover my face with a pink hoodie, avoiding all eye contact.

And I'd step on the scale every morning to see how my constant efforts had (or, more likely, *hadn't*) paid off. But surely this was all healthy, right? I was keeping my metabolism fueled! I was embracing low fat like it was Johnny Depp! I wasn't overeating! Then why wasn't the scale budging . . . and why were my hours of cardio at the gym doing, well, nothing?

So I soldiered on, trying anything and everything I could get my stomach on. I bought into countless ever-new, recycled fad diets, thinking perhaps *this* time I'd find some revolutionary tidbit of information not mentioned in the vast graveyard of similar claims, where tombstones bore epitaphs of HE RAN MORE and SHE ATE LESS. I built up stores of diet pills and thermogenics, which provided a nice caffeine boost and placebo effect, if nothing else. One time, shortly after I had ordered one such specific concoction, I received an email asking me to return the recently recalled product. Seeing this as the *ultimate* testament to its fat-burning power, I stored the sacred bottle away for "special times." I remember telling my best friend, Jason, between belts of "A Whole New World" en route to Disneyland, how I hadn't eaten in twenty-four hours, thanks to the magic pills. (As this was before my intermittent fasting days, this was sort of a big deal.) He responded with, "Melanie, maybe you should stop taking those." Maybe I should have listened, Jason. Maybe I should have listened.

A more serious weight-loss endeavor involved a cookie diet. You heard me right: Cookie. Diet. For around two hundred dollars a month, I received a shipment of specially formulated diet "cookies," in oatmeal raisin, chocolate, and blueberry flavors. The protocol called for eating six cookies spread over breakfast and lunch, followed by a healthy dinner. In reality, I usually ended up eating all the cookies all at once—with perhaps an extra thrown in—and the boxes rarely lasted the full thirty days. Diet. Fail. (This was clearly in my pre-

Paleo days, as I now grimace at the idea of willingly ingesting such processed concoctions, with their long list of grainy ingredients. Yikes.)

Then there was the obligatory fling with the ultimate playboy in the dieting world: Mr. Vegetarianism. For our marriage ceremony at a newly opened restaurant by USC, I carefully selected an appropriate dinner salad, drawn to the fittingly romantic "Green Goddess" dressing. My attempted meat abstinence was embarrassingly short-lived—I lasted maybe a week, at most. I don't even remember when I decided to once again let animal flesh grace my lips. As a self-proclaimed lover of *moments*, such amnesia is telling. (To my vegetarian readers, I still love you! I'm just an omnivore at heart.)

I even ventured into the world of hCG drops, sublingually administering the human chorionic gonadotropin hormone while following a severely calorie-restricted diet. The idea was to convince my body it was pregnant, encouraging it to willingly tap into stored body fat to support a (nonexistent) baby. I'll leave it at that. Ridiculously low-calorie intake aside, the diet was essentially whole foods in nature, since I basically just ate chicken and lettuce, with the occasional apple. My appetite did, in fact, diminish, though I'm not sure if that was due to the drops or the placebo effect. In any case, I did lose some weight on the protocol, though I suppose it's hard *not* to on 500 calories a day!

THE LOW-CARB WORLD

One night late sophomore year, I stumbled upon a concept called *ketosis* in the depths of a low-carb forum. At this point, a lone memory defined "low-carb" for me. In high school, on the way to play practice for *It's a Wonderful Life* (I played Violet), my dear friend Katie had explained the stupidity of the low-carb Atkins diet, in which she could eat a steak but not a carrot. I remember thinking to myself, *Yep, that's pretty stupid.*

Yet as I read on the forum about the sciencey mechanisms at play, the whole "low-carb" thing seemed a *smidge* less stupid. According to the logic, weight loss wasn't so much about calories as it is about macronutrients. Drastically reducing carbs could make the body go into a nebulous fat-burning state of ketosis, distinguished by the body's production of ketones for fuel. You could even roughly gauge the level of ketones in your system with some spiffy urine analysis strips—like scientifically measuring your fat burning! I found this ridiculously tempting. Who needed questionable body-weight scales when I could get such *telling* results? And so I committed, ordered the Ketostix, and kissed carbohydrates a momentary (or so I thought) goodbye.

Something clicked.

As I entered this elusive "fat-burning" state, evidenced by dark pink analysis strips, my body seemed to finally *get it*. Lack of calorie counting aside, I just *felt* like I was finally tapping into stored fat. My appetite dwindled. I no longer hungrily awaited meals. Unlike with previous diets, my energy levels, mood, and even my skin improved. I gained enough confidence to go out in public *without* makeup. (This is huge.) Perhaps there was something to the whole "diet" thing beyond dieting? It was like seeing the forest for the trees, whereas before I'd been fixating on squirrels.

Despite my narrow weight-loss focus widening to a more science-based view of metabolism, a new neurosis arose: Carb counting slyly replaced calorie counting. I continued to judge food by its label, now identifying grams of sugar rather than number of calories. While I didn't give a second thought to ingesting *hundreds* of grams of fat, I'd break a sweat at the idea of consuming an extra carb or two, convinced that such actions would throw my body into sugar-burning mode and reroute my meals into fat storage.

INTERMITTENT FASTING

One night junior year, my all-too-familiar Internetland procrastinations (now often replete with low-carb research) led me to a life-changing page: Rusty Moore's "Lose Body Fat by Eating Just One Meal Per Day?" The blog post explored a radical idea of eating the majority (if not all) of one's daily sustenance in the evening for weight loss, as originally discussed in Ori Hofmekler's *The Warrior Diet*. Hundreds of reader comments testified success. (I literally read each and every one at the time.)

This idea was a bit absurd. After all, everyone knew breakfast was the most important meal of the day! Whenever I went too long between meals, I felt guilty. If my appetite oddly vanished, I took it as a sign that my metabolism had abandoned ship. Yet after reading this post, I reevaluated such actions with newfound perspective. After all, calorie counting was the first lesson of Dieting 101, and that hadn't exactly panned out. On the other hand, my low-carb regimen rich in "unhealthy" fat was granting me an insane amount of success. Why not continue flying in the face of common wisdom? So despite my skepticism, I committed, resolving to consume one giant meal per day, for a week. I could do anything for a week, right? What harm could it bring?

For my first date with the stranger I would soon know as intermittent fasting, I selected a day I'd be busy on the film set of my talented friend Carmen. I devoured a large preparatory meal the night before, and awoke to a new dawn, armed with a hunger-combating arsenal of coffee and adrenaline. On set, I took a silent pride in willingly forgoing the catered pizza, instead sipping on one (or ten) teas from crafty—film lingo for the perpetual snack station. Oddly enough, I survived. I went home that evening and ate to my heart's content, laying my head to rest with the satisfaction of a diet job well done.

As the week continued, my intermittent fasting acquaintance morphed into the dietary pal "IF." While I had never been much of a breakfast person, aside from the processed pleasures of Pop-Tarts and a weird, brief obsession with instant cheesy mashed potatoes and cherry Coke Zero, I soon found similar ease in forgoing lunch as well. I liked how my day was no longer needlessly interrupted by food. Rather than furiously biking to my apartment between classes for rushed meals I'd barely taste, I spent the time tackling film readings, contentedly looking forward to the night's cathartic feast. When I hit my one-week goal, I saw no logical reason to stop. So I didn't. Instead, I dove headfirst into the scientific literature, seeking explanations for why bits of fasting were inviting not only weight loss but feelings of vitality.

Yet intermittent fasting hid its own demon. Unlike low-carb, which I'd gladly explain to interested third parties, I felt the need to keep IF a secret, fearing ostracizing accusations of disordered eating. Thankfully, my go-to diet buddy, Ben, decided to try IF as well, and the partnership replaced self-stamped brands of #loner with #team. My glowing skin and newfound energy supplied further validation, as visits to the campus health center dissipated, and weight loss accelerated. All the tricky little blips on my body, the ones I'd simply accepted as part of my constitution, began to evanesce, creating the intangible difference between feeling thinner and feeling *lean*.

The longer I continued intermittent fasting, the more confident I felt uttering its name. The more days I put behind me, the more my testimony seemed somewhat valid, since clearly I wasn't (to my knowledge) falling over dead from starvation. One semester became many semesters, and many semesters became a lifestyle.

PALEO

Intermittent fasting carried me smoothly through my upperclassman years, graduation, and initiation into adult life. As I settled into my first post-USC apartment in Hollywood (Yes, I *literally* lived in Hollywood), I beamed with the overwhelming excitement of finally pursuing my acting dreams "for real." On one warm afternoon that summer, my aforementioned diet pal Ben texted me about the Paleo diet. Though I had occasionally encountered the concept when it overlapped with the low-carb and IF communities, I had never really considered it, figuring that my low-carb fasting was "good enough."

The Paleo diet, however, took things a step further, advocating complete whole-foods consumption, to mimic the diet of humans before the advent of agriculture, when, supposedly, everything went a bit south. Going Paleo would mean forgoing all grains, legumes, processed foods, and potentially dairy, which apparently encouraged inflammation and disease in the body. I'd have to bid farewell to such pleasures as artificial sweeteners, processed low-carb goodies, and the divine beauty of cream cheese. Honestly, I didn't see how cutting out such items could make *that* much of a difference, as I'd bestowed the majority of the blame for ill health upon sugar. Many Paleo people also consumed carb levels way beyond my comfort zone. Yet this Paleo carrot was just too tempting, so in the name of self-experimentation, I once again decided to #commit. I promptly picked up a copy of Robb Wolf's *The Paleo Solution*, constructed a Mulan-themed poster outlining the approach (gotta love that beginning transformation scene!), tacked it to my refrigerator, and dove in.

If low-carb opened my eyes and IF bought me contacts, Paleo was like getting Lasik eye surgery. My energy further improved, any remaining headaches vanished, and my skin began to truly shine. Better yet, the Paleo paradigm gifted me with, ironically, a freer approach to food, compared to my strictly low-carb days. I welcomed back more veggies and fruit into what had become an incredibly meat- and coconut-oil-reliant diet. Eradicating processed Frankenfoods widened my palate to newfound flavor appreciation. I no longer sought seasonings for satisfaction, as seemingly plain whole foods began tasting glorious. While low-carb eradicated the fear of calories and IF killed the fear of weight troubles, Paleo bestowed an invaluable feeling of intuition as I began to understand how certain foods made me *feel*.

There was no going back.

WINE

Of course, there was one more piece of the puzzle to come! Ya see, a miserable night of accidental overindulgence at Film School Prom near the end of my USC years had left me unable to partake of the stiffer stuff for a good six months. While the smell of hard alcohol still conjures feelings of nausea in me to this day, I did begin enjoying a glass of red wine here and there. (I was raised in a wine-appreciating family—shout-out to my dad!) I initially saw such activity as a "cheat" in my diet protocol. However, after extensive research, I realized there truly were a myriad of benefits from red wine consumption, arguably outweighing abstinence. Why cloud something with fear or doubt when it can just be an awesome life enhancer? I'm now a red wine girl through and through! My heart is won with wine, not chocolate.

THE SOCIAL WOES

And so I continued in my Paleo-eating, intermittent-fasting, wine-drinking ways. The dietary outfit particularly suited my initial postgraduation "job": six months working as a background actor on basically every TV show known to mankind, playing everything from a Cheerio cheerleader on *Glee* to an insane patient on *Criminal Minds*. The fasted state perfectly fueled hours of fake talking, silent dancing, mock waitressing, and actual running. (Oh hey, shark-filled tornadoes!) It also assailed the gratuitous food temptations of set life. While lower-budget sets might feature collections of water and peanuts, mainstream TV shows and movies displayed stunning arrays of produce, cheese, meat, sandwiches, cakes, cookies, fruit-infused water coolers, and even the occasional vitamin pack. One set I visited had a shrimp ice sculpture. Shrimp. Ice. Sculpture. And that's just the snacks! Actual set meals were buffet-style, featuring elaborate salad stations, an array of entrées (oh hi, salmon and filet mignon!), as well as many a delectable side. Thankfully, IF nipped this recipe for weight gain in the bud. Freed from appetite, I'd visit crafty, pick up a bottle (or five) of water, and walk away without a second thought. (Though background actors were often sternly reminded that crafy was for snacking, not shopping, I justified my stocking up of water bottles by my lack of food consumption. Of course, I now shudder at all that *plastic*, but such is another issue entirely.) Come actual mealtimes, I'd only partake in "lunch" (so called regardless of whether it was at 9:00 a.m. or 9:00 p.m—which *did* happen) when it aligned with dinner.

Being on set 24/7 also meant interacting with new people for long periods of time, occasionally forming long-lasting friendships in the process. (Here's looking at you, Kellie!) Both fortunately and unfortunately, my meal choices often became evident, especially on the all-too-common days that crept near the sixteen-hour mark (officially known in the film world as "golden time" thanks to *über* boosted pay rates!) near the end of my fast.

THE CULMINATING EFFECT

While I loved discussing Paleo and intermittent fasting with interested parties, I didn't love my vague "Well, studies show that . . ." response. I needed a solid reference. I was also becoming a bit worn out by the skeptics, especially those accusing souls *convinced* I was engaging in lunatic behavior, and who made it their temporary goal to right my ways. So I resolved to research everything and set proverbial pen to paper, the incarnation of which became the initial, self-published form of this book, *The What When Wine Diet: Paleo and Intermittent Fasting for Health and Weight Loss.* I was overjoyed with the overwhelmingly positive reader feedback. I was no longer alone in my diet journey!

That was a few years ago, and the passing time, growing audience, new-found experiences, and expanding research—coupled with signing with my dream literary agent (the first time I ever *actually* cried from happiness; the second time will likely be if I ever sign with CAA)—collectively lead to where I am now: creating this updated dream version of the book, with a dream publisher and dream editor. While not much has changed for me foundationally since writing the original version (I'm still a wine-loving, Paleo, intermittent-faster gal!), some of my opinions have evolved. I pray that I never become locked in my ways, and always welcome new research, ideas, and findings with open arms. This resulting *What When Wine* features about 80 percent new content (basically a new book!), expanding substantially on all the topics and addressing common questions I've received since the original version.

But enough about me. Let's jump into the nitty-gritty of the power of food, so we can make it work for *you*! I hope you may find some clarity between these pages, as well as a lifestyle that perfectly suits your fancy. You are your own self-experimenter with your own colorful diet history, and only *you* can know what works best for *your* body. So raise a glass to your health and waistline! You got this!

How It All Went Awry

The average person stores enough body fat to fuel a walk of one thousand miles. Unless you're Vanessa Carlton, that seems pretty far to me. This invites the question: With all this fat just waiting around to be used, why is it so difficult to actually burn the stuff?

This fat-burning perplexity arises from our body's intrinsic preference for both fat use and fat storage, which developed in a time of alternating feast and famine. While I don't want to go super loincloth-sporting, out of left field with proclamations of "We are cavemen!" I *would* like to point out the vast difference between how humankind *used* to acquire, eat, store, and burn food, and how humankind *now* acquires, eats, stores, and burns food. This foundational shift not only spells immediate trouble for our health and waistlines, it also elucidates why your potential weight struggles are totally not your fault.

A HISTORICAL PERSPECTIVE

Don't worry, this book isn't a history textbook in disguise—I promise! I just want to briefly show where your body is coming from, so you can adjust where it's going. In the generally accepted evolutionary timeline, humans solidified their genotype somewhere between 600,000 and 25,000 BC.[2] The whole "genotype" thing involves the foundational blueprint for how the body functions, including its interactions with food and the environment. As hunter-gatherers during this genotype-determining era, we spent a great amount of time hunting and gathering our food, appropriately enough. We also oscillated between times of food scarcity and food aplenty.[3] Without a predictable supply of food,[4] our bodies developed mechanisms for body-fat storage. We could eat food (in the form of animals, fruits, nuts, and root veggies), store the leftovers as body fat, and be prepared for times when food wasn't readily available. Yay us!

During this time, our brains neurologically adapted to encourage consumption of energy-rich foods, such as sugar and fat. We didn't have to worry about "overeating," since food simply wasn't available in massive, easily accessible quantities *to* overeat. At the same time, our fat deposits were not unsightly blemishes to be erased at all cost, but rather, valued supplies of energy necessary for survival. We were on #teambodyfat, which was not a burden but a backup battery!

TODAY

Today's environment warps our body's good intentions for fat storage. We are now surrounded by easily accessible, hyperpalatable foods that require no substantial time or energy to attain, yet which supply a vast amount of energy. Though meal composition and availability have changed, our genetic preferences for what to *do* with this food have not. Our bodies, unaware of mealtime's now-perpetual nature, readily store food as body fat, while still keeping us hankering for more . . . for our "survival." No good deed goes unpunished! Even worse, many of these "foods" distress our digestive systems or are even toxic in nature, leading to inflammation, deteriorating health, and weight gain.

THE CURSE OF HYPERPALATABILITY

In *Charlie and the Chocolate Factory*, a magical candy factory churns out glistening pieces of addiction in colorful wrappers. You may remember the ill-fated nincompoop Augustus Gloop—an obese child whose greedy appetite led to his demise, when (spoiler alert!) he could not resist the forbidden chocolate river . . . and its purification tubes. And so we're left with the Oompa Loompas' piercingly telling dirge, *For who could hate or bear a grudge / Against a luscious bit of fudge?* As the rest of the children succumb to the factory's temptations, their lack of control—despite the promise of inheriting the *entire* factory if they can just resist—illustrates the allure of modern food treats. (Although perhaps the children's health was ultimately spared by *not* inheriting this colorful candy world, but such theses are for another day!)

Indeed, processed food goodies can be ridiculously hard to resist, encouraging consumption even at the expense of one's vitality. Trust me, I'm with you all the way to the concession stand! Is it any wonder, then, that the rise of such concoctions mirrors the rise of the obesity epidemic,[5] with Americans growing fatter and fatter in the presence of more delicious instant food choices, microwave meals, and fast-food chains, all fueled by fervent advertising? Sugar consumption has also notably tripled from 4 percent to 12 percent of Americans' diets in a mere few generations.

The sweetened, refined nature of processed foods, coupled with chemicals added to "enhance" flavor, generate addictive properties rivaling those of illegal drugs, triggering cravings, loss of control, and compulsive overuse despite negative ramifications. They stimulate the release of feel-good neurotransmitters and hormones such as dopamine and opioids in the mesocorticolimbic reward center of our brain, encouraging us to ravenously reach for another hit, even in the absence of any actual hunger, and even when we know we'll feel like manure in a few hours. (Shout-out to that moment when you're totally stuffed, yet all of the sudden "magically" have room for dessert!) Some studies even observe that rodents prefer sweetened sugar solutions to cocaine (including rodents who used to *love* them some cocaine!), while other rodents willingly chow down on hyperpalatable foods despite being shocked.

Since we're biologically predisposed to seek out high-calorie sweet and fatty foods in preparation for "starvation," we're kinda screwed[6] when we're surrounded by these addicting goods 24/7,[7] as our bodies simply aren't equipped to judge the large number of highly absorbable, nutrientless calories they provide.[8] When we taste a soft drink/soda/pop (depending on your geographic location), our body proclaims, "Sweet thing! Good for us! Drink more!" as though it were a nutritious apple, unaware that we're actually ingesting around 140 calories, 39 grams of sugar, and nothing good besides fleeting happy feelings. With no nutrition attained (think vitamins, protein, healthy fats, etc.), our bodies keep demanding more, encouraging increased snacking, larger portion sizes, and growing bellies. We do, effectively, eat ourselves to death.

THE CURSE OF ACCESSIBILITY

Not only are we surrounded by yummy food 24/7, we also expend negligible energy to get it. Consider eating a steak. As a hunter-gatherer, you'd seek out an animal, chase it down, kill it, and construct a fire to roast it. That's a pretty big task. As a modern human, you order a steak at a restaurant, perfectly prepared to your liking, and wait for it while sipping on wine with friends. Or perhaps you exert a *smidge* more effort and pick up a raw steak from the store. If you want to get really rustic, you might go camping and grill it or something.

Or consider the vegetarian side of things. As a hunter-gatherer, you'd invest a considerable amount of time and energy picking fruit, digging up root vegetables, or gathering and shelling nuts. (It takes a *lot* of nut shelling to produce even a small handful of nuts—just saying.) You were also restricted to whatever fruits and nuts were actually in season. As for grains? They were inedible fields, not loaves of bread.

What happens today? You walk into a magical place called the grocery store, with its radiant display of produce, oblivious to the seasons, and naked nuts asleep in glistening plastic packages. The fields of grains have magically transformed into packages of refined flour. The effort to acquire all these plants involves swiping a credit card. Not much pain for a *whole lot of gain*.

THE CURSE OF ENTERTAINMENT

Food has also transitioned from nutrition to fuel life's activities to an activity in and of itself. For evidence of our growing fixation with food, look no further than art and popular culture. A 2010 quantitative study of fifty-two artistic depictions of Leonardo da Vinci's *The Last Supper* found that the *food* in the pictures has increased in size by 68 percent over the last decade.[9] Instagram accounts parade photos of #foodporn. In the popular bath-and-body industry, products once scented with inedible flowers and ocean breezes now emit aromas of birthday cake and tiramisu.

Yep, food is the cool kid on the block. We use it to entertain ourselves, deal with stress, self-medicate, make friends, and express love. We eat brownies rather than meditate, placate noisy children with treats, center celebrations around fanciful cakes, and pick out restaurants like movies.

CURING THE ADDICTION

Thankfully, despite all the curses, a cure exists! Adopting historical dietary patterns of food choices (Paleo-style whole foods) and/or timing of meals (intermittent fasting) can revert the body to its natural fat-burning state. This frees up fat stores, and frees *you* from the curse of cravings. You may be surprised at how quickly your body adapts to the way it was always meant to function, as hunger fades away and body fat bids farewell. Are you excited? I know I am!

The Calorie Conundrum

Oh, calories. The bane of existence. And yet the fuel of existence. Such irony. In the grand scheme of Paleo and fasting things, calories shouldn't even *be* a thing. However, since calorie fixation runs rampant, I'd like to tackle the issue right from the get-go, so we can move on to more pressing matters. Yes, calories do matter. But no, a calorie is not a calorie.

WHAT IS A CALORIE?

We tend to massively oversimplify the concept of calories. We read the calorie section of a nutrition label like it holds the secret to the food's ultimate destination after we eat it. In reality, the colloquial "calorie" is a misleading concept for a complicated process.

A calorie signifies a unit of heat, and refers to how much energy a food provides. Common diet wisdom chants, "Calories in versus calories out!" Translation: Eat fewer calories than you burn, and you will lose weight; eat more calories than you burn, and you will gain weight. True, when all's said and done, weight gain and weight loss *does* involve whether you burned or stored your calories—what determines such burning and storing is another beast entirely.

Let us reflect on the first law of thermodynamics, which you may remember from high school chemistry. (Shout-out to Coach V!) According to this conservation law, energy cannot be created or destroyed. In other words, the energy from calories has to *go* somewhere; it cannot simply "disappear." No arguments there. This means, as discussed, that if you take in more energy (calories) than you burn, you will gain weight. If you burn more energy (calories) than you take in, you will lose weight. Simple, right?

Well . . . not so much.

If it were *only* a matter of counting calories, then calorie-restricted diets would *always* produce the calculated weight change. We really would be able to achieve our intended weight via the latest calorie-counting app. Yet calorie-restricted diets rarely result in the predicted weight loss. Studies (not to mention life) show that people often lose very small amounts of weight despite severe calorie restriction, and people may gain weight with little, if any, overconsumption.[10]

A tightly controlled 2003 pilot study[11] compared three groups:

1. Men who ate 1,800 calories and women who ate 1,500 calories on a low-fat diet.
2. Men who ate 1,800 calories and women who ate 1,500 calories on a low-carb diet.
3. Men who ate 2,100 calories and women who ate 1,800 calories on a low-carb diet.

Now, if all calories were equal, then the low-carb and low-fat diets of identical calorie amounts (#1 and #2) should have yielded the same amount of weight loss, and the higher-calorie, low-carb diet (#3) should have resulted in less weight loss, right? But what actually happened? The low-fat group (#1) lost an average of 17 pounds, the low-carb group that ate the same number of calories (#2) lost an average of 23 pounds, and the higher-calorie low-carb group (#3) lost an average of 20 pounds.

What gives?

While "a calorie is a calorie" doesn't violate the first law of thermodynamics, it *does* muddle the second law of thermodynamics. This law, involving entropy, basically says that in a chemical reaction, an unpredictable amount of energy will be lost as heat. It doesn't disappear; it just goes somewhere else. Simply stating that "a calorie is a calorie" does not account for all the many places the energy from a calorie may *go*, which aren't always fat stores.

FACTORS AFFECTING CALORIES

To further demystify things, let's look at a few of the many factors potentially affecting calorie destination.

TYPES OF CALORIES

While technically all calories are equal, not all calories are equal *in the way our bodies see them*. The "version" in which calories exist in different foods affects their ultimate level of assimilation in the body, referred to as their *metabolic advantage*,[12] and includes the thermic effect of food—the amount of energy required to process calories in the first place.[13] Around 20 to 30 percent of protein calories, 10 to 30 percent of alcohol calories, 5 to 10 percent of carbohydrate calories, and 0 to 3 percent of fat calories are "burned" just from digestion. This means if you ate a 500-calorie meal of *pure* protein, you'd likely end up with fewer calories available for fat storage than if you ate a 500-calorie meal of *pure* carbohydrates. The calories don't disappear; the body simply requires the use of more calories for digestion and assimilation.

Certain calories can also be unlikely candidates for fat storage. Though you may ingest a certain amount of calories from fiber, for example, your body may not *absorb* any of them. On the flip side, you may believe you're taking in a large number of "free" calories via fiber, but your gut bacteria may transform some (or even a lot) of them into butyrate, a type of energy that *is* usable by the body.[14] It all depends on a lot of stuff going on inside us about which we, quite frankly, have little clue at present.

Protein calories are also unlikely fat-storage candidates, since they're preferentially broken down into amino acids used for growth and repair, rather than fuel storage. A 2014 study found that weight-lifting individuals who consumed an average of eight hundred *extra* calories per day in the form of protein *did not gain weight*.[15] While excess dietary protein can be converted into glucose (blood sugar) via gluconeogenesis, the process is costly.[16] Plus, the resulting glucose tends to enter the bloodstream or refill liver glycogen rather than build up fat stores. Given the complexities of macronutrient energy extraction, a 2004 *Nutrition Journal* review even concluded that viewing protein and carbs as similar energy sources is downright contradictory.

Or consider calories from alcohol, which we shall analyze in detail in the "Wine?" section. (So excited!) Despite alcohol calories being viewed as diet busters, studies consistently show that these calories themselves do *not* readily contribute to weight gain, even when added in excess. While the energy from such calories does not "disappear," it can clearly go somewhere other than fat stores.

BODY "SET POINT"

In addition to calorie composition, a number of other uncontrollable controlling factors influence how our meals are used and stored in the body. Despite fluctuating calorie intakes and energy expenditure, the body tends to cling to a certain weight, or "body set point." Over a few months, a person's weight typically fluctuates by a super low 0.5 percent. Longer periods of time tend to show similarly little change in weight. In the body, homeostasis is the name of the game, number of calories consumed aside.

While this set point is not completely understood, many factors may influence it, including fluctuations in insulin sensitivity, activity in the central nervous system, regulation by the hypothalamus,[17] and concentrations of various hormones (like ghrelin and leptin) and genetics.[18] One study found that when multiple pairs of twins were fed the same number of excess calories, the amount of weight gained varied dramatically between different pairs of twins (by around 8 to 30 pounds!), yet was very similar within pairs of twins.[19]

The body may also initiate metabolic processes to maintain an energy balance. Controlled-calorie studies find that underfeeding can decrease physical activity, the resting metabolic rate, and even the thermic effect of meals. On the flip side, overfeeding can decrease appetite while increasing total energy expenditure, thermogenesis, and a drive toward more physical activity. (By the way, the body does tend to more adamantly safeguard against weight loss than weight gain, making conventional dieting all the more difficult.)

NEAT

Nonexercise activity thermogenesis refers to all the unconscious movement you do as a part of daily life. (Basically, any movement that isn't "exercise.") Examples include fidgeting, laughing, standing up straight, or just walking around with energy and purpose! A 1986 metabolic-ward study estimated that NEAT could account for 100 to 800 calories burned per day,[20] while a 2014 study reckoned this could reach up to 2,000 calories per day in lucky individuals![21] People who have epic NEAT regulation may resist weight gain, even when overeating, by increased NEAT. Due to its vague nature, NEAT throws a wrench in calculating a person's calories burned for the day.

THE GUT MICROBIOME

As a final frontier, the gut microbiome may radically influence things, creating intestinal conditions that extract more or fewer calories from food. For example, studies suggest that both rats and humans with more Firmicutes bacteria in their gut tend to weigh more than those with more Bacteroides bacteria.[22] Transferring gut bacteria from obese mice to lean mice can even make the lean mice gain weight, with no change in calorie intake! Of course, studies are at times conflicting, and we know very little about the intricate inner workings of gut bacteria populations, but I think it's safe to say that such gut bugs play a role in how our bodies process calories, for better or worse.

THE TAKEAWAY

The number of calories you technically consume says very little about how the body *actually* uses the calories, or how many calories are even in the running for fat storage. A pessimist might view this as confirmation of the hopelessness of dieting, in which the body resists all valiant efforts at weight loss. (If we could just count calories, things would be so easy!) On the contrary, I prefer an optimist's interpretation. Given the varying effects of calories and the body's metabolic responses to them, why fixate on the whole business in the first place? It's a red herring, misdirecting vital focus and taking away your power. To gain control, you simply must change your approach by choosing foods that support metabolism and energy expenditure, and hormonally set up your body to burn fat on a cellular level. Your body will want to burn fat, and you'll break up with calories like they were never a thing. (Cue Taylor Swift song.)

WHAT?

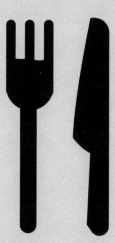

WHAT IS PALEO?

The "what" of *What When Wine* refers to the semi-new (but quickly aging) celeb diet on the block masquerading by the svelte name of "Paleo." Yes, the Paleo diet *does* refer to the prehistoric Paleolithic era. But no, it is *not* an anachronistic historical reenactment in which you live your life like a caveman (unless that's your thing, of course).

Paleo does not mandate sticking to a definite food type, calorie number, or macro list, or only eating things available to a girl or guy who was alive 2.5 million years ago. Rather, a Paleo approach helps you identify the foods that are simply incompatible with your body, yielding a toxic effect (however sly it may be) that deteriorates health and invites degenerative disease. While some foods tend to do this across the board (hi, grains!), others depend on one's personal constitution, thanks to a myriad of factors to be discussed. So despite the implications of skeptical news reports and increasingly commercialized Paleo goodies, Paleo is not a diet fad but rather a lifestyle—a holistic approach to health, seeking the whole foods on which our bodies thrive.

What does this entail? In general, a Paleo template embraces an abundance of hearty, delicious whole foods, while eliminating inflammatory grains, added sugars, and processed or refined foods. More questionable Paleo categories include dairy, legumes, plants such as nightshades, and alcohol. (Although I'm obviously slightly on board with that last one.) To simplify things, think natural. If it's an animal, then it's Paleo. If it's a plant or vegetable naturally existing in the wild and you can pick it and eat it without any problem, then it's probably Paleo. Otherwise . . . debatably not Paleo. If it contains unpronounceable ingredients sounding like they came from a lab . . . definitely not Paleo.

Now that we've got the basics out of the way, let's jump into the logic and scientific reasoning for the Paleo diet! Blind faith can be dangerous, and it'd be a farce if I just presented you with a food list with no explanation or reasoning. Time to explore *why* what you eat matters . . . because it truly does!

THE HISTORY STUFF

Around ten thousand years ago with the Neolithic Revolution came a concept called agriculture. On the plus side, this signaled awesome advancements for mankind. With a more reliable, grain-based food supply, we humans could now settle down from our previous hunter-gatherer ways and invest our energy in wondrous technological and lifestyle advances. #Winning.

But dark things accompanied our new table setting. We stopped hunting and gathering whole foods we'd been consuming for thousands of years, and began chowing down on foods foreign to our bodies.[1] Despite this relatively abrupt shift in diet from the Paleolithic period, our bodies have developed minimal genetic adaptations for the consumption of these new food sources.[2] As a result, we ingest things that often don't register as food but rather as toxins, heralding many of the health concerns we have today: degenerative diseases and autoimmune conditions, diabetes and obesity, heart disease, arthritis, and even cancer. To name a few.

How can what we eat encourage disease? Many non-Paleo "foods" can wreak havoc on our digestive system, inhibiting nutrient absorption and instigating systemic inflammation. This plunges the body into a state of panic, resulting in autoimmune diseases in which the body confuses "invader" proteins with its *own* proteins and creates antibodies against itself. (Talk about shooting yourself in the foot!) Many non-Paleo foods can also cause insulin levels to skyrocket, which promotes fat storage, diabetes, obesity, and all the problems that arrive with them.

Let's break things down a bit, shall we? (No pun intended.)

WHAT IS DISEASE?

Disease refers to maladies suffered by the body, and it includes infectious diseases, from external sources, and degenerative diseases, which originate within the body.

Infectious diseases come from pesky pathogens such as viruses, bacteria, and fungi, with examples including the common cold, flu, measles, and chicken pox. (If you want to get dark and historical, think the bubonic plague.) Infectious diseases may be prevented and treated with vaccines (though I realize that's a touchy subject), as well as a properly functioning immune system.

While infectious diseases are like obvious threats, degenerative diseases are more like double agents: sneaky kryptonite within your own body. In this case, cells, tissues, and organs stop functioning correctly. Ironically, degenerative diseases can actually be exacerbated by an overactive immune system. (More on that later.) We can discourage degenerative diseases via preventative lifestyle measures, to ensure the equipment doesn't break in the first place. Common degenerative diseases include arthritis, diabetes, Alzheimer's, and heart disease. A prime example is cancer, in which malignant cells with genetic defects reproduce at an expedited rate, overwhelming the body and interfering with essential functions. Only a small percentage of cancer cases are inherited, while 90 to 95 percent of cancer occurrences are linked to lifestyle choices. Some 30 to 35 percent of deaths from cancer are linked specifically to diet.

But I'm getting ahead of myself.

THE CONNECTION BETWEEN FOOD AND DISEASE

Observational studies indicate degenerative diseases likely stem from lifestyle choices rather than genetics. For example, chronic illness is influenced more by the country in which one currently lives rather than by one's birth country. Twin studies also indicate that environment, rather than genes, often determines degenerative illness. This is motivating! It means you're not necessarily "born with" a future of disease; rather, your choices in life (including diet, exercise, and environment) may be the defining factor. As they say, "Genetics loads the gun; lifestyle pulls the trigger."

In today's society, we like to apply the infectious-disease model to all bodily dysfunction. We readily attribute health problems to some third-party invader, fixed by popping a third-party pill. This interprets our *symptoms* as the problem to be fixed. (Stop the pain, and we're all good!) In contrast, a holistic Paleo view of the body and disease interprets the majority of ailments as signs of a deeper problem. (Stop what's *causing* the pain, and we're all good!) The source problem, whatever it may be, is often inflammatory and autoimmune in nature—a state created by the body reacting to foreign, toxic substances in our diet.

WHAT IS INFLAMMATION?

Inflammation gets a bad rap all around, although it bears good intentions. The word *inflammation* comes from the Latin *inflammare*, meaning "to set on fire" . . . which is kind of what it does. Inflammation is the body's reaction to trouble. When reactive proteins in the body called pattern recognition receptors (PRRs) sense an injury or pathogen, they initiate the inflamed state you likely know well: redness, swelling, increased temperature, reduced function, and pain. Fun times. Levels of inflammation can materialize in blood tests as high levels of a PRR called C-reactive protein.

Although unpleasant to experience, acute inflammation is actually a protective process. Inflamed tissue allows defense chemicals to enter the area and do their cleanup job. The yucky swelling actually prevents the damage from spreading, kicking out pathogens and debris and prepping the site for healing. It'd be like if an intruder snuck into your house in the middle of the night, and your super protective dad/brother/neighbor/dog started screaming/attacking/running around the room. While they may scare away the invader, they might create a bit of a mess in the process. That's inflammation.

Things go terribly wrong when we shift from injury-based acute inflammation (like a stubbed toe) to prolonged chronic inflammation. This occurs when the body enters a perpetually inflamed state and begins needlessly instigating prolonged inflammatory responses, seemingly unable to get rid of the "invader." It'd be like if your protective dad/brother/neighbor/dog ran around the room chasing the invader . . . and never stopped! Talk about chaos!

Chronic inflammation can range from the unpleasant but relatively benign, such as skin rashes or irritable bowel syndrome (though I could talk for hours about the woes of IBS), to the more serious and even life-threatening, such as rheumatoid arthritis, celiac disease, or heart disease. Even cancer is linked to inflammation.[3] Today's autoimmune diseases occur when the immune system marks foreign proteins from food or the environment as dangerous, and enters the state of attack, attacking its own proteins in the process.

So acute inflammation from a stubbed toe = good. Chronic inflammation from anything else = not so good. More like downright nasty. What's even nastier? How we often deal with inflammation these days . . .

PILLS, PILLS, PILLS

Whenever I was given a pain pill for miscellaneous aches as a kindergartener, my suspicions were on par with my doubts about the Easter Bunny. How could *one* pill miraculously fix *any* painful ailment? How could *one* bunny bring all those eggs to so many people? Something fishy was going on. Shouldn't there be *separate* headache pills, stubbed-toe pills, and soreness pills? Although I'd ask grown-ups this question, I never received a satisfactory answer. Until now.

Over-the-counter pain pills such as Advil and Aleve are categorized as NSAIDs: nonsteroidal anti-inflammatory drugs. NSAIDs work by blocking enzymes (such as COX-1 and COX-2) in charge of releasing the hormones that green-light inflammation, discouraging the inflammatory response from occurring in the first place. While seemingly great as a temporary fix, NSAIDs only mask the problem. They do not solve nor, dare I say, even address it.

Popping a pill to calm down inflammation doesn't fix the actual issue— the "why" of the situation. Wouldn't it be better to stop the cause of inflammation in the first place, rather than silence the body's response to it? To make things worse, NSAIDs increase intestinal permeability within twenty-four hours of ingestion, which actually *encourages* inflammation. Short-term studies have found that NSAIDs create erythema (redness from inflammation) and potential ulcers, while long-term studies have found bleeding stomach ulcers and greater inflammation of the intestines. Such irony.

FOOD AND INFLAMMATION

How does what we eat factor into the inflammation thing? As it turns out, modern food choices can majorly encourage the body's overreactive inflammatory state. Next up, we'll tackle Paleo's inflammatory no-no's in detail, all of which became food sources in relatively recent human industries: grains (which contain problematic proteins and toxic antinutrients), refined sugar (which is highly inflammatory and spikes insulin, encouraging fat storage), and processed foods (which contain straight-up toxins). The time has come, my friends, to lift the veil!

GRAINY PROBLEMS

Ask any version of pre-nineteen-year-old Melanie her favorite food, and you'd be greeted with a resounding "Pasta, cookies, cake, forever and ever Amen!" Some of my fondest memories include breakfast cereals featuring leprechauns, toucans, and cardboard-box activities, and using bread to pretend I was *Alice in Wonderland*, plucking off bits of a caterpillar-topped mushroom, growing smaller or bigger with each bite. I never could have imagined my life without grains . . . and yet here we are.

Americans currently consume around 85 percent of their daily carbohydrates from grains, especially refined versions. As the foundation of the world's food, this highly economical food source has supported the industrial and technological achievements of mankind, since you arguably must eat to do productive things. So that's good.

Except that's where the good ends.

Historically, hunter-gatherers likely consumed *no* grains, and were arguably much better off for it. There's a lot going on in these little grainy guys, so let's just jump in, shall we?

WHAT IS A GRAIN?

Grains are the seeds of grasses and include three of the world's top crops (rice, wheat, and maize), as well as others such as oats, barley, cornmeal, millet, and sorghum. Composition-wise, a living embryo, dubbed the *germ*, contains most of the grain's nutrients. It's surrounded by the endosperm, providing structural protein and starch for energy, which is in turn protected by the outer bran, featuring fiber and B vitamins.

Whole grains, such as whole-wheat flour and brown rice, contain the germ, endosperm, and bran. Removing the bran and germ leaves us with only the starchy endosperm, à la refined grains, such as white flour and white rice. Whole grains are touted as "healthy," since they contain the original vitamins, minerals, and fiber found in the germ and bran. That said, they also contain more of the plant's antinutrients, which we shall discuss.

NATURE'S DEFENSIVE NATURE

When facing danger, living things typically either offensively fight back or defensively run away. But plants are in a pickle, since they can't attack or run away. (Please let me know if you catch your vegetables sneaking out the back door.) So what's a plant to do? Simple. Become super passive-aggressive.

In order to discourage being consumed, plants contain antinutrient compounds, which serve as a silent but deadly defense mechanism: You eat the plant and experience bad things![4] Defensive compounds in plants can do things such as attach to the proteins of bacteria, fungi, or *your* gut and wreak havoc, all while helping protect the seed from being digested. Double win for the plant. Though the plant perishes in the process, it may leave a great enough impression that some species learn to leave the little guys alone. (Note: Fruits are a slight exception, as they allure with their sweetness and *count* on being eaten to spread their seeds. As such, they often feature fewer antinutrients than grains, legumes, and many vegetables.)

Antinutrient compounds particularly abundant in grains include gluten, lectins, and phytates.[5] Other problematic plant compounds include saponins, goitrogens, oxalates, and protease inhibitors, to name a few. By the way, the whole "soaking" and "sprouting" thing is an effort to deactivate the toxic parts of the grain. Now you can walk by the sprouted section at your local health food store with a smug knowingness!

GLUTEN

Chances are, you've heard a bit about an oddly popular and nefariously vague substance called gluten. When I personally found out I was allergic to wheat, I jumped for joy. It was like my official invitation to the gluten-free club. I was no longer the poser I'd felt like until that point. ("Hi! I don't eat gluten because . . . umm . . . it's bad. Can I sit with you guys?")

Gluten is a large structural protein found in grains and is quite resilient in nature. Many of today's wheat products have been technologically engineered to contain more protein, and thus more gluten along with it. Yikes. Used as a stabilizing agent, gluten also sneaks its way into most processed foods, even those seemingly free of grains. "I didn't know BBQ sauce would have gluten," said my sister, when I offered her some gluten-free BBQ sauce. Yep. If it comes in a package and doesn't say "gluten-free," just assume a bit of gluten lurks inside. (Even if it says "gluten-free," I'm not making any promises!)

Gluten is quite difficult for the body to digest, and it contains at least 50 epitopes—protein segment "targets" for our bodies' antibodies—which harbor potential to spark an immune response and consequently encourage gut permeability.[6] In this condition, known as leaky gut syndrome, food particles and toxins can leak into the bloodstream. Gluten also stimulates the release of a protein called *zonulin*.[7] While zonulin actually serves a well-intentioned purpose of opening the gut barrier to allow nutrients into our body, too much zonulin allows bacteria and food particles to enter into circulation as well, encouraging inflammation and immune responses. It'd be like if, instead of just unlocking the door for your friend, you opened all the doors and windows in your house. Think of everything that could get in, from humidity to thieves! And if you're eating a diet high in processed and/or allergenic foods, it'd be like opening all those doors and windows in a super shady neighborhood to boot!

The gluten protein itself also easily sparks an immune response, in which the body attacks the gluten and potentially itself in the process. The impaired digestion, immune responses, and/or leaky gut from gluten exposure can consequently instigate digestive issues, skin problems, fatigue, and irritability on the more benign end (though none of that stuff is fun!); and rheumatoid arthritis, osteoporosis, and even cancer on the more serious side. Gluten has also been linked to psychiatric and neurological diseases such as depression, dementia, autism, epilepsy, and schizophrenia. As well as just straight-up "brain fog."

If that weren't all bad enough, gluten also contains a particularly toxic and resistant compound called *gliadin*, which can wreak havoc on cells even before any allergic or immune response. Studies show gliadin can inhibit cell growth, increase intestinal permeability, rearrange the cytoskeleton, alter enzymes in the esophagus, and even instigate apoptosis, or cell suicide, of cells you want to keep![8] These gliadin peptides can also silently attack the brain, leading to a substantial loss of brain matter and breakdown of synapses.[9]

Gluten nomenclature varies widely. In general, a *wheat allergy* indicates an IgE antibody immune response to wheat, with symptoms typically occurring immediately.[10] And while criteria is vague, up to 6 percent of the U.S. population is officially estimated to be *nonceliac gluten sensitive*,[11] meaning they suffer a negative reaction to gluten without an apparent allergic or autoimmune component. That said, around 30 percent of Americans believe they are intolerant of gluten (and I bet rightly so!).[12] Those sensitive to gluten may experience a range of symptoms hours to days after exposure, though the main ones tend to include digestive issues, brain fog, anxiety, and fatigue.

For the most severe gluten reaction, we've got *celiac disease*, an autoimmune condition officially affecting approximately 1 percent of the population, though the percentage appears to be on the rise. In celiacs, the body mounts a super intense immune response to gluten, attacking the small intestine as a result. It typically takes weeks to years after gluten exposure for the effects to become apparent, although some celiac patients do react immediately, with diarrhea, nausea, or other digestive problems. An inflamed intestine can inhibit nutrient absorption and result in diarrhea, gas, bloating, vomiting, and constipation, as well as extra-intestinal symptoms such as weight loss, malnutrition, fatigue, skin problems, anemia, osteoporosis, neurological disturbances, memory problems, infertility, cancer, and even death. While a 2016 government review deemed the tests for celiac disease to be generally accurate,[13] individuals on gluten-free diets may experience false negatives, as you must be consuming gluten in order to generate the gluten antibodies registered by the test.

But never fear! Knowledge is power, and a Paleo diet, which eschews grains and processed foods, is by nature gluten-free! Speaking of, gluten-free is increasingly gaining popularity, with 2015 global market sales reaching almost $2.8 billion, projected to rise beyond 7 billion by 2020.[14] With the current zeitgeist labeling gluten-free in vogue, you can confidently parade around the store with your gluten-free-content-laden cart, to the envy of onlookers! (Although I don't encourage the consumption of gluten-free processed goodies and grains.)

LECTINS

As the Scarecrow says en route to Oz, "I think it'll get darker before it gets lighter." That's right, folks: If the whole gluten thing was making you a little nervous about grains, it gets worse! Time to meet gluten's nefarious cousin lurking in the corner, named *lectin*. Everyone introduce yourself!

Like gluten, lectins are also a protein found in plants that function as a part of the plant's natural defense mechanism. They're particularly concentrated in grains, but also found in legumes and tubers such as potatoes, beans, and soy.

Oh, and a lectin's sole purpose is to destroy you. Kind of.

The word *lectin* comes from the Latin word *legere*, meaning "to select." Lectins are particularly sticky proteins that can bind to the sugary membranes of attacking bacteria, viruses, or fungi, in order to deter and destroy them.[15] Of course, if *you* ingest lectins, they don't lose their tendency to stick to sugars, which is bad news for your digestive tract and its intestinal wall of sugars!

Lectins can strip away the protective mucous layer in your stomach and intestines, stimulate acid secretion, encourage bacterial overgrowth, bind to immune cells, and inhibit repair of damaged cells in general. They can do this damage directly to cells: no prior allergy, intolerance, or autoimmune condition required! Lectins can also prevent absorption of *actual* nutrients, stealing your own supplies while they attack you! If this were a war (which it sort of is), you might want to be on team lectin.

And it doesn't end there. Lectins can also create holes in the digestive tract, allowing bacteria and bits of food to enter the bloodstream, yielding the afore-mentioned leaky gut syndrome. When the body senses these leaked foreign invaders, it creates antibodies and mounts an immune response, often injuring itself in the process and leading to a slew of issues, such as allergies, fatigue, skin rashes, and joint inflammation. When in the bloodstream, the lectins can continue binding to #allthethings, leaching minerals and creating systemic inflammation. With their resilient maliciousness, it's no surprise that lectins are linked to digestive issues, metabolic syndrome, obesity, arthritis, and other chronic diseases. Lectins can also bind to the thyroid and cross the blood-brain barrier, leading to neurological problems.

Just consider one particularly nasty and abundant lectin: wheat germ agglutinin (WGA). In clinical trials, WGA has been shown to bind to the cells throughout the gut, alter metabolism, permeate the intestinal wall, integrate into blood vessel walls, bind to immune cells, instigate pro-inflammatory cytokines, atrophy the thymus, inhibit nuclear DNA replication, bind to nerve fibers, and affect the central nervous system. WGA can inflict this harm even if the person is neither allergic to nor sensitive to wheat. Unfortunately, WGA is so efficient at destroying invaders that wheat is currently being engineered to *increase* WGA content, in order to function as a "natural" pesticide. {Sigh.}

OTHER GRAINY PROBLEMS

Grain's issues don't stop at gluten and lectins. Here's more to consider:

PHYTATES

Found primarily in grains, legumes, nuts, and seeds, phytates prevent a plant's seeds from growing prematurely. On the plus side, phytates can function as antioxidants in the human body, with potential anticancer properties. However, phytic acid (the main component of a phytate) can bind to minerals in the body, including calcium, magnesium, iron, phosphorous, and particularly zinc, significantly preventing their absorption, while also inhibiting digestive enzymes. While phytates may be problematic only if you're consuming large amounts of beans and/or whole grains (as many do!), I vote erring on the side of less.

EXORPHIN ADDICTION

When broken down by the body, gluten can create addictive gluten exorphins, similar to opioid-mediating meds such as morphine. While such pain-relieving potential may seem like a positive, these analgesic effects can mask the pain caused by gluten's injury to the intestines. It's like gluten shoots you, drugs you so you *don't even realize*, and makes you want more to boot! Umm . . . no thank you? These exorphins may be a key player in asymptomatic celiac disease, in which celiacs suffer injury to their intestines despite no apparent symptoms. The opioid-like effect of grains has also been linked to neurological disease, including schizophrenia, which is around thirty times more prevalent in celiacs.

DIGESTIVE ENZYME INHIBITORS

Some compounds found in wheat can be real party poopers when it comes to digestion. Take, for example, alpha-amylase inhibitors, which serve as yet another defense mechanism in grains, particularly against insects. In addition to being a major allergen, amylase inhibitors block starch-digesting enzymes produced by the pancreas, potentially affecting the pancreas's performance over the long term. (Ironically, some people willingly ingest alpha-amylase inhibitors via diet pills created to "block carbs." I may or may not have ingested my fair share of these in my pre-Paleo, low-carb days. Oops.)

Like alpha-amylase inhibitors, protease inhibitors also inhibit digestive enzymes, specifically one called trypsin, for protein. Trust me, the last thing you want is to have undigested proteins floating around your system. (Oh hey, autoimmune reactions!) Studies have also found that protease inhibitors can cause the pancreas to have a slight panic attack as it tries to overcompensate, which can lead to an unhealthy enlargement of the pancreas, encouraging cancer.

As a foundational food source, grains are, for lack of a better word, shoddy. They average less protein content than meat, and, unlike meat's status as a complete protein, grains feature insufficient amounts of the amino acids lysine and threonine. This means you need to consume even *more* grains to provide adequate protein in a grain-based diet.

On the micronutrient side of things, grains lack vitamins A, C, and B_{12}, and are low in antioxidants. Nutrient deficiencies associated with increased grain consumption include biotin, niacin, the amino acid tryptophan, and thiamin, while studies also show that high grain intake inhibits vitamin D metabolism, though the mechanisms are unclear. Though whole grains do feature other B vitamins, iron, zinc, and copper, their bioavailability is low, due to fiber and phytate content.

Although one can argue for obtaining these missing nutrients from other food sources, grains tend to *replace* meat, fruit, and vegetables in one's diet, rather than *supplement* them, so even though many grain products are now "fortified" with vitamins, many studies link grain-based diets to nutritional deficiencies. And, while whole grains may contain more nutrients than refined grains, they also contain more antinutrients. Ya just can't win.

WHAT ABOUT FIBER?

Fiber refers to indigestible carbohydrates found in the cell walls of plants. It adds no real nutritional value to food, but it can serve as a bulking agent (filling you up, so to speak), regulate digestion, and feed gut flora. Fiber can be either *soluble*, meaning it dissolves in water, or *insoluble*, meaning it does not. Soluble fiber bulks up in your system, while insoluble fiber basically passes through unchanged.

Though Paleolithic hunter-gatherers likely consumed more dietary fiber than we do today, such fiber came from fruits and vegetables, supporting healthy fermentation in the gut microbiome, unlike grain-based fiber, which is often injurious to the GI tract and at odds with gut bacteria. In fact, today's "eat more fiber" thing may be a bit misleading, and you might want to think twice before popping that fiber supplement.

I like to think of fiber as a reality TV star: quite famous, but of questionable merit. Fiber first joined the popular crowd in the 1960s. While studying lymphoma cancer affecting children in East Africa, British surgeon Dennis Burkitt noticed that certain cancers prevalent in Western civilizations were absent in poor, third-world countries. He compared the indigenous populations' whole-foods diets, featuring fibrous fruit and vegetables, to the Western diet of refined flour and sugar, and concluded it was the *lack of fiber* in the latter that was causing colon cancer, rather than any other difference. (Perhaps the *addition* of refined sugar and carbohydrates?) Burkitt wrote a book on his findings (with no concrete supportive studies), and fiber became a legend.

But even if fiber's rise to fame was based on an assumption, surely studies later confirmed its health benefits, right?

Not so much.

A 2000 *New England Journal of Medicine* trial evaluating 2,079 patients found that increasing dietary fiber does *not* mitigate colon cancer risk,[16] while another study that same year featuring 1,429 patients revealed similar findings. A follow-up study in 2002 reevaluated 1,208 of these original patients, just in case they weren't *actually* eating enough fiber (some ideas die hard!) . . . and reached the same conclusion. Likewise, a 2007 review of fiber studies to date concluded that the relation between fiber and colon cancer has not been adequately addressed, with further trials and research needed.[17] That's a lot of gray area for an "eat more fiber" mantra saturating a nation and fueling the sale of commercial products. (Shout-out to all those fiber supplements I'd chew in my pre-Paleo, low-carb days, because they tasted like candy, even though they felt like a rock in my intestines and made me intolerably gassy.)

To further convolute the matter, excess fiber (especially from grains) may even be detrimental. While debates rage on, and a multitude of factors are likely involved, certain types of excess fiber may potentially bind to some minerals in the body, making them less absorbable. This is particularly problematic in the context of grains, which contain high amounts of phytic acid further reducing mineral bioavailability. One study published in the *American Journal of Clinical Nutrition* even found that, while a high-animal-protein diet bore no effect on colon cancer as suspected, adding fiber actually increased calcium excretion, despite an increase in calcium intake.[18]

In young children, excess fiber can encourage maldigestion, malabsorption, and stunted growth. While a 2003 *Journal of Pediatric Gastroenterology and Nutrition* article notes that fiber may encourage insulin sensitivity and discourage childhood obesity, it reasons this because adding fiber may *displace* high-calorie, sugar- and fat-laden, processed foods. As in Burkitt's theory, the fact that fiber appears "protective" may simply be due to the fact that it's eaten instead of refined foods, which are actually causing the problems.

And for people with gut dysbiosis, rampant in today's antibiotic-heavy society, excess fiber may exacerbate bacterial overgrowth, or encourage fermentation in the wrong place (such as the small intestine rather than the colon), leading to an array of digestive issues.

As a 2007 *World Journal of Gastroenterology* review nicely concludes:

> *Whilst it is not the intention of the authors to totally discourage fiber in the diet and the use of fiber supplements, there does not seem to be much use for fiber in colorectal diseases. We, however, want to emphasize that what we have all been made to believe about fiber needs a second look. We often choose to believe a lie, as a lie repeated often enough by enough people becomes accepted as the truth. . . . While there are some benefits of a diet high in natural fiber, one must know the exact indications before recommending such a diet. Myths about fiber must be debunked and truth installed.[19]*

I, as well, am not saying that fiber is a bad thing, as natural fiber from fruits and veggies likely supports gut health, evident from ancestral humans. But consuming fiber as a supplement and considering it as a quota to fill? That may be hype more than anything else.

Of course, if you're still worried about getting enough fiber on a Paleo diet, there's no need to fret! Calorie for calorie, the amount of fiber in green vegetables far outweighs that in grains, and it's the "good" kind of fiber, at that! Other Paleo foods high in fiber include squash, sweet potatoes, avocados, and fruits such as apples and berries. (Side note: Stripping fruits of their fiber via juicing or dehydration can result in high amounts of sugar, causing insulin spikes, which we'll discuss in the next chapter.)

THE TAKEAWAY?

Whew! Who knew there was so much going on in that slice of bread! We tackled a lot in this section, so here's a brief recap. Basically, grains are disagreeable for two main reasons:

1. Grains wreak havoc on your gut, leading to a myriad of diseases.
2. By forming the foundation of a diet, grains replace much more nutritious food and encourage deficiencies.

With everything bad going for them, grains just don't have much good going for them. They're cheap and economical. That's pretty much it. Given their toxic nature and lack of benefits, it's no surprise that a grain-based diet poses quite a few problems. I'm looking at you, FDA food pyramid! (Though, granted, the current ChooseMyPlate.gov may be a step in the right direction.)

SWEET PROBLEMS

We're hardwired for sweets. Evolutionarily speaking, the sweetness found naturally in energy-rich fruits, tubers, and honey indicates easy-breezy energy. While this supported our Paleolithic ancestors in times of food scarcity, the same does not apply today, as sugary concoctions entice us from commercials, food counters, and pantries.

To start things off, sugars found in carbohydrates can be great for our bodies. Contrary to popular belief, Paleo does *not* necessitate a low-carb or high-fat ketogenic approach (though you can surely entertain these approaches if you like!). Recent research indicates most hunter-gatherer societies likely consumed anywhere from 35 to 65 percent carbohydrates. While current U.S. consumption averages a comparable rate of 50 percent carbohydrates, the type of carb-containing foods contrasts sharply. Stone Age carbs came from fibrous, nutrient-rich, blood-sugar-controlling fruits and vegetables, with maybe a percent or two from the "added sugar" of honey. Today, we consume most of our carbohydrates via insulin-spiking, inflammatory grains and processed foods, with around 15 percent added sugars, most coupled with refined fat to boot! The time has come, my friends, to tackle the sugar demon once and for all!

WHAT IS SUGAR?

Sugar is the popular term for the sweet, starchy, and/or fibrous macronutrients known as carbohydrates. Simple carbohydrates are single or double molecules of sugar (monosaccharides or disaccharides), and include glucose, fructose, sucrose (a combination of glucose and fructose), lactose, and the less common maltose (a combination of two glucose molecules). While found in various concentrations in almost all foods, glucose constitutes a large percentage of the sugars in vegetables, nuts, and grains, while fructose is more prevalent in fruit. Sucrose, akin to white table sugar, is usually produced from refined sugarcane or beets. Lactose is found in milk and dairy products, while the more uncommon maltose appears in things such as cooked sweet potatoes and malted beer.

Simple carbohydrates break down rather quickly in the body, and tend to encourage a more immediate release of insulin—the hormone responsible for nutrient assimilation and fat storage. Complex carbohydrates, on the other hand, are chains of sugar molecules found in starches such as tubers and whole grains, and take longer for the body to break down. Lastly, carbohydrates from fiber are inaccessible to the body, but can be broken down by the gut microbiome.

There is no actual *requirement* for dietary carbohydrates. While a typical carb burner's brain does utilize around 120 grams of glucose per day, a lower-carb diet, ketogenic diet, or even ketone and/or MCT oil supplementation can provide alternative (and arguably superior) energy substrates for the brain. This can drastically reduce the amount of one's daily "required" glucose by up to 50 to 75 percent at the extreme end.[20] Our bodies can also generate the minimal amount of glucose from protein and fat (if necessary) via a process called gluconeogenesis. (I tell you this *not* to make you avoid carbs, but rather to assure you that you will *not* die if you cut down your intake of them, even significantly.)

THE PROBLEM WITH SUGAR

The body ultimately converts most carbohydrates we ingest, both simple and complex, into glucose molecules. (Fiber is an exception, and things also get a bit funky with fructose, which is processed by the liver. See "Fake Problems" on page 39 for the lowdown on fructose!) This glucose, whether it originally came from your spinach or your muffin, ultimately becomes blood sugar in the body. Now glucose is a fuel, which is a good thing. (Yay energy!) On the flip side, too much glucose is actually toxic to the body.

Think about the sugar you're likely most familiar with: white table sugar. It's sticky stuff, right? Not surprisingly, excess sugar can gunk up the blood, sticking to red blood cells and proteins, in a process called *glycation*. This can interfere with circulation, generate inflammatory cytokines, cause the fat molecule cholesterol to rise (though cholesterol is not inherently a bad thing, as we'll discuss in "Fat Problems" on page 28), and increase free radicals fifty-fold.[21] (Free radicals run around the body and react with cells, damaging their membranes, proteins, and genes, and encouraging oxidative stress, aging, and deterioration.) At the same time, sugar can disable the body's cleanup system by halting phagocytosis, in which white blood cells "eat" and expunge toxic particles, bacteria, and invaders.[22]

Given all this information, is it any surprise that sugar intake is strongly correlated with many forms of degenerative disease[23] and cancer?[24] If I were to say that too many carbs = death, that would seem like crazy talk. Except they kinda do. But perhaps sugar's biggest issue, especially in our refined-carbohydrate-fueled society, involves that aforementioned little hormone called insulin.

THE ROLE OF INSULIN

Insulin is a hormone in the body responsible for transporting nutrients from your food into cells. It is also the primary regulator of fat storage. As discussed, when you eat carbs, the resulting glucose elevates your blood sugar levels. The pancreas then produces insulin to move the sugar into cells throughout the body, so it can't do damage in your bloodstream. Even though it stops fat burning, insulin beneficially lowers blood sugar and assimilates nutrients. But things get tricky. (Don't they always?) Insulin works "correctly" when we eat whole foods, which moderately affect blood sugar levels, keeping all hormones and functions in check. Blood sugar rises after a meal, insulin takes care of it, and everyone's a happy camper! Modern processed foods high in refined sugar, however, *rapidly* raise blood sugar, encouraging insulin release far beyond levels to which the body is accustomed. From there, things just get gnarly.

Ya see, when initially summoned by the pancreas, insulin first ushers glucose into the liver and muscles to be stored as glycogen. The liver can store around 100 grams of glycogen, while the muscles can store around 350 to 700 grams of glycogen, depending on one's personal constitution. While these glycogen stores adequately suit a whole-foods diet, the same cannot be said for today's high-carbohydrate intake and often-sedentary lifestyles. If the liver and muscle glycogen stores are full, insulin escorts glucose to the backup plan: fat stores! Yep. Sugar can become fat—along with any other fat consumed with the meal.

And here comes the *real* problem. After a while, the body's cells can become tired of being hit with insulin all the time, and consequently downregulate their insulin receptors, in a condition called *insulin resistance*. It'd be like if your mom regularly brought you dinner. You'd be like, "Thanks, Mom!" and life would go on. But what if she started bringing you food *all the time*? Morning, noon, and night, and all the moments in between? At first you might suck it up and politely bite into the casserole, but after a while, you might get a little annoyed. If she kept showing up, eventually you might close your doors and pretend you weren't home. You'd just be like, "No, Mom."

That's what happens with insulin resistance. Since the blood sugar can't get into the cells, blood sugar remains elevated. And since elevated blood sugar is toxic, the pancreas is like, "OMG! Toxic blood sugar is still high!" and produces *more* insulin to lower blood sugar, until the blood sugar is forced into the cells. (Basically, Mom breaks down your door, horror-movie- or black-comedy-style, depending on your genre preference.) Because insulin instigates fat storage, these increasingly high levels put the body into a constant fat-storing mode. Even worse, since the cells are resisting glucose, the brain may launch a ravenous appetite to eat *more*, even when too much has already been consumed. You can be eating a *ton*, and the cells can even become *full* of fat, yet the body still believes it's starving! Hello, never-ending spiral into simultaneous hunger and fat gain, as well as metabolic syndrome and obesity!

All this wear and tear on the pancreas from constant insulin production can notably result in the lifestyle-associated type 2 diabetes, in which the body does not properly utilize insulin.[25] (By comparison, type 1 diabetes is typically genetic, and occurs when the person lacks the ability to produce insulin in the first place.) In fact, an extensive 2013 epidemiological study found that sugar consumption alone, regardless of other factors (including weight, social ties, economics, and exercise), correlated strongest to diabetes.[26]

WHOLE FOODS AND INSULIN

Proper control of blood sugar is vital if you want to avoid the blood sugar roller coaster, prolong health, and deter disease. Thankfully, a whole-foods, Paleo diet helps control blood sugar levels by eradicating insulin-spiking, sugar-laden processed foods. Consuming protein, healthy fats, and minimal to moderate carbohydrates from fruits and vegetables welcomes a state of insulin sensitivity. This means the pancreas and insulin do their job properly, efficiently utilizing sugar and nutrients from food, without endless appetite, fat gain, and the problems arising from such. In this state, the body also relies more on steady fat stores for fuel, which is awesome for body composition and health in general. (To be discussed!)

But don't just take my word for it! Many studies have confirmed the blood sugar and insulin benefits of a Paleo-style diet. Back in 1984, researchers found that switching the modern diet of diabetic Australian aborigines to one that mimicked their ancestral diet significantly improved their blood sugar and insulin responses. More recently, a 2009 study found that a Paleo-style diet instigated beneficial blood glucose and insulin responses in nine healthy individuals in a mere ten days.[27]

Perhaps most revelatory are studies that compare the Paleo diet to other "healthy" diets. A 2007 randomized, controlled trial compared a Paleo diet (lean meat, fish, vegetables, fruit, nuts, tubers, and eggs) to the Mediterranean diet (whole grains, low-fat dairy, fish, vegetables, fruits, oils, and margarine) in twenty-nine individuals with heart disease, diabetes, or glucose intolerance.[28] It found the Paleo diet reduced glucose AUC (which refers to the body's glycemic response) by 26 percent, compared to a paltry 7 percent on the Mediterranean diet! In the same vein, a 2009 randomized, controlled crossover study of thirteen diabetic patients compared a similar Paleo diet to a diet recommended by the American Diabetes Association (whole-grain bread, cereals, fiber, vegetables, tubers, fruits, and decreased fats).[29] It found that the Paleo diet produced better results than the ADA diet for managing diabetes and improving glycemic control.

Despite the small sample sizes, I find these studies indicative that a Paleo-style diet is pretty great for blood sugar control. Not too long ago, I would have left things at that. However, recent research has rendered things a *smidge* more complicated. The time has come to throw another wrench in the matter!

PERSONAL GLYCEMIC RESPONSES

As discussed, whenever we eat carbohydrates in any form, they are ultimately converted to blood sugar. Even if you eat a piece of broccoli, that broccoli will partly become blood sugar, albeit a relatively negligible bit. The rate at which various carbohydrates supposedly affect blood sugar is measured by the glycemic index: a scale of 0 to 100. Higher-glycemic-index foods spike blood sugar (and therefore insulin) faster, whereas lower-glycemic-index foods raise blood sugar more slowly. Simple carbohydrates have higher glycemic indexes, while complex carbohydrates fall lower on the scale. Anything that speeds up digestion will raise glycemic index (such as refining flour, dehydrating fruit, or juicing vegetables), while fat and protein tend to lower glycemic index, although high carbohydrate content in a meal can override that.

While the glycemic index provides a starting point for blood sugar control, it notably only works for foods in isolation, and most people don't tend to eat "mono" meals. Glycemic index can also be influenced by a ton of factors: Did you add condiments? Chew longer? Eat recently? Eat more? Byeeee glycemic index! Furthermore, recent research indicates that individual blood sugar responses to foods vary widely, to the point that we arguably can't make any generalizations about glycemic responses.[30] Oh hi, aforementioned wrench!

An elaborate 2015 research project meticulously monitored the postprandial (translation: after-meal) glycemic (translation: blood sugar) response levels in eight hundred people for one week, via glucose monitors embedded in the skin. These recorded a whopping 1.5 million glucose measurements, 46,898 meals, and around 10,000,000 calories. Oh my. The researchers also analyzed the participants' lifestyles, physical activity, and gut microbiomes.[31]

At the risk of sounding sensationalist, the results were pretty shocking, with different people reacting *completely* differently to the same foods. Almost every single food sparked a range of reactions. I kid you not. For example, while white bread has an official (high) glycemic index of 70, some people experienced small blood sugar responses (like 15), while others featured much higher reactions (like 80). Some reacted intensely to bananas, but not to cookies, while others would do just the opposite. Though certain foods did cause average lower blood glucose responses (such as chocolate and ice cream) and others higher (such as cereal and rice), the ranges were still all over the map. (Pita and pizza in particular showed extremely large variances.)

While there weren't any certainties in blood sugar responses, there were a few trends. Increasing the amount of carbohydrates tended to increase blood glucose responses (not good), while increasing fat, alcohol, or water content in a meal tended to decrease the response (good). But again, that didn't go for everyone. Salt intake, being awake for a long time, high cholesterol levels, and age also bore negative effects. Certain gut bacteria (such as proteobacteria and enterobacteria) also correlated to higher responses. In any case, high blood sugar responses to meals typically led to higher markers of inflammation.

Given this information, the researchers developed an algorithm based on 137 factors that could potentially determine the "right" foods for an individual's ideal blood sugar control. These meals could potentially include anything from apples to ice cream to salad to salmon to cheesecake to veggies to beer—it all just depended on the person! The researchers found that when the new participants adopted their personalized diet for a week, they consistently experienced not only better blood glucose responses but shifts in their gut microbiomes to match!

The takeaway? Although a person's blood sugar response to food is super important, we likely can't determine it by counting carbs or looking at any one list. Rather, a myriad of factors involving individual hormones, diet, lifestyle, genetics, and gut microbes play a key role. This means you've got to find what works for *you* personally, in *your* whole-foods, Paleo template.

How to do this? Self-experimentation and intuition are key! You can take a casual approach, and go by how you feel: Meals should leave you pleasantly satisfied for a good amount of time, not hankering for more shortly afterward. If eating a certain type of carbohydrate makes you crash or feel foggy headed, chances are it's not doing good things to your blood sugar.

If you desire more certainty (oh hi, me!), you can measure your actual blood glucose response to certain foods. I cannot recommend enough that you check out Robb Wolf's most recent book, *Wired to Eat*, which goes into great detail about this whole topic and provides a specific protocol for determining the best foods for your blood sugar.

As a final note, I hope you don't interpret this study as license to go gung-ho on processed goodies. Even if it turns out that a certain cookie, cake, or candy doesn't *technically* spike your blood sugar, such foods do much more harm than good, instigating inflammation and stripping away our health, as we'll look at in the upcoming "Fake Problems." I encourage you to apply these principles to the various whole-food carbohydrate sources, in a Paleo-style approach. You may be a fruit lover, for example, or perhaps sweet potatoes are more your thing. Heck, you might even thrive in Paleo gray areas, such as legumes, lentils, and white rice. In any case, do you, in the way that does you best!

FAT PROBLEMS

The title of this chapter is a bit misleading, since the main problem with dietary fat isn't dietary fat itself; rather, it's a problem that people *think* it's a problem. If you follow me. Eating fat is not what automatically makes you fat. Yet how often do I find myself at a restaurant, debating between the New York strip and filet mignon, when my salivations are interrupted by a friend's lament:

"Oh, I want the steak, but I'll be good and get the low-fat veggie pasta."

Back in my standard American diet (SAD) days, I'd eye my companion with a sort of envy, resenting her self-control, as I apparently had none. Today, however, I simply bite my tongue, issue a soft sigh, and think to myself, "Get the steak. It's fine." The dinner table is no place for a debate on food politics, even though politics have defined its current manifestation. Old habits die hard. Old dietary dogma based on myths? That may just be immortal.

THE DEFAMATION OF FAT

There's a very complicated and twisted history to the vilification of dietary fat. If you want a fascinating perspective of the full story, consider reading *The Big Fat*

Surprise: Why Butter, Meat and Cheese Belong in a Healthy Diet by Nina Teicholz, or *Good Calories, Bad Calories: Fats, Carbs, and the Controversial Science of Diet and Health* by Gary Taubes. (Taubes is an acclaimed science writer, though I will note that some critics disagree with his lengthy analysis, as oft happens in the political health wars.) In any case, I shall attempt a brief summary. History lesson time!

It all started in the 1950s, when a scientist by the name of Ancel Keys theorized that high amounts of saturated fat found naturally in animal products increased cholesterol and thereby promoted heart disease. In support of this idea, he published an extensive "Seven Countries Study" showing that countries with diets low in saturated fat experienced less heart disease. In 1961, Keys achieved celebrity status when he graced the cover of *Time* magazine, proclaiming the evils of saturated fat. In 1977, the government joined the crusade, publishing its first "Dietary Goals for the United States," which advocated increased carbohydrate intake and decreased fat intake for heart health—the first government publication regarding diet risk factors. The low-fat diet for health paradigm was born!

The problem? As discussed by Taubes, this colossal cultural shift potentially rested on a vast assumption of medical advice based on inconclusive and skewed evidence. For starters, Keys's uncontrolled "Seven Countries Study" looked at broad trends easily involving a myriad of factors, rather than cause-and-effect data. And though Keys gathered data for twenty-one countries, he picked seven that supported his theory, omitting those with high dietary fat but low heart disease (such as France, Germany, Holland, and Switzerland), as well as Chile, a country with low dietary fat but high levels of heart disease. Contradictions were also dismissed, such as in Finland, whose eastern population featured significantly more heart disease than its western population, despite equivalent fat intakes. Pick seven *different* countries from Keys's data, and the saturated fat–heart disease link disappears.

Problems also brewed in Keys's keystone (pun intended) country: the Mediterranean island of Crete. Keys surveyed the island during an anomalous time of dietary hardship from World War II, as well as during Lent, which minimized the residents' normal meat and cheese consumption. As such, the low-fat dietary data Keys collected from this island of "low" heart disease did not represent the country's normal, fattier diet.

Actual controlled studies of fat in patient diets at the time were overwhelmingly inconclusive, ultimately favoring no saturated fat–heart disease connection. As Taubes notes, only two trials actually looked at a low-fat diet's effect on heart disease (as opposed to the effect of a polyunsaturated versus saturated fat diet on heart disease): One study indicated that a low-fat diet reduced heart disease rates; the other indicated that it did not. That means there were two studies in total addressing the efficacy of a low-fat diet when it became #thething . . . and they contradicted each other.

The studies looking at replacing saturated fat with polyunsaturated fat were even less supportive. Some showed that diets rich in polyunsaturated fat reduced heart disease, but increased death rates overall (kind of defeating the purpose). Others simply showed no correlation. In fact, a 2010 meta-analysis of twenty-one related studies found that there is no satisfactory evidence to conclude that saturated fat directly encourages heart disease.[32]

Ironically, those inaugural 1977 government dietary goals were sort of on-point in spirit. The preface noted, "Major health problems are diet related. Most all of the health problems underlying the leading causes of death in the United States could be modified by improvements in diet." I couldn't agree more! Yet while the guidelines advocated a lower sugar intake, they focused on decreasing fat intake and increasing carbohydrate intake, which indirectly increases sugar intake. Why was fat demonized rather than sugar? Why did a low-fat diet strike the nation, rather than a low-sugar one? (Though I could leave this rhetorical, I will mention that documents uncovered in 2016 revealed the sugar industry's secret role in paying off scientists for sugar-absolving, fat-damning studies, Godfather-style. I suggest you google *The New York Times* article "How The Sugar Industry Shifted Blame To Fat," if you fancy some conspiracy theories more concrete than crop circles.)

A LOOK AT CHOLESTEROL

What about Keys's original thesis involving dietary fats and cholesterol? Cholesterol is a waxy lipid substance in the body vital for health, as it builds cell membranes, assimilates vitamins, and synthesizes hormones. We now know that dietary cholesterol minimally affects blood cholesterol, meaning the cholesterol you eat does *not* automatically pop up as cholesterol in your bloodstream. Just consider the fact that Paleolithic people consumed an estimated 480 milligrams of cholesterol per day, compared to 260 milligrams for Americans today, yet had lower cholesterol levels and were largely free of cardiovascular disease.

Furthermore, cholesterol is divided into two main types: LDL and HDL. In excess, LDL, or "bad cholesterol," can form plaque on artery walls, which restricts blood flow and *does* encourage heart disease. HDL, or "good cholesterol," helps remove excess LDL from the bloodstream. While dietary saturated fats can slightly raise LDL, they simultaneously raise HDL, meaning they insignificantly affect total cholesterol levels. (In fact, the saturated fatty acid stearic acid may actually lower overall cholesterol.) Fats also tend to encourage a more benign (and potentially protective) form of LDL, while carbs tend to raise a more dangerous, dense version. The type of dietary fat that *does* specifically raise bad cholesterol and lower good cholesterol is *trans fat*, which was included in food products largely in response to the demonization of saturated fat. (Oh hey, most low-fat margarines!) Such irony.

THE FAT-FEARING ZEITGEIST

As discussed in *Good Calories, Bad Calories*, despite the utter lack of scientific evidence to reduce fat intake in the 1950s to 1970s, Americans were ready to accept any heart disease theory offered, as officials were proclaiming heart disease strikingly "on the rise." (Scare tactics are great for making people listen.) In actuality, this "rise" was likely due to a few slightly misleading factors, such as the decline of deaths from infectious diseases, which left older humans susceptible to degenerative disease. The year 1949 also saw the addition of "arteriosclerotic heart disease" as a category on death certificates. This is huge. After its inclusion, heart disease rates "rose" by 20 to 35 percent within the year, since it could now be cited as a cause of death. Furthermore, the 1948 National Heart Act, as well as the creation of the National Heart Institute, signified a major influx of government funding into heart disease awareness and prevention, beginning with an unprecedented $9 million for heart research. President Eisenhower's heart attack in 1955 sealed the deal for the new fear of heart disease.

And so, advised to lower fat intake at all costs despite a lack of legitimate supporting evidence, Americans eagerly turned to high-carb, low-fat diets featuring grains, sugar, and processed foods. Food manufacturers jumped on board, churning out polyunsaturated margarines to replace butter, and "healthy" low-fat fake fats. The damage was done. Meals became more sugary, more fake, and arguably less satisfying. Heart disease rates continued to rise. Oh, and we welcomed the beginning of the obesity epidemic and the rise in diabetes as a bonus!

DIETARY FAT AND HEALTH

Now that we've analyzed dietary fat's frustrating political context, let's see what *actually* goes down when you eat fat. For starters, it is lamentable that we use a single word (*fat*) to describe both dietary fat *and* body fat, which are not exactly the same thing. Yes, dietary fat can become body fat. But it doesn't have to. At the same time, carbohydrates can become dietary fat, yet we don't call *them* fat. In any case, it is *excess food* that becomes fat, regardless of the form. Additionally, it is carbs that spike insulin and "tell" your body to store fat, whereas dietary fat alone bears no such effect.

Unlike carbs, you actually need fat. Yes, the stuff is actually good for you. Shocker. (I say that in jest, yet I know many, if not most, *do* find that shocking.) The historical Paleolithic diet on which our genome developed likely featured around 35 percent fat—comparable to the high end of today's fat intake in the United States. (More on the composition of that fat in a bit!) While both carbs and fats can be used as energy for the body, fats provide essential nutritional building blocks: Around 20 to 80 percent of the brain is fat.[33] Fat is also vital for vitamin assimilation, with the fat-soluble vitamins

A, D, E, and K all stored in fat. The essential fatty acids (EFAs) must also be obtained from food.

What about the "essential" carbs, you ask? Wait for it . . . there are none. As discussed in "Sweet Problems" on page 20, even if you ate *no* carbs, the body can generate glucose from fat and protein, via a process called gluconeogenesis. I admittedly did this for a good six months or so my last year of college. My neighborhood grocery store would mark down the rotisserie chickens to three dollars each night, so I just ate an entire chicken with coconut oil every evening. It was a pretty fantastic, albeit pre-Paleo, passing phase. I now favor many more fruits and vegetables, and many fewer additives, thank goodness.

TYPES OF FAT

The time has come to demystify what we actually *mean* by all these fatty labels, which often invoke generalized (erroneous) assumptions about health benefits or concerns. Though the various dietary fats are similarly composed of carbon, hydrogen, and oxygen atoms, not all fats are created equal. The number of hydrogen atoms in a given fat determines the number of bonds between its carbon atoms, which determines the "type" of fat. Stick with me here. (Pun intended.)

There are two parent categories of fats: saturated and unsaturated. In saturated fats, all the carbons are fully "saturated" by hydrogen atoms, and each carbon is only connected to others by a single bond. Unsaturated fats, on the other hand, feature fewer hydrogen atoms, which the carbons make up for by forming double bonds with fellow carbons. One double bond creates a mono-unsaturated fat, while multiple double bonds create a polyunsaturated fat. These bonds are like bendy places in the fat chain, and fats with more bonds tend to be more fluid. Double bonds are also less stable and easily react with oxygen, or *oxidize*, meaning they go rancid (*not* a good thing).

Let's look at the various types of fats in a bit more detail. Please keep in mind that while we often categorize dietary fats as a single type (e.g. animal fat is "saturated" and olive oil is "monounsaturated"), most foods typically feature multiple types of fat.

SATURATED FATS

Saturated fats are found mostly in butter and animal fats. They contain no double bonds: All the carbons in the fatty acids are saturated in hydrogen atoms. As such, they are solid at room temperature and very stable. This is a good thing, as it means you don't have to worry so much about them spoiling or oxidizing, including in your body. Saturated fats make up 50 percent of the body's cell membranes, and support calcium, vitamin, and essential fatty acid synthesis. In whole-foods form, they typically bring fat-soluble vitamins such as K, A, and D to the table. While saturated fats do elevate cholesterol, as previously discussed, they raise both HDL and LDL, rendering their influence on cholesterol benign in the grand scheme of things.

MONOUNSATURATED FATS

Monounsaturated fats are found in many nut, seed, and fruit oils, including olive, sesame seed, and safflower oil. They also constitute a good percentage of animal fat, forming about 30 percent of butter and around half of bacon fat (lard) and beef fat (tallow).

Monounsaturated fats contain one double bond between fatty acids and are typically liquid at room temperature, but may gel or solidify when cooled. While not as stable as saturated fats, monounsaturated fats don't go rancid as easily as polyunsaturated fats. They may support good cholesterol levels and reduce risk of breast cancer, heart disease, and stroke.

As a side note, I've found that monounsaturated fats are often ignored in the Paleosphere, which often focuses on defending saturated fat and highlighting the damage done by omega-6 polyunsaturated fats. As such, monounsaturated fats often fall by the wayside, despite their nutritious nature.

POLYUNSATURATED FATS

Polyunsaturated fats are abundant in fish, nuts, and grains. They contain more than one double bond between fatty acids, and favor a liquid state that easily oxidizes. Polyunsaturated fats are a double-edged sword in that they can be both super awesome and super damaging. The body cannot synthesize two specific types of these polyunsaturated fats, which must be obtained from diet: the essential fatty acids (EFAs), linoleic acid (LA) found in omega-6s, and alpha-linolenic acid (ALA) found in omega-3s. These EFAs make up cell membranes throughout the body, from immune cells to red blood cells to cardiac and neural tissue, and affect cells' flexibility, fluidity, and activity. Omega-3 deficiency in particular may encourage skin rashes, vision problems, stunted growth, dampened immune system, arthritis, heart problems, diabetes, inflammatory bowel disease, declined cognitive functioning, depression, and even cancer.

While both omega-3s and omega-6s are required by the body, omega-6s tend to be inflammatory, while omega-3s tend to be anti-inflammatory. We need them in the proper balance, and historically consumed them in a beneficial omega-6-to-omega-3 ratio of around one-to-one or two-to-one. Omega-6s are abundant in seed and vegetable oils (such as corn, peanut, and soybean oil), grains, and processed foods, while omega-3s are found in flaxseed, walnuts, and fatty fish. Conventional meats contain more omega-6s, while grass-fed meats feature more omega-3s. Our modern diet can yield an omega-6-to-omega-3 ratio of up to twenty-to-one! Scary stuff. To make things worse, too much omega-6 can interfere with proper assimilation of omega-3, further skewing the ratio.

Since the cells of our body are *literally* made of EFAs, this high omega-6 intake shifts the body toward a cellular foundation of inflammation, encouraging a myriad of health issues, including cardiovascular problems, autoimmune diseases, and cancer. Omega-3s, on the other hand, are anti-inflammatory and protective against such conditions. They may mitigate inflammatory conditions and decrease mortality rates in general. The brain in particular requires adequate omega-3 levels, and deficiencies have been linked to Alzheimer's,[34] bipolar disorder,[35] depression,[36] and schizophrenia.[37] In fact, pregnant women may experience postpartum depression because the unborn child utilizes the mother's omega-3 fatty acids for developing brain and nervous tissue.

It is prudent to maximize omega-3 intake and minimize omega-6 intake. (The ratio is so off in today's diet that it is unlikely you'll achieve a ratio too high in omega-3s.) It's also important to note that fatty fish contain omega-3s in the form of EPA (eicosapentaenoic acid) and DHA (docosahexaenoic acid), which are much more bioavailable and provide greater health benefits than the ALA form found in vegetarian sources. In fact, the body likely converts less than 5 percent of ALA to DHA. DHA is particularly important for vision and brain function, and is critical for infant development. Women even preferentially store DHA in their thigh fat, which is reserved for pregnancy, to nurture the child.

Please know that it can take months to adjust the omega-6-to-omega-3 ratio within your cells. The fats within blood cells, for example, change approximately every 120 days. This means you can't fix your ratio overnight: Long-term, consistent dietary changes are key! That said, while I traditionally advocated consuming omega-3s via fish oil supplements, I am no longer a fan of this approach. Even though omega-3s are beneficial, they are very unstable, and isolated pill versions harbor the potential to instigate oxidative damage, regardless of manufacturer safety claims. As such, I encourage addressing your omega-6-to-omega-3 ratio by minimizing processed foods, oils, and grains, and eating low-toxin, wild-caught fatty fish. You can check out the Environmental Defense Fund's "Seafood Selector" for the best current sources of low-toxin fish high in omega-3s.

If all of that was confusing, here's a quick recap! The typically liquid polyunsaturated essentially fatty acids (EFAs) must be consumed through one's diet. These include omega-6 fats, which tend to be inflammatory, and omega-3 fats, which tend to be anti-inflammatory. Because we eat way too much omega-6 today, we should focus on minimizing omega-6 intake while adding more omega-3s. These omega-3s appear in the form of ALA in plant foods, such as flaxseed and walnuts, and EPA and DHA in fatty fish—the ideal form for health. So if you take away nothing else from this section, know that eating some low-toxin fatty fish can be a great step in your health journey!

MEDIUM-CHAIN TRIGLYCERIDES (MCTS)

Medium-chain triglycerides are a special type of saturated fat common in coconut and palm oil. They're the darling of the Paleo world, with a seemingly never-ending list of stunning benefits. Unlike other fats, which must be broken down in the intestines, MCTs are sent directly to the liver for energy, providing instant fuel in a manner similar to carbohydrates, yet without the insulin spike! MCTs also encourage the production of ketones—an energy substrate that supports the body, and particularly the brain. MCTs may discourage fat gain and decrease appetite, upregulate fatty acids for energy use, enhance thermogenesis, and regulate insulin. They can support the immune system, act as antioxidants, benefit cholesterol ratios, and potentially protect against a myriad of diseases, such as cirrhosis and cardiovascular disease.

Plus, coconut oil tastes delicious! You can add it to salads, veggies, or meats, or even eat it plain! I like the virgin, unrefined versions.

TRANS FATS

Trans fats are found naturally in small, beneficial amounts in breast milk, as well as the meat of some herbivores. Their modern, bastardized form abundant in processed foods, baked goods, and low-fat/fake-fat foods (such as margarine), however, constitutes approximately 2.6 percent of the modern diet, which spells bad news for our health. To create trans fats, normally liquid vegetable fats are solidified via hydrogenation, meaning their hydrogen atoms are tweaked to make them more shelf stable, resistant to spoilage, and tolerant of higher temperatures.

The problem? Trans fats basically do all the bad stuff saturated fats were supposed to do. They raise bad cholesterol, lower good cholesterol, and harm endothelial function. They encourage inflammation and increase blood levels of inflammatory biomarkers such as C-reactive protein (CRP). (One study found that CRP levels were a whopping 73 percent higher in women who consumed larger doses of trans fats!) And unlike saturated fats, trans fats actually *do* increase risks of heart disease, insulin resistance, and diabetes. In fact, processed trans fats are the only "food" I can think of that pretty much everyone agrees is bad for your health. Like really.

While trans fats are listed on food labels, a serving size can legally contain up to 0.5 grams and still be called zero. In products with small serving sizes (such as in condiments and sauces), "zero" trans fats can add up quite quickly, and even small amounts can be harmful. Thankfully, a Paleo diet effectively frees you from these sneaky devils, so you shouldn't have to worry about them!

THEN VERSUS NOW

Though fats are a vital and healthy macronutrient *not* to be feared, context is everything. Hunter-gatherers likely ingested up to 35 percent of their diet as fat, but the composition of their diet departed strikingly from today. These Paleo peeps dined on game meats featuring more mono- and polyunsaturated fats than current commercial meat, resulting in around 7 to 8 percent saturated fat, compared to around 12 percent today. They also likely consumed way more beneficial omega-3s, and way less detrimental trans fat. Basically, they ate the good fats, in the right amounts, and without insulin-spiking refined carbohydrates alongside.

I encourage you to seek out a similar fat profile in your diet, which you can do by embracing grass-fed meats, and potentially pastured eggs if tolerated. Eschew inflammatory omega-6s abundant in grains and seed oils in favor of omega-3-rich fatty fish, as well as monounsaturated fats in foods such as avocados. Try to consume your fat from whole-food sources, rather than slathering foods in oil. Lastly, remember that combining sugar and fats together, especially when refined, can be a bit problematic. (Yes, if you eat a ton of fat with sugar, you *will* probably store that fat!)

Most important, I hope you may transcend politics and lose your fear of this lamentably demonized macronutrient. Your body and health will thank you!

FAKE PROBLEMS

Today's processed foods are delightfully delicious and deliriously deadly. Their rainbow of chemicals, preservatives, and flavorings developed by food scientists hack our hardwired, unconscious predispositions to seek out energy-rich foods. Constant access to these modern temptations has resulted in slavery to appetite and burgeoning waistlines, even though their ingredients often have toxic effects and instigate immune responses, so you feel more crème-de-la-crap than crème brûlée. It's not your fault you want them, and saying no may seem daunting, but, speaking as a former addict, it *can* be done!

FOOD ADDICTION

Ever had that moment when you simply *had* to eat another one of those prepackaged chips or cookies, even though you weren't *really* hungry, or it didn't even taste *that* amazing? Guess what—it's not all in your mind!

Well, it is . . . but that's the point.

Processed foods are highly addictive, and not in a casual, hard-to-resist way. Nope. They're *literally* addictive: scientifically designed to trigger the mesolimbic dopaminergic "reward section" of our brain—the same neural circuits activated in drug or alcohol addiction. Like these drugs, processed foods can trigger cravings, feelings of loss of control, withdrawal, and continued use despite the problems that result from ingesting them.

In theory, a person's appetite should adequately moderate energy intake and deficits, making you feel hungry when you actually *need* food and full when you do not. Yet modern foods disrupt this system, increasing hunger while decreasing satiety signals, even though they should technically suppress appetite due to their typically high calorie content. Tapping into our hedonistic pathways, these hyperpalatable foods provide a "hit" of pleasure, while raising the threshold for that pleasure. More and more of the substance is then required to achieve the same effect.

In the 1970s, researchers discovered that rats would happily gorge on Froot Loops, even at the expense of their safety.[38] In follow-up experiments, feeding the little guys other grocery store goodies, such as chocolate chip cookies and condensed milk, could fatten them up in a matter of weeks, more so than the high-fat rat chow intended to do the same. This led to the development of the "cafeteria diet," which mimics the processed stuff humans eat.[39] Studies found that the cafeteria diet quickly encouraged inflammation, glucose intolerance, binge eating, and "exaggerated obesity" in rats (as if obesity weren't bad enough).[40]

Other studies find that sucrose (refined sugar) consumption stimulates the release of dopamine: a feel-good chemical that motivates us to continue engaging in a behavior. When rats are conditioned to associate sucrose with the cue of pushing a lever, they will eventually experience dopamine hits as soon as they press the lever, even *before* the sucrose is actually delivered, and even if *no* sucrose is delivered at all. The presence of sugar in the small intestine can also stimulate dopamine, conditioning us to crave whatever food we're eating at that time. This is bad news, since most processed foods typically add some sort of sugar to the mix, even when you'd least expect it.

And the culprits don't end with sugar. Consider umami—one of our five food tastes. Umami naturally comes from glutamate found in things such as mushrooms, meat broths, and fermented foods. Modern foods often concentrate the umami flavor in the form of monosodium glutamate (MSG), which activates our addictive neural pathways. While we don't typically crave umami by itself, umami added to foods renders them bingeworthy in our brain. Sneaky!

We've also got the ever-vague "natural and artificial flavors," the fourth most prevalent food ingredient after sugar, salt, and water, which can be derived from almost anything. (McDonald's french fries, for example, contain "natural beef flavor" made of hydrolyzed wheat and milk. Because *obviously*.) These flavors are specifically engineered to tap into our cravings, while being more potent and addictive than actual food. They also have a brief life span, so you constantly reach for more. (Ever had that moment where you quickly chewed your way through a pack of gum? #Guilty.)

Alterations to the brain's natural cravings for these foods can even begin in the womb. One study found that when pregnant rats were fed highly palatable junk food, their baby rats were more inclined to seek out those same foods and become obese. This is especially troublesome, given that, as of 2016, around 40 percent of U.S. women are estimated to be obese.[41] In other words, a majority of children born today may be programmed from the beginning to crave junk food.

WHY, WHY, WHY . . .

Despite how it may appear, our brain is actually not trying to screw us over: It's trying to protect us! Go figure. Our craving for processed foods involves the central governing system of the hypothalamus, which developed in a time of food scarcity and is in charge of making sure we've got enough energy reserves to live, so we can ultimately reproduce. (Since you have to live to reproduce, this also means hunger cravings take precedence over reproductive cravings. Translation: Your lover may have nothing on chocolate cake!)

Thanks to the hypothalamus, we crave things that indicate energy and nutrition. Our bodies associate sweetness with energy-rich fruit, umami with protein-rich meats, and fat with energy-rich calories in general. In the old days, indulging these senses was self-limiting: We could only gather so much produce or hunt so much meat at any one time. These whole foods also required a great deal of digestion, while providing a whopping load of nutrition. Today however, these same taste cues are attached to easily accessible and digestible, highly caloric, nutrient*less* foods.

Also keep in mind that in nature, sugar and fat are typically not found together. (You're either eating fruit *or* you're eating your latest kill.) This minimizes the potential problem of insulin release from sugar encouraging epic fat storage of the fat. Modern food, on the other hand, *loves* to parade high-sugar, high-fat combinations, writing an instant recipe for weight gain. (The sugar tells your body to store the fat . . . and you store the fat.)

A historical perspective also explains why most people don't crave vegetables: They provide very few calories, especially considering the effort required to gather and prepare them. It's also possible we don't crave micronutrients and minerals because they were naturally present in the whole foods of the hunter-gatherer diet. While vital for health, such vitamins also aren't as necessary for reproduction as energy from fat and sugar. (Ever heard someone say, "OMG, I would kill for some potassium"? Yeah, me neither.)

Unfortunately for the ladies, the odds are not so much in our favor in the craving department. As we are the gender responsible for the energetically costly process of childbearing, our bodies tend to crave these hyperpalatable foods more fervently than men's do. Female rats, for example, tend to lap up more sugary drinks than male rats,[42] while studies suggest that women are more likely to become "addicted" to food, supported by global obesity rate demographics.[43]

I could go on and on about this whole-food craving issue, but I bet you get the point. If you want to go deeper into the science of food cravings and the workings of our brain, I suggest checking out Stephan Guyenet's *The Hungry Brain: Outsmarting the Instincts That Make Us Overeat.*

FOOD ADDITIVES

Beyond the addictive potential of processed foods, we've got a whole 'nother issue to consider: toxins and autoimmunity. More than three thousand food additives (many of which are banned in other countries) overwhelmingly color today's boxed and canned goodies, both figuratively and literally. I'm talking things such as solvents, preservatives, nitrates, nitrosamines, pesticides, carrageenan, dioxins, and food dyes. (My mother always insisted Kool-Aid would "turn your insides blue!") And don't even get me started on trans fats, which we looked at in "Fat Problems" on page 28. Some of these compounds are literally toxic. BPA and propylene glycol, for example, can disrupt hormones. BHA, artificial colors from petroleum, and synthetic hormones found in dairy products can act as carcinogens. And bromine and BHT compounds may encourage hypothyroidism and organ damage.

Even additives that are not "officially" deleterious to health can register as foreign substances in the body, resulting in digestive distress, inflammation, and immune "confusion," as the body begins attacking its own tissue in response. Before Paleo, I didn't think cutting out additives would make *that* much of a difference, but boy was I wrong! Doing so was the key to eradicating lingering skin issues, joint pains, and headaches. When they tell you the "small" amounts of these compounds don't matter, ask them if they'd like to drink a "small" amount of arsenic.

HIGH-FRUCTOSE CORN SYRUP

Refined fructose may be especially problematic for our health and waistlines. Unlike glucose, which quickly becomes blood sugar and encourages insulin release upon ingestion, fructose is shuttled to the liver for processing and minimally affects blood sugar in the short term, which initially granted it a "healthy" label.

But things are not as they appear. In the liver, fructose can be processed into fat and shipped out on proteins, raising triglyceride levels and encouraging the formation of advanced glycation end products (AGEs), which accelerate aging. Fructose also does not raise leptin levels which regulate satiety, and thus does not easily quell the appetite. Studies link high fructose intake to nonalcoholic fatty liver disease, pancreatic cancer, metabolic syndrome, high cholesterol, and weight gain. People intolerant to fructose may also experience digestive distress such as gas and bloating, as malabsorption leads to fermentation.

Fructose's damaging effects are heightened in its *refined* form, such as in high-fructose corn syrup (HFCS)—the premier sweetener of processed foods and beverages. Between 1970 and 1990, HFCS consumption increased more than 1,000 percent, mirroring the rise of the obesity epidemic.[44] Present today in everything from soft drinks to meat (yes, meat), HFCS constitutes more than 40 percent of added caloric sweeteners in the United States, with Americans consuming an average of around *60 pounds* per year.

HFCS yields close to a one-to-one ratio of glucose and fructose, but in liquid form, making it essentially liquid sucrose. Herein lies a major potential problem. Readily available to the body in liquid form, the glucose in HFCS spikes blood sugar and insulin, while the fructose can promote triglyceride formation and fat storage. Talk about the perfect storm! Not surprisingly, HFCS is strongly correlated with diabetes, obesity, and all the problems arising from such. In fact, rats with access to HFCS gain significantly more weight than those with access to sucrose, even when they consume *the same number of calories.* (So much for "a calorie is a calorie"!)

That said, the studies damning fructose typically involve high amounts in refined form (such as HFCS), which radically departs from the smaller amounts of fructose found naturally in fruits, accompanied by water, fiber, and vitamins. Fructose-related weight gain in our present society may primarily stem from the vast calorie overconsumption from HFCS, since people tend to *add* HFCS-sweetened foods and drinks to their diet, rather than *replace* food with it. On the contrary, fructose added via fruit promotes fullness and typically leads to a similar or even lower number of overall calories consumed, which may explain why recent analyses suggest that fructose in whole-foods form (Paleo-style!) likely does *not* encourage weight gain.[45] So, choose the apple over the apple-flavored HFCS treat, and you're good to go!

ARTIFICIAL SWEETENERS

Not gonna lie, I went through *quite* the artificial-sweetener phase to wean off sugar. I conditioned myself to forsake Coke in favor of Diet Coke—a drink I had originally disliked. I opted for sugar-free dressings and marinades, and popped zero-calorie mints like candy. All the while, I defended my habit, citing lack of scientific support for deleterious effects.

At first glance, artificial sweeteners *seem* like the perfect solution to our sugar cravings, allowing us to indulge our sweet tooth, sans calories. It all started in the 1800s with saccharin, now masquerading as the pink packet of Sweet'N Low. Chemically derived from petroleum, saccharin is three hundred times sweeter than table sugar, and not metabolized by the body. Next came aspartame in 1965 (Equal's blue packet), which is two hundred times sweeter than table sugar, and actually is broken down by the body into amino acids and methanol. Most recently, we got yellow Splenda, chemically modified sucralose—a sucrose molecule, which is six hundred times sweeter than sugar, and not metabolized by the body.

Despite technically being "zero" calories, artificial sweeteners are often linked to weight gain, like in a 1980s study of almost 80,000 women,[46] a 1990s study of 31,940 women,[47] and a 2008 study of 3,682 individuals.[48] (And, it seems that the more artificial sweeteners you ingest, the fatter you may get!) Though the mechanisms aren't quite clear, artificial sweeteners often promote overconsumption, possibly by tapping into sweet cravings to increase appetite. Rats eating saccharin tend to eat more and gain more weight.[49] And one human study found that tasting aspartame increased appetite, while swallowing it in pill form did not.[50] It's also possible that, in tasting the sweetness with no actual *substance* behind it, our bodies encourage us to eat more to make up for the lack of calories. Studies have also found that when patients unknowingly ingest artificial sweeteners, they ingest fewer calories.[51] But when they *know* they're using artificial sweeteners, they eat more calories.[52] This indicates that perhaps we overcompensate with other calories in response to being "good" with artificially sweetened foods.

As for artificial sweeteners and insulin release, the findings are mixed. Some studies find that artificial sweeteners encourage an insulin response, while others don't. I personally think if an artificial sweetener makes you hungrier or increases cravings, something funky is probably going on.

Perhaps most significantly, recent research indicates that artificial sweeteners may encourage weight gain (as well as a host of other sinister problems) via the gut microbiome. In a 2014 study, mice given artificial sweeteners developed obesity, glucose intolerance, and diabetes, unlike mice given glucose or sucrose, despite similar food intake and activity levels.[53] The artificial sweeteners (particularly saccharin) increased the rodents' Bacteroides bacteria and decreased their Firmicutes bacteria, a foundational shift that can increase metabolism of starch, sugars, and fatty acids. Basically, these bacteria may make you extract more calories from your food! When the artificially sweetened, glucose-intolerant mice were given antibiotics to wipe out their changed gut population, their issues resolved. Transferring the gut bacteria from the saccharin mice to bacteria-free mice instigated similar problems of glucose intolerance in the latter.

The researchers also examined nutritional data from 381 humans, and found that those who ingest artificial sweeteners become overweight and glucose intolerant, with elevated liver enzymes to boot. The researchers also performed a small control test, in which seven healthy non-artificial-sweetener users ingested saccharin for less than a week. Four of the participants experienced glucose intolerance as a result, with similar negative changes in their gut microbiome. The three who *didn't* experience problems also didn't experience gut microbiome shifts. So artificial sweeteners *might* affect your gut microbiome, and if they do, that could spell trouble for your waistline!

WHAT TO DO??

I sincerely hope you're not panicking at this point. I even more sincerely hope you're not attempting to quell said panic with a soothing (sugar-free?) Oreo. And to be honest, even though I've been Paleo for almost half a decade, I still feel tempted by certain food products. Anything advertised by that deviously cuddlelicious Pillsbury Doughboy really gets to me, like some ex-lover you never quite forgot. (Debating whether I should provide the names of said boys? Editor, please stop me!)

But the thing is, even though I *sort of* want that Funfetti cake or ex-crush, I actually *can* move on. I haven't *actually* eaten any slice-and-bake cookies in years (or texted any exes). And my life is not worse for it, nor do I feel like I'm denying myself, as doubters doth protest. Though I occasionally hanker for the neon-sprinkled cake or a certain *boy*, I know even a minuscule taste will only make me want them *that much more*. So, as with any drug, I just say no! Instead of thinking about what I "can't" have (even though I *can* if I really want!), I think about all the delicious, nourishing, satisfying foods I *can* have. Speaking of . . . Oh hey, "Personal Paleo Guide" up next!

PERSONAL PALEO GUIDE

Here we are! Your personal Paleo template! Hopefully in reading the preceding chapters, you now understand *why* choosing certain foods is key for health. As a been-there, done-that girl, I honestly believe jumping all-in is the best and ultimately easiest approach to starting Paleo. True adherence eliminates cravings, which can linger when you keep around crave-worthy chemical substitutes or cheat meals. It's like seeing your ex every day, compared to moving away and never seeing him or her again. Which situation is easier for getting over the whole shebang? An extended period of strict adherence is also vital for complete elimination of problematic foods, as even seemingly small exposures (mere milligrams) can ignite negative reactions and inflammation in certain individuals. Once you begin experiencing enhanced energy, health, and vitality (not to mention weight loss!), Paleo quickly becomes a breeze. Cravings for toxic foods vanish as you begin desiring just the good stuff.

I advocate complete commitment to a thirty-day trial run. (Plus, my Paleo approach includes wine, so how hard can it be?) I encourage you to eliminate the "No-No!" list for good, as well as the "Maybe!" list for the first thirty days. After that, you can begin experimenting for yourself, individually testing the "Maybe!" foods to see how you react.

Please keep in mind that we are all unique snowflakes, and there is no one perfect diet for everyone. (Wouldn't it be easy if there were?) Aided by this book and your own intuitive self-experimentation, I ultimately encourage you to determine which foods work best for *your* perfect Paleo lifestyle, which is likely not *my* perfect Paleo lifestyle. What's more, your perfect Paleo yesterday may not be your perfect Paleo tomorrow. So take things one step at a time, and be prepared to embrace new food experiences. You got this!

PALEO FOOD LIST

Please see the considerations which follow for more details. Check out Melanie Avalon.com/recommendations for Paleo-friendly commercial versions when applicable.

YES!	
MEAT ANY! FRESH, NOT PROCESSED. PREFERABLY GRASS-FED, PASTURED, ORGANIC.	**Poultry**: Chicken, Duck, Quail, Turkey, etc. **Red Meat**: Beef, Bacon (No Additives, Nitrates, Sugar, etc.), Lamb, Pork **Game Meat**: Bison, Buffalo, Deer, Elk, Rabbit, etc.
SEAFOOD MUCH! NO PRESERVATIVES. PREFERABLY WILD-CAUGHT, UNLESS RESPONSIBLY FARMED WITHOUT ANTIBIOTICS. CHOOSE FISH LOW IN MERCURY AND TOXINS. SEE THE ENVIRONMENTAL DEFENSE FUND'S "SEAFOOD SELECTOR."	**Fish**: Barramundi, Cod, Flounder, Mahi Mahi, Salmon, Tilapia, Trout, etc. **Shellfish**: Clams, Lobster, Oysters, Shrimp, Scallops, etc.
VEGETABLES MOST! PREFERABLY ORGANIC, ESPECIALLY IF CONSUMING THE SKIN. SEE THE ENVIRONMENTAL WORKING GROUP FOR CURRENT PESTICIDE CONCENTRATIONS.	**Cruciferous Veggies**: Bok Choy, Broccoli, Brussels Sprouts, Cauliflower, Kale, Turnip, etc. **Leafy Greens**: Arugula, Collards, Iceberg, Lettuce, Mustard Greens, Romaine, Spinach, Turnip Greens, etc. **Sea Vegetables:** Arame, Dulse, Kelp, Nori, etc. **Summer Squash:** Yellow, Zucchini, etc. **Other:** Artichoke, Asparagus, Beets, Carrots, Celeriac, Celery, Cucumbers, Mushrooms, Olives, Onions, Radish, Rhubarb, Watercress, etc.
STARCHES SOME! PREFERABLY ORGANIC, ESPECIALLY FOR ROOT VEGGIES.	**Sweet Potatoes**: Okinawan, Orange, Purple, etc. **Winter Squash**: Acorn, Butternut, Pumpkin, Spaghetti, etc. **Other**: Jicama, Parsnips, Plantains, Rutabaga, Taro, Yam, Yuca, etc

FRUITS	**Berries**: Blackberries, Blueberries, Cranberries, Raspberries, Strawberries, etc.
ALMOST ALL! PREFERABLY ORGANIC, ESPECIALLY IF CONSUMING THE SKIN.	**Citrus**: Lemon, Lime, etc. **Melons**: Cantaloupe, Honeydew, Watermelon, etc. **Other**: Apple, Apricot, Avocado, Banana, Cherimoya, Cherries, Coconut, Figs, Grapefruit, Grapes, Guava, Kiwi, Lychee, Nectarine, Orange, Papaya, Passion Fruit, Peaches, Pears, Plums, Pomegranates, Tangerine, etc.
NUTS AND SEEDS TONS! PREFERABLY ORGANIC, SOAKED.	Almonds, Brazil Nuts, Cashews, Hazelnuts, Macadamias, Pecans, Pine Nuts, Pistachios, Pumpkin Seeds, Sesame Seeds, Sunflower Seeds, Walnuts
PLANT OILS NUMEROUS! PREFERABLY ORGANIC, COLD-PRESSED.	Avocado, Coconut, Flaxseed, Macadamia, MCT Oil, Olive, Palm, Walnut
DAIRY THESE! PREFERABLY ORGANIC, PASTURED.	Clarified Butter, Eggs, Ghee
ANIMAL FATS LOTS! PREFERABLY ORGANIC, GRASS-FED.	Duck Fat, Lard, Schmaltz (Chicken, Goose), Tallow
NATURAL SWEETENERS JUST A FEW! PREFERABLY ORGANIC.	Coconut Sugar, Nectar, Honey (Raw, Unpasteurized)
OTHER A HANDFUL! PREFERABLY ORGANIC WHEN APPLICABLE. NO ADDITIVES.	**Chocolate**: Cocoa, Cacao **Salt**: Celtic Sea Salt, Pink Himalayan, Redmond **Spices**: All, Except Chili Flakes, Cayenne, Nutmeg, Paprika **Vinegar**: Gluten-Free, With No Sugar Added: Apple Cider Vinegar, Red Wine, etc. **Other**: Coconut Aminos, Fish Sauce, Nutritional Yeast, Vanilla Extract
BEVERAGES A BIT! PREFERABLY ORGANIC. NO ADDITIVES.	Tea, Coffee, Nut Milks (Almond, Cashew, Coconut, etc.), Water, Wine

MAYBE!	
ALCOHOL	Clear, Hard (Gluten-Free Vodka, Gin, Tequila, etc.)
DAIRY	Butter, Kefir, Yogurt (No Additives, Grass-Fed, Raw, Unpasteurized, A2)
LEGUMES	Green Peas, Green Beans
NIGHTSHADES	Eggplant, Goji Berry, Sweet/Hot Peppers (Black Pepper Is Okay), Tomatoes, White Potatoes
SOY	Fermented (Miso, Natto, Tempeh, etc.)
SWEETENERS	"Natural" Noncaloric (Monk Fruit, Stevia, Sugar Alcohols, etc.)
OTHER	White Rice

NO-NO!	
IN ADDITION TO THE BELOW, AVOID ANYTHING PACKAGED, PROCESSED, OR WITH CHEMICAL ADDITIVES.	
ALCOHOL	With Added Sugar, Colors, Additives, Gluten (Most Colored Rums/Tequilas, Most Whiskeys, Liqueurs, etc.)
ARTIFICIAL SWEETENERS	Aspartame, Saccharin, Sucralose, etc.
CHOCOLATE	Milk With Additives
GRAINS	All, Including "Gluten-Free" Ones (Amaranth, Barley, Buckwheat, Cereal, Corn, Oats, Rice, Rye, Wheat, White Flour, Whole Grain Flour, etc.)
LEGUMES	Alfalfa, Black Beans, Black-Eyed Peas, Chickpeas, Chili Beans, Garbanzo Beans, Kidney Beans, Lentils, Lima Beans, Navy Beans, Pinot Beans, Peanuts, etc.
OILS	Refined, Hydrogenated, Processed (Canola, Corn, Safflower, Soybean, Sunflower, Vegetable, etc.)
SOY	Processed (Tofu, Soy Additives, Soy Sauce, etc.)
SUGARS	Added, Refined (Agave Nectar, Cane Sugar, White Table Sugar, etc.)
OTHER	"Junk Food," Quinoa, Trans-Fats

THE "YES!" LIST CONSIDERATIONS

NUTS AND SEEDS

Nuts and seeds are quite Paleo. That said, these little gems of protein and fat feature phytic acid and enzyme inhibitors that can bind to their (and your) nutrients, making them less bioavailable. You can soak your nuts and seeds for around seven hours or so to combat this effect. Keep in mind that consuming nuts and seeds in whole form is more Paleo in spirit than spooning your way through nut butters, as it's shockingly easy to go overboard on those. Due to pesticides, you also *definitely* want to go organic. And avoid peanuts, which are actually legumes (sneaky). They're often contaminated with carcinogenic mycotoxins, and are very allergenic, with the highest rates of food-induced fatality.

PLANT OILS

Plant oils can be a great source of healthy fats, nutrition, and flavor, and they are excellent for cooking, baking, marinades, and salad dressings. That said, they are nevertheless refined, with many commercial forms being prone to oxidation. When using plant-based oils, favor organic, cold-pressed, unrefined forms, and avoid heating them at super high temperatures. (Check out the "Recipes" section on page 269 for appropriate baking temperatures.) I suggest embracing the antimicrobial, ketone-boosting coconut oil. (If you don't like its coconuty flavor, you can try cold-pressed, refined versions.) In any case, I encourage you to get your plant fats from whole foods whenever possible, such as nuts, seeds, olives, coconut, and avocado.

ANIMAL FATS

Like plant oils, rendered animal fats (such as tallow, lard, and ghee) are also refined versions of whole foods—except this time, meat! But unlike most plant oils, animals fats are highly stable and do not easily oxidize. Contrary to popular belief, they're also not 100 percent saturated fat: Most are almost half monounsaturated fats! (Not that saturated fat is a bad thing, as we discussed in "Fat Problems" on page 28. I encourage you to favor animal fats in whole-foods form (such as a nice steak!), using small amounts of rendered grass-fed animal fats in cooking if you so desire. (Save going super crazy for a specifically ketogenic approach.)

EGGS

Think of pastured eggs as nature's multivitamin! They're rich in eighteen fat-soluble vitamins and minerals (including A, D, E, K, and B_{12}, as well as the elusive zinc, selenium, and choline), protein, omega-3s, monounsaturated fats, DHA, and lecithin. Contrary to popular belief, recent studies suggest that eggs do not negatively affect cholesterol, nor do they increase cardiovascular risk.[54] In fact, eggs may help prevent cardiovascular disease, as well as many other infectious and degenerative conditions, thanks to their antioxidant, antimicrobial, immune-mediating power.[55] That said, some people are allergic to egg proteins, and may need to exclude them from their personal Paleo template. Since most of these allergenic proteins (such as ovomucoid, ovalbumin, and lysozyme) reside in the egg white, egg yolks may be less problematic. If you do include eggs, favor the pastured version for richer nutrition.

CLARIFIED BUTTER/GHEE

Oh gee, what is ghee? (Too much?) Unlike normal butter, which contains around 5 percent milk solids, clarified butter and ghee are almost pure forms of butterfat. Their saturation and extremely high smoke points (~485°F) makes them great for cooking. Ghee tends to have a nuttier flavor than clarified butter, due to caramelized milk solids (which are ultimately removed).

When obtained from grass-fed sources, ghee and clarified butter are rich in fat-soluble vitamins and minerals (including A, E, and the elusive K_2), carotenoids, antioxidants, and an array of healthy saturated, monounsaturated, and polyunsaturated essential fatty acids, including the EPA and DHA forms of omega-3. Ghee has been shown to discourage fat oxidation in the body, benefit cholesterol levels, and discourage heart disease.[56]

Since these fat sources feature few proteins that may spark an immune response, they're often well tolerated, even by those who react to "normal" butter. That said, those with super sensitive immune systems or autoimmune conditions may want to exclude them.

"NATURAL" SUGARS

I generally don't advocate isolated sweetness, which can sustain sugar cravings, spike blood sugar, hinder weight loss, and exacerbate the all-too-common problem of food addiction. That said, sometimes you need to bake a Paleo cake, or just fancy something sweet, and I'd much rather you use a Paleo-friendly "natural" sugar than refined sugar. Plus, some of these may even provide a few health benefits!

Honey

I can't say honey isn't Paleo, because, well, it's *literally* Paleo. Historically, hunter-gatherers likely consumed an estimated 2 to 3 percent of their daily calories from honey. That said, honey is the most calorically dense food substrate found naturally in the wild, sort of like a more nutritious Paleo equivalent to refined sugar (refined by bees!). While honey was likely quite beneficial in Paleolithic days when a cavegirl's just trying to survive, the same argument is harder to make in today's world of easily accessible foods, as Americans fill up to 15 percent (if not more) of their diet with added sugars. Braving your way through a honeycomb at the expense of angry bee stings is also *slightly* different than selecting prepackaged honey from air-conditioned grocery store aisles.

That said, raw honey can be high in B vitamins, minerals, enzymes, amino acids, and antioxidants. It's great for wound healing, and may support GI and dental health.[57] Consuming small amounts of local, raw honey can benefit allergies. Honey is also antibacterial and beneficial for the immune system, due to its hydrogen peroxide content, low water ratio, and other (likely undiscovered) compounds.

For those who can justify its price tag {sigh}, the highly studied Manuka honey from New Zealand contains nonperoxide activity compounds with über-potent antimicrobial properties. A 2016 study found that Manuka honey could successfully inhibit *all* pathogens in vitro tested to date, encompassing more than fifty buggers, including *Helicobacter pylori* and resistant bacteria.[58] Researchers were even unable to create bacteria resistant to Manuka when they *tried*! Manuka honey can notably target tricky biofilms (the mucous protective matrixes where bacteria camp out and laugh in your face), and may be selectively toxic to bacteria, but not to us!

That said, while small amounts of honey may taste yummy, provide some nutrition, and even be therapeutic, context and one's personal tolerance is key. Having a tablespoon of honey is not the same as exploring your inner Winnie the Pooh. And even though honey may potentially aid blood glucose control, it probably won't eradicate your sweet tooth. I recommend using honey smartly and sparingly, and favor getting your staple sweetness from whole-food sources such as fruit. Keep in mind that, despite any adorable honey bear bottles, conventionally refined versions of honey are often denatured to the point that they're essentially nutrientless quick hits of sugar. Favor raw, unpasteurized forms.

Coconut Sugar/Nectar
Like honey, coconut nectar is arguably "Paleo" in nature, as hunter-gatherers may have lapped up sweet coconut sap. Refined coconut sugar is more Neolithic, but still may be better than conventional table sugar. These coconut sweeteners do

contain a bit of nutrition, such as iron, zinc, calcium, potassium, the prebiotic inulin, and polyphenols. That said, you can easily acquire these benefits from whole foods, so save coconut sweeteners for special treats, recipes, or occasions.

CHOCOLATE

At the expense of sounding incredibly bland, I've always been more of a vanilla person myself, but I know many people are total chocolate lovers! After all, chocolate is the most craved food in the United States, with 40 percent of women hankering for it.[59] On the plus side, chocolate's inner spirit—cacao—is super rich in flavanols, antioxidants, and magnesium, and may support cardiovascular health,[60] blood pressure,[61] cholesterol, and insulin levels.[62] It's also been "scientifically" shown to boost mood and reduce stress levels.[63]

Unfortunately, most chocolate manifests as processed, refined commercial forms filled with added dairy, fat, and sugar. Chocolate's health benefits also come from its *dark* side, and dark cacao powder is not the same as chocolate goodies with foil-wrapped promises of golden tickets. It's not even the same as the more prevalent *cocoa* powder—a more processed and heated form (#mindblown moment).

Though studies have shown that the marked cacao/cocoa percentages on commercial chocolate products tend to accurately reflect their antioxidant potential, that doesn't mean you should reach for any bar labeled with a high cacao/cocoa content.[64] Be wary of additives. If what you really love about chocolate is the sugar and/or dairy riding along with it, then Houston, we have a problem. But if small amounts of rich, bitter dark chocolate make you feel good without instigating cravings, then we're onto something!

SPICES

Not only do spices boost flavor in dishes and generate instant variety, they can also provide an array of health benefits, including antioxidants, antimicrobial powers, and cancer prevention. From oregano to garlic to ginger, go with what you like and what makes you happy! You definitely want to get organic spices without fillers, to avoid toxic pesticides and additives, and you may want to avoid chili flakes and paprika if you're sensitive to nightshades.

VINEGAR

Vinegar is created by fermenting previously fermented carb-containing foods, such as fruits or rice, resulting in a sour taste from acetic acid. (Think about how wine becomes vinegary when left out too long.) While absent in Paleolithic days, vinegar's polyphenol-rich, antimicrobial powers can provide flavor and health benefits, like blood sugar and blood pressure control, free radical scavenging, and support of a healthy weight. Apple cider vinegar is often available in raw, unpasteurized form, and features health benefits from its cloudy probiotic substance called "the mother." Avoid vinegars with added sugars or gluten, such as malt vinegar and many balsamic vinegars.

TEA AND COFFEE

Additive-free teas and coffees are definitely Paleo-friendly, and come with a myriad of health benefits. Since teas and coffees are quite prone to pesticides and mold toxins, favor organic, mold-free forms. Also know that instant coffee has been shown to cross-react with gluten in particularly sensitive individuals.[65]

WINE

I diverge from many Paleo gurus in advocating wine right from the get-go! Since we've got a whole section dedicated to this topic, I'll keep matters brief. I believe including wine in moderation is great for living and loving life, while bestowing a myriad of health benefits to boot. Of course, you don't *have* to drink wine, and also might want to exclude it if you're sensitive to histamines or sulfites, not already a drinker, or want to try a hard-core liver-loving reset.

SUPER important note: Government regulations make it nearly impossible to know just what is in any given wine. If you react negatively to wine, you might actually be reacting to its additives (sugar, sulfites, stabilizers, colorizers, fining agents, etc.), pesticides (which are particularly concentrated in conventional grapes), and/or mycotoxins. For this reason, I strongly encourage you to purchase organic or biodynamic wines, which are available at decent prices at Trader Joe's, Whole Foods, and Sprouts.

That said, many wineries implement organic practices without the certification, due to financial costs, lack of need, or even the stigma of "organic" wines. I wholeheartedly recommend you check out Dry Farm Wines. They travel the world and conduct lab tests to find small, sustainable wineries that produce all natural, organic wines with no additives or pesticides, and which are low-alcohol (<12.5%), sugar-free (<1 g/L), and mold-free! I personally sought to partner with them for readers of this book. Check out DryFarmWines.com/melanieavalon for more information, and to get a bottle for a penny with your first subscription, shipped straight to your door! #wine #winning

THE "MAYBE!" LIST CONSIDERATIONS

DAIRY

Dairy sparks heated debate in the Paleosphere, and for good reason. After all, what other food source is actually a *hormonal* food with the purpose of modulating immune systems and growing offspring? While dairy brims with potential for nourishment and health benefits, it also may encourage GI distress, inflammation, allergies, and addiction. Some people do well with dairy, others not so much. In any case, the type and source of dairy may be a factor.

Starting with the dark side, dairy is a Neolithic food, as historical hunter-gatherers only consumed it via breast milk. Dairy is intended for newborns in the early days of their personal timeline, and last time I checked, you weren't a newborn. (If you are, and you're reading this . . . wow.) This means dairy can be intensely insulinogenic and growth promoting, which may benefit bodybuilders, but not so much the general public.

Many people are sensitive to dairy, for a variety of reasons. Some people lack adequate amounts of the lactase enzyme, necessary to break down milk's lactose sugar. (Though studies suggest true lactose intolerance is rare, and negative reactions to dairy often involve other factors.) Others may experience immune reactions to the proteins in milk: casein, casomorphin, butyrophilin, and whey. These dairy proteins have also been shown to cross-react with gluten, so gluten-sensitive individuals may experience negative immune and intestinal reactions.

Dairy also harbors addictive potential, thanks to opioid-like casomorphin peptides, which likely serve a purpose of encouraging mother/child bonding and restful sleep, among other things. (I don't know about you, but I seriously can't stop eating cheese after the first bite, which is particularly high in these compounds.) Opioid compounds can also slow gut motility, explaining why dairy causes constipation and bloating in many people.

Of particular note, today's cow milk can be either of the A1 or A2 variety (or a blend of both).[66] The A2 variety is the "original" form of milk prevalent before domestication, and the same type as human breast milk. A genetic muta-tion around five to ten thousand years ago, however, bred a new type of milk, A1, in European cattle. Studies show that A1 milk can be more difficult to digest than A2, exacerbate GI distress and inflammation, encourage the release of more addictive opioid peptides, slow gut motility, disrupt gut bacteria, and ramp up mucus production in many individuals. While a small amount of mucus is helpful in the gut, an excess can disrupt gut function and encourage bacterial dysbiosis. (Plus it makes me feel gross, and who likes breakouts?)

Whew—that was a lot of grimy stuff with dairy! However, there *is* poten-tial for dairy in your personal Paleo template, as organic, grass-fed, unpas-teurized forms in the A2 variety (including goat's milk) might not yield an inflammatory response. (Studies have notably found that organic versions of dairy reduce allergic skin disorders such as eczema, compared to conventional dairy.)[67] Raw cultured dairy with live cultures, à la yogurt and kefir, also con-tain fewer inflammatory opioid peptides and sugars (which are hydrolyzed by the bacteria), and may actually support digestion and GI health.

You can experiment with dairy after thirty days of strict Paleo to see how you react. I realize raw, grass-fed, organic, A2, and cultured is a lot of qualifiers, but you can increasingly find a number of products satisfying many of these criteria at natural food stores, and even in some conventional grocery stores.

Grass-Fed Butter

Due to its concentrated fat content low in proteins and sugar, butter lacks many of dairy's problems. In fact, butter contains around four hundred types of fatty acids (including short-, medium-, and long-chain forms of saturated, monounsaturated, and polyunsaturated fats),[68] making it quite a "complicated" fat, indeed! When from grass-fed cows, butter features an anti-inflammatory profile rich in the EPA and DHA forms of omega-3, the antioxidant CLA, and fat-soluble vitamins A and K_2. That said, some people may react to butter's residual milk proteins. You may be able to tolerate clarified butter or ghee, or you may want to omit butter entirely.

LEGUMES

Legumes are typically excluded in Paleo approaches, due to their lectins, which can injure the gut, and phytates, which can bind to nutrients, making them less absorbable. (See "Grainy Problems" on page 9 for more on this.) That said, legumes lack the more damaging antinutrients prevalent in grains (such as gluten and gliadin), while featuring more nutrients. I'd construct the legume cost/benefit hierarchy as follows: green beans > green peas > all other beans and peas > peanuts. (Avoid peanuts, which are highly allergenic and sometimes moldy!)

The following preparations may reduce some legume antinutrients:

- Soak legumes for twelve to twenty-four hours before cooking. The wetness tricks the legumes into thinking they've been planted, and thus release their antinutrient compounds.
- Utilize moist heat, such as boiling or steaming.
- Cook at high temperatures, above 176°F.
- Pressure-cooking is great!
- Fermentation can reduce lectin activity. (Avoid tofu, but tempeh *might* be okay for you.)

NIGHTSHADES

Edible nightshades include white (not sweet) potatoes, sweet and hot peppers, tomatoes, and eggplant. They contain naturally occurring chemical alkaloids, which serve as protective mechanisms against invaders. These problematic compounds include the spicy capsaicin found in peppers, as well as soapy saponins, which get their name from the soapwort plant used to make soap.

Nightshade compounds may irritate the respiratory and digestive tract, inhibit digestive enzymes and nutrient uptake, encourage leaky gut, and yield an immune response and inflammation, particularly arthritis. Not everyone reacts negatively to nightshades (oh hey, pepper lovers!), but those who do often *really* do (oh hey, pepper haters!). Cooking nightshades can help neutralize negative effects.

WHITE POTATOES

Many Paleo peeps readily parade the benefits of sweet potatoes and yams while branding white potatoes the devil, without knowing why. Here's why!

Potatoes feature a very high starch content, which may be problematic for those who function best on lower-carb diets. That said, sweet potatoes are comparably high in carbohydrates, and some people do thrive on more carbs, so I think we can throw that argument out the window. Contrary to popular belief, both white and sweet potatoes are pretty high in nutrients (although sweet potatoes feature strikingly more beta-carotene, the precursor to vitamin A). So there goes that argument as well.

A tater's primary quandary likely involves lineage. While sweet potatoes belong to the Convolvulaceae (morning glory) family, and yams to the Dioscoreaceae (yam) family, white potatoes call the ominous Solanaceae (nightshade) family home. As discussed, nightshades contain protective plant compounds that can spark intense immune reactions in some people. White potatoes can be particularly high in the glycoalkaloid saponin known as *solanine*, which can rapidly enter the bloodstream and encourage intestinal permeability and inflammation, along with other unpleasant effects. The proteins in potatoes may also cross-react with gluten in some individuals.

The takeaway? White potatoes may or may not work for you, depending on your personal constitution, particularly your relationship with nightshades. (I recently ate a dinner solely composed of white potatoes, after not having had them in years, as my own potato tolerance test. At 3:00 a.m., I was crying from the muscle spasm pain, in an *I just might die, I need my mother* type way.) Also consider your carbohydrate tolerance. If you do well with starch, these guys may work for you. Or you may belong to the camp that experiences blood sugar swings, insulin spikes, fatigue, foggy mind, and/or gut dysbiosis from starch (like me). As always, feel free to experiment with white potatoes after thirty days of a stricter Paleo approach.

WHITE RICE

A grain on the "Maybe!" list?? Gasp! Before you summon thoughts of *sham!* let's take a closer look at the affair. When you think about it, white rice (if organic) is essentially stripped of everything that makes it "grainy," since its antinutrients reside in its (dearly departed) outer bran and hull. If you soak your white rice and cook it for a good length of time at high temperatures, you're basically left with a glutinously gluten-free glob of starch. Of course, while this makes white rice low in toxins, it also makes it low in nutrients.

While I definitely don't advocate rice right from the get-go, it may provide a benign source of (cheap!) energy. And with essentially all glucose and almost no fiber, white rice can be easily digestible, especially for some individuals with gut dysbiosis or fructose intolerance. That said, the proteins in rice may cross-react with gluten, so proceed with caution.[69] You can check out the "Recipes" section for a gentle form of slow-cooked rice porridge called congee (page 325).

FERMENTED SOY PRODUCTS

Non-GMO fermented soy products such as tempeh, miso, and nattō may potentially inhabit a place in your personal Paleo template, providing a healthy source of complete protein and beneficial bacteria. That said, please see the "No-No!" list considerations on page 64 for a complete discussion of these foods.

CALORIE-FREE "NATURAL" SWEETENER SUBSTITUTES

I'm not certain that consuming substances that taste very similar to sugar, yet without the calories, is the best idea, as doing so can send false signals to your body. (See "Fake Problems" on page 39 for more on that.) The goal here is to eradicate, not substitute, our sugary indulgences. That said, there are a few potentially friendly options out there, especially when flexing your Paleo baking skills.

Stevia

A South American herb in the daisy family, stevia's primary extracts, stevioside and rebaudioside, are about 250 to 300 times sweeter than table sugar. With zero calories, a glycemic index of 0, a lack of accumulation in the body, and satiety rates similar to sucrose, stevia has a lot going for it. It also may provide a few health benefits, such as blood sugar, insulin, blood pressure, and cholesterol control. Stevia also boasts antimicrobial and anti-inflammatory properties, can discourage tooth decay, may benefit the liver and GI system, and might even protect against cancer.

So why am I not proclaiming, "Use stevia all the timmmeeee!"? As per usual, it boils down to context and intention. Refined stevia simply isn't a whole food, and may sustain sweet cravings—something I'd much prefer you supplant via the natural carbs found in fruits and veggies. If you're eating stevia by the gallon as a surrogate for sugar, then we've got some problems. On the other hand, I think it's likely fine to use a bit of stevia here and there, if it works for you. As always, look for organic stevia without additional additives.

Sugar Alcohols

Common sugar alcohols include xylitol, erythritol, sorbitol, and maltitol. They contain a low glycemic index with a minute fraction of the calories of table sugar, but with similar perceived sweetness. Studies indicate they negligibly affect blood sugar and insulin, if at all.

Discovered in 1891 and commercially in use since the 1960s, the sweetest and most commercially prevalent sugar alcohol, xylitol, is derived from hardwood. It's particularly beneficial for oral health and preventing cavities, and has thus become sugar-free gum's shining star. Erythritol, with its lower calories and glycemic index, is also gaining popularity, and may be easier on the GI tract than xylitol, which is where things get tricky . . .

On the plus side, sugar alcohols may serve as beneficial prebiotics for gut bacteria, depending on what your personal microbiome fancies for dinner. However, this bacterial fermentation can also promote gas, bloating, and a laxative effect, particularly for those sensitive to FODMAPs: fermentable oligosaccharides, disaccharides, monosaccharides, and polyols. (I'm having flashbacks to my gas-filled days of chewing my way through xylitol-sweetened gum. So. Much. Pain.) Studies also suggest sugar alcohols may change gut flora composition,[70] which makes me quite nervous.

While sugar alcohols occur naturally in small amounts in some stone fruits (such as berries, cherries, and melons), vegetables (such as cauliflower), and mushrooms, you'd be hard-pressed to find a hunter-gatherer snacking on some sugar-free gum or stirring Truvia into his tea. I encourage you to analyze your intentions. A pinch of sugar alcohols may fit nicely into your template, but be wary of sustaining sugar cravings or going crazy, and heed your gut reactions (literally) in the process. (P.S.: A 2014 study found that erythritol can actually function as a natural pesticide . . . sugar-free food for thought right there.)[71]

HARD ALCOHOL

While I can make an argument for wine being Paleo, hard alcohol is a different story. Though we humans *do* feature genetic adaptations to process alcohol, distilled alcohol is essentially the refined form of the more "natural" and health-benefiting wine (oh hey, fermented fruit!), and potentially the root of health problems related to the category.

That said, moderate alcohol intake (wine or no) is consistently linked to a myriad of health benefits, specifically heart health and longevity. If you can include occasional hard alcohol in your personal Paleo template, and ultimately walk away all the happier (and maybe even healthier), then why not? Choose clear versions of liquor, such as gin, vodka, or tequila, which are less likely to contain troublesome additives. (Annoying government regulations make it difficult to ascertain exactly *what* is in any given spirit.) Opt for gluten-free spirits (beer is a definite no-go!), and sip them straight up, or with inoffensive mixers, such as club soda and lime. Robb Wolf's NorCal Margarita is a popular drink in Paleoland, consisting of tequila, lime juice and pulp, and club soda.

For extensive details on alcohol metabolism, health benefits, risks, and factors to consider regarding consumption, check out the "Wine?" section on page 143!

THE "NO-NO!" LIST CONSIDERATIONS

SOY

Soy is tricky business. A complete plant protein, soy first became a popular U.S. vegetarian option in the 1970s. Then things got real in the 1980s and '90s, when correlational studies began linking Asian women's soy intake to health benefits, particularly reduced breast cancer.[72] Hungry to capitalize on these findings, the food industry catapulted soy into the mainstream, aided by growing whispers that soy could benefit other health conditions as well, including postmenopausal symptoms, osteoporosis, and cardiovascular disease. That said, the scientific support for soy is a bit splotchy, with many studies revealing a potential dark side, including cognitive, immune, thyroid, and reproductive dysfunction, as well as increased cancer risk.

Soy's seemingly simultaneous benefits and problems boil down to a common trait. As a potent phytoestrogen, soy mimics the hormone estrogen in the body. This means it can attach to estrogen receptors, though it may or may not function as well as real estrogen, and can send confusing signals to the body. Think of it like trying to get the cheaper off-brand of an iPhone cord or printer cartridge: It may work smashingly (Amazon Basics, I love you!), or it may cause your device to freak out. (How does the printer *knowwww?*) For women with fluctuating hormonal issues, phytoestrogens such as soy may effectively alleviate symptoms, or they may just make things worse. It's very individual, very hard to predict, and very hard to gauge long-term effects.

Soy's estrogen-mimicking nature makes it notably relevant for breast cancer, which often involves estrogen stores. The problem? Some studies suggest soy may discourage cancer, while others find it may encourage it.[73] Yikes! As for the findings regarding Asian women and breast cancer, the association is quite likely influenced by lifestyle and environment. When Asian women relocate to the West, their offspring's risk of breast cancer mirrors that of their new neighbors. Moreover, consistently consuming moderate amounts of soy in whole and fermented form throughout one's life, as in the Asian template, may work on a beneficial epigenetic level. In contrast, suddenly slamming huge amounts of (likely processed) soy later in life, in the common "OMG, soy is so great, let me start eating all the soy now!"-type way, might alarm the body a bit.

To further darken soy's prospects, as of 2016, a shocking 94 percent of U.S. soy is genetically modified, meaning it contains manufactured proteins foreign to our system. This spells trouble for autoimmune conditions, allergies, and particularly cancer. Studies even suggest that GMO foods may alter the DNA of our gut bacteria, encouraging continued production of foreign proteins in your system, even *after* you cut out the stuff.[74] Processed soy also often includes problematic additives, and nonorganic forms are rich in pesticides. In 2015, 96 percent of nonorganic soy was sprayed with herbicides, particularly glyphosate,[75] a potential cytotoxin carcinogen and endocrine disruptor.[76] Soy also contains natural protease and trypsin inhibitors, as well as phytic acid (in more resilient forms than other legumes), which can impair digestion and nutrient assimilation.

The form of soy, however, may be key. Women in Asian countries tend to consume soy in the whole form of edamame, as well as fermented forms such as nattō, miso, and tempeh. These forms may mitigate antinutrients, while benefiting the gut microbiome. On the other hand, modern processed soy is arguably a bastardized GMO-rich, hormone-messing protein, abundant in everything from tofu to dairy to fake meats, and all the other Frankenfoods.

The takeaway? I just don't believe we know enough about how soy interacts with the body to make a call one way or the other regarding its health benefits. Like with dairy, I find it difficult to universally parade the consumption of a food (often in colossal amounts) that so clearly affects the body hormonally, especially in processed form. (I shudder thinking about feeding infants soy milk!) I suggest you avoid processed forms of soy at all costs.

AGAVE

I'd like to touch briefly on the health food poser known as agave nectar. This highly concentrated sweetener produced from the blue agave plant can yield a shocking nine-to-one fructose-to-glucose ratio. (High-fructose corn syrup, by comparison, is only half fructose.) As discussed in "Sweet Problems" on page 20, this spells bad news for your liver, waistline, and health in general. And unlike honey, agave is devoid of any nutrients, while featuring the soapy antinutrient saponins to boot! Please avoid agave. Your body doesn't care that it was once a plant. It's basically just refined liquid fructose.

PROCESSED "PALEO" GOODIES?

Paleo's commercial rise to fame has promoted a slew of processed goodies labeled "Paleo," which may or (more often) may not qualify as such. Beyond their potentially debatable additives and refined nature, processed Paleo goods can easily become kryptonite in our quest to free ourselves from the chains of modern food addiction. While you may eradicate some inflammation in switching out your typical candy bar for a "Paleo" candy bar, you're still unlikely to achieve optimal blood sugar control from such. Weight loss, if that is your goal, may also be more difficult.

I encourage you to eschew processed Paleo goodies whenever possible. If you do want to occasionally indulge (oh hey, birthday party cakes, special occasions, or just some well-deserved me time!), then consider making and baking your own versions, such as the ones provided in "Recipes" on page 269. Embrace the culinary adventure of cooking with nut flours, coconut sugar, honey, and the like. You'll have fun, you'll be creative, you'll expend energy, you'll know *exactly* what you're getting, and you'll infuse your food with more love.

ON SENSITIVITY VERSIONS

AUTOIMMUNE PALEO (AIP)

While many people thrive simply eating most whole foods, people with particularly sensitive immune systems may nevertheless react to certain Paleo items. If you find you still struggle with inflammation and/or autoimmune conditions even after adopting a general Paleo approach, you may want to consider an Autoimmune Paleo (AIP) approach, which can omit unexpected potential problems, such as nuts and seeds and all dairy, among others.

For more on AIP, please visit MelanieAvalon.com. Recipes in this book that are AIP-friendly are noted as such.

LOW FODMAP

The fortunate ones among us have particularly resilient and epic gut microbiomes, and can indulge in seemingly everything without passing a thought or gas. Others (myself included) struggle for reals in the bacteria department, thanks to an onslaught of antibiotics, processed foods, pesticides, and food poisoning, among other factors. If meals make you gassy and bloated, or you struggle with constipation, diarrhea, or both, you may want to try a low-FODMAP (fermentable oligosaccharides, disaccharides, monosaccharides, and polyols) approach. This may relieve symptoms by eliminating fermentable carbohydrates, which are difficult to absorb in the small intestine. After following a low-FODMAP approach for a bit, you just may heal your gut and adjust your microbiome (which is *quite* changeable!), and eventually introduce more foods.

For a free color-coded chart comparing the FODMAP status of 300-plus foods, please visit MelanieAvalon.com/guides. Recipes in this book that are FODMAP-friendly are noted as such.

PALEO Q&A

WHAT MACRONUTRIENT RATIO SHOULD I CONSUME?

Historically, most hunter-gatherers likely consumed an average macronutrient profile of around 35 to 40 percent carbohydrate, 25 to 30 percent protein, and 20 to 35 percent fat. That said, you are not a hunter-gatherer, and your personal perfect Paleo protocol depends on *your* own constitution. Don't lock yourself into any one macronutrient breakdown, and don't fear any of the macros either. The goal is to eat the foods that provide the tools necessary for energy, growth, renewal, and vitality. Ultimately, we'd like to achieve a state of *metabolic flexibility*: the capability to utilize the full spectrum of fuel substrates.

I encourage you in the beginning to eat Paleo whole foods according to your hankerings, letting the macronutrient ratio fall as it may. Down the road, you can experiment with specific protein-fat-carb configurations depending on your goals. Keep in mind that your ideal macronutrient composition may vary: Sometimes you may function better on higher carb, other times lower. Don't fall into the trap of thinking that, because a certain approach worked for you at one time, you are married to it for life. You can always try new things! That's part of the beauty of our wondrously flexible bodies!

HOW MANY CARBS SHOULD I EAT?

I used to be a hard-core low-carb roadie. For reals. I believed carbs were potentially the devil in disguise, and fruit- and tuber-loving peeps were slaves to sugar addiction, blind to the benefits of eschewing all sweetness.

I've since reevaluated things a bit.

While some people flourish on very low-carb or ketogenic diets, others thrive on higher-carb approaches. Neither makes you a better or worse person, and either can potentially support health and longevity. (That said, some people are more "carbohydrate sensitive," while others are more "carbohydrate insensitive." It's a real thing, influenced by factors such as genetics and the gut microbiome.) In any case, while hunter-gatherers averaged 35 to 40 percent carbohydrates, that may have inched closer to 65 percent in some populations.

I recommend a moderate-carb approach to start: up to around 150 grams per day. That said, you can totally eat less, and might even eat more. Do what makes you feel best, with the understanding that what makes you feel best may change! (Some people, for example, find they do better with lower-carb in the winter and higher-carb in the summer.) Your body is smart. Trust it. If you want the apple or the sweet potato, please eat the apple or the sweet potato. If you want to go days without eating a single carb, that's totally fine too! (You'll grow more intuitive in distinguishing carb needs from cravings after you've regulated blood sugar levels by eliminating refined sugar and processed foods.)

WHAT TYPE OF CARBS SHOULD I EAT?

As if the whole carbohydrate thing weren't confusing enough, we've also got the *type* of carbs to consider. As discussed in "Sweet Problems" on page 20, carbs can be either simple or complex. Simple carbs naturally tend to pop up more in fruits, while complex carbs dominate starches. You might function better on one type or the other, based on your genetics, gut microbiome, or who knows what else. People with more copies of the AMY1 gene, for example, tend to have higher levels of starch-digesting enzymes in their spit.[77] Experiment for yourself, and eat the type of carbs that make you feel energetic, without bloatedness or crashing. (Or maybe you're the lucky person who can do *any* type of carbs! Jealous!)

WHAT IS THE KETOGENIC APPROACH TO PALEO?

Now that we've discussed carbs, time for the flip side of the equation! By going very low-carb (generally around 20 to 50 net carbs per day), moderate(ish) protein, and high(er) fat, you can enter a state of ketosis, in which your body switches to an almost completely fat-burning mode, and begins generating supplemental ketones: an alternative (and arguably superior) energy substrate for the body, with a host of benefits. You can measure your level of ketones via various urine strips and blood meters. We'll look at ketosis more in the "When?" section on page 77, as daily fasting instigates the ketogenic state as well, which is how I personally like to get my daily keto!

CAN I DO PALEO AS A VEGETARIAN OR VEGAN?

I do not personally thrive on a vegetarian approach, and I do not believe it is ideal for health in most cases. Our genome developed on a diet inclusive of animal sustenance, which is rich in complete, bioavailable nutrition (when appropriately sourced). Vegetarian diets, on the other hand, can lack adequate amounts of omega-3 fats (specifically EPA and DHA), iron, zinc, calcium, and vitamins D and B_{12}. Furthermore, many nutrients in legumes and grains are inaccessible, thanks to plant antinutrients, while a vegetarian's typically high-fiber intake can further reduce absorption rates. Some studies also suggest all-cause mortality tends to be comparable in vegetarians versus nonvegetarians.[78]

Of course, vegetarians do experience their fair share of health benefits, such as typically lower weights, cholesterol, blood sugar levels, blood pressure, and rates of death from heart disease. And while the diets of most centenarian populations include some sort of animal component, one can point to the plant-based diets of the long-lived Seventh-day Adventists. Recent 2017 research on the dental work of El Sidrón Neanderthals from northern Spain also suggests they may have been vegetarian, dining on a diet of bark, moss, pine nuts, and mushrooms.[79] Yum! And of course, matters of animal treatment, sustainability, and the environment are *essential* topics to consider, though such discussions constitute a subject for another book entirely!

In any case, I completely respect people's food choices. Paleo *can* be done vegetarian-style, it just may be a bit tricky. A Paleo vegetarian approach forgoes "staple" items of grains and soy to instead embrace some combination of tubers, fruits, potentially legumes (see the "Maybe!" list considerations on page 57 for more on that), as well as plant-based fats, like coconut, olive, and avocado. I've included some delicious vegetarian dishes in the "Recipes" section on page 269. If you do decide to wed Paleo and vegetarianism, here are my other suggestions:

EAT REAL FOODS: Don't fall prey to the many vegetarian Frankenfoods designed to get well-intentioned animal abstainers to open their wallets; these foods typically feature an array of fillers and additives. Please don't eat the meat substitutes. Just please. Check out "Fake Problems" on page 39 for more on this.

LACTO AND OVO AND VEGAN, OH MY!: Many studies find that including dairy and/or eggs in a vegetarian diet significantly decreases mortality rates and health biomarkers. Grass-fed dairy may provide a great source of protein, fats, vitamins, and probiotics (if fermented), while pasture-raised eggs are vitamin superstars, with protein and omega-3 fats to boot![80] See the "Yes!" and "Maybe!" list considerations on pages 51–57 for all the deets!

AVOID (MOST) SOY: While many vegetarians turn to soy as a staple protein replacement, too much soy (especially its modern processed incarnations) can potentially function as an endocrine disrupter and cancer promoter. Most tofu, I'm sorry to say, is a processed yucky GMO no-go. Instead, favor fermented soy products, such as tempeh, miso, and nattō, which feature more bioavailable nutrients (B_{12}!) with beneficial gut bacteria to boot.

SHELLFISH: I recently discovered scallops and my life changed. (Such yummy deliciousness nutritiousness!) Perhaps you can justify consuming shellfish, which lack a central nervous system and arguably a "consciousness." If so, full speed ahead!

Scallops, clams, and oysters are overwhelmingly rich in the vegetarian-elusive zinc and B vitamins, and provide a great source of complete protein and healthy fats.

OMEGA-3 FATS: Given their common foundation of seeds, nuts, and grains, vegetarian diets tend to be quite high in omega-6 fats, which support a cellular basis of inflammation. You need omega-3 fats for cell membranes, brain health, and a host of other things! Unfortunately, the form of omega-3 fats found in plants, ALA, must be converted into the body's preferred form of EPA and DHA. The body's conversion rate may be a shockingly low 2 to 10 percent, and some people harbor genetic mutations that further limit this conversion. Consider minimizing omega-6 fats (which can compete with omega-3 concentrations), eating sea veggies (which contain a little bit of omega-3), and potentially using algae-based omega-3 supplements.

B VITAMINS: This is a biggie! A vegetarian diet naturally lacks the vital vitamin B_{12}. B_{12} is key for proper energy production and cellular metabolism, red blood cell formation, the nervous system, synthesis of DNA, and cellular detox. A deficiency can result in low energy, fatigue, cognitive dysfunction, memory loss, oxidative stress, inflammatory homocysteine, and an inability to properly detox, among other issues.

B_{12} is found primarily in meat and dairy products, though many omnivores still experience deficiencies, so imagine what happens on the vegetarian side of things! Even lacto-ovo vegetarians can be hard-pressed to get enough. A 2014 review of vegetarians revealed B_{12} deficiencies of up to 33 percent in children, 45 percent in infants, 39 percent in pregnant women, and 86.5 percent in adults,[81] with the worst rates in vegans.[82] In forgoing B_{12} for extended periods of time, vegetarians are also at risk of losing their ability to properly metabolize the vitamin in their GI tract—a condition called *pernicious anemia*.[83]

Certain mushrooms, sea vegetables, nutritional yeast (avoid versions with added folic acid!), and some fermented foods (nattō, tempeh, and some sauerkrauts) contain various levels of B_{12}, though still likely inadequate amounts.

So what's a B-desiring vegetarian to do? You can try methylated forms of B vitamins, without added fillers, while avoiding folic acid at all costs.

SHOULD I TAKE SUPPLEMENTS?

In a perfect world, a whole-foods diet would provide all the nutrients we need. But this is not a perfect world. A conglomeration of toxins, antibiotics, skewed omega-6-to-omega-3 ratios, high grain intakes, and the chronic stress of modern life have collectively promoted damaged guts less adept at assimilating nutrients. Even natural food sources tend to be less nutritious than in the past, thanks to soil depletion and modern growing practices. Smart supplementation may help fill in gaps, enhance performance, and increase vitality in general.

That said, there are *many* supplements out there, and despite what my supplement graveyard might insinuate, I now err on the side of less rather than more. We are all unique, and it is difficult to ascertain if a given supplement will help (or even hinder) a person, so I don't feel comfortable making blanket recommendations. Instead, I encourage you to eat whole foods for foundational nutrition, embracing an array of grass-fed animal products, colorful produce, and superfoods, such as pastured egg yolks and beef liver. That said, I shall address a few commonly deficient vital categories, and let you be the smart researcher you are for your own specific approach. If you do supplement, please look for versions with no problematic additives or fillers. You can visit MelanieAvalon.com for more detailed information.

OMEGA-3S: As discussed throughout this book, the omega-6-to-omega-3 ratio is highly off in today's society. That said, I don't like recommending fish oil omega-3 supplements, because some studies indicate that many (if not most) are oxidized to some extent.[84] In fact, there are even debates about whether high polyunsaturated fat intake is actually harmful, as proposed by Ray Peat. I suggest addressing your omega-6-to-omega-3 ratio by minimizing omega-6-rich grains and vegetable oils, and embracing omega-3s in their natural form, via wild-caught, low-toxin fish. (Check out the Environmental Defense Fund's "Seafood Selector" for more on that!) Vegetarians and omnivores alike can also purchase omega-3 supplements derived from algae.

PROBIOTICS: It is without a doubt that I say the gut microbiome is *key* for health. That said, we know *so* little, and there are *so* many different bacteria and *so* many influencing factors and individual differences, that I could never make a blanket recommendation. I encourage you to get your bacteria buddies in whole-foods form, from fermented veggies (unpasteurized sauerkrauts), dairy (kefir and yogurt), and even soy (tempeh and nattō), depending on what you tolerate. Feel free to research and experiment with different strains beyond that. (I personally have benefited from soil-based organisms.)

VITAMIN D: Almost half of the U.S. population may be deficient in vitamin D, a hormone that the body synthesizes from sunlight, and which is vital for the immune system, heart, blood pressure, brain, and mood. I'd love for you to get your D from sunlight, without slathering yourself in potentially toxic chemical sunscreens. (Check out The Environmental Working Group's "Guide to Sunscreens" for the best sunscreen options.) But since modern indoor life can make adequate sun exposure difficult, supplementing with a liquid vitamin D may help address deficiencies.

MAGNESIUM: Our modern diet is often deficient in the mineral magnesium, which is involved with all enzymes in the body that use ATP for energy, and is vital for a healthy heart, gut, bones, digestion, immune system, and life in general! Supplementing with magnesium, either orally or transdermally with an oil or lotion, can aid sleep, stress, and energy, among a host of other things.

DIGESTIVE SUPPORT: Proper digestion is key for health, yet our digestion often becomes distressed due to modern food choices, gut dysbiosis, leaky gut, antibiotics, stress, and PPIs. Various digestive enzymes and/or hydrochloric acid (HCL), which is naturally produced in the stomach to break down protein and fat, may greatly enhance digestion in some individuals.[85]

CAN I DO JUICING?

Raw juice cleanses may be great temporary methods of cleansing, due to their inevitable calorie restriction, maximization of nutrient absorption, and minimization of toxins. That said, stripping fruits and veggies of their fiber results in a *lot* of quick-hitting carbs. Even if you drink *only* green juices, that is still a lot of simple sugar, which may not be best for your insulin levels. Although the inevitable calorie deficit may negate deleterious effects (as the sugar is burned more immediately, leaving less room for damage), I still prefer complete fasting, à la intermittent fasting, to be discussed in the next section! When it comes to fruit and vegetables, I advocate embracing their whole, natural form.

CAN I HAVE CHEAT DAYS? WHAT IF I MESS UP?

Although I've admittedly indulged in my fair share of them (especially in my early Paleo days), I strongly advise against cheat meals as a "written" part of your protocol, and preferably not at all in the initial thirty days. Cheating tends to keep cravings present, postponing your ultimate freedom from grain and sugar addiction. Furthermore, a substantial introduction period is vital to eliminate all inflammatory aspects of your diet, as seemingly minor exposures to problematic foods can yield allergic and immune responses.

But if you do indeed cheat, don't beat yourself up! You're only human! Don't fall into the "I just had a cookie, so I might as well eat *everything* I can, since I already messed up" mindset. You'll feel better the day after a minor slip than a major one. If you broke your arm, would you say, "Well, might as well break every other limb, since I'm already broken"? I'd honestly rather you cheat majorly and not give it a second thought than have a minor cheat and become overwhelmed with regret and worry. Love, forgiveness, health, and healing beautifully support each other. Don't be hard on yourself! You're doing the best you can given your circumstances. Remember that.

WHAT ABOUT WATER?

Before Paleo, I'd wonder if I was drinking enough water. Now the question seems almost odd. When you replace sodium-rich processed foods with hydrating produce, you don't have to stress about fulfilling some magical water quota. Drink so you don't feel thirsty. And if you're thirsty, drink water! Unlike hunger signals, our thirst signals don't tend to get screwed up.

Note: You may require more water on lower-carb versions of Paleo, especially if ketogenic. Though glucose is stored with water as glycogen, fat tends to be hydrophobic. So for all my keto-ers, drink up! Fluctuating water stores often explain seemingly drastic shifts in weight when adjusting carb intakes.

SALT AND IODINE

Historical hunter-gatherers consumed potassium and salt in around a 5-to-1 ratio. Today, our sodium intake *far* exceeds our potassium intake, leading to a host of health problems. Replacing processed foods with whole foods will drastically decrease your salt intake, and help address your sodium-to-potassium ratio, while likely slashing water retention to boot! You also may find you gain more clarity in the sodium department, and can simply salt food to taste. (Those following a ketogenic approach may require more salt.) All that said, the salt situation is still a bit complicated. Check out James DiNicolantonio's book, *The Salt Fix*, for a nuanced perspective.

I recommend replacing standard commercial salt, which often contains anticaking agents and the corn sugar dextrose, with pink, Himalayan, and sea salts, which also feature trace minerals. That said, modern commercial salt contains added iodine, a key nutrient vital for neurological and thyroid health.[86] Our increasing modern exposure to compounds such as bromine and fluoride compete with iodine receptors, encouraging deficiency. This can also be exacerbated by plant-based diets, since many veggies (such as the cruciferous variety) contain goitrogens, which can inhibit proper iodine utilization. Make sure you get adequate iodine from whole-food sources, such as wild-caught, low-toxin fish, sea vegetables, cranberries, and strawberries.

WHEN?

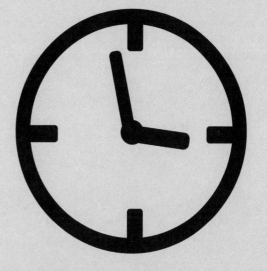

WHAT IS INTERMITTENT FASTING?

The "when" of *What When Wine* carries us to the temporal realm, where the magic lies not so much in what we *do*, but rather in what we *don't* do. And it's shocking what a bit of not doing can do! Conventional eating patterns often feel like those dreams where you're running but just can't move. You dutifully eat your 500-calorie meals like clockwork and log every *thought* of a bite in your food journal, yet the accumulating bodily evidence of prior meals remains. Indeed, beneath any ego-driven perception of willpower lies complicated cellular processes that truly control body composition. But have no fear! In embracing a way of eating that is foreign to our modern selves yet familiar to our bodies, you can finally awaken from the nightmare!

Intermittent fasting, colloquially known as IF, is a pattern of eating in which you restrict the hours you eat each day, rather than the amount of food you eat. It is not so much a diet as a diet pattern. Eating constantly throughout the day conditions the body to wait around for snacks and meals, rather than tapping into its own substantial reserves. IF reverts your body to the fat-burning beast it's meant to be! When I first started intermittent fasting, it was like a lightbulb went on: Suddenly weight loss wasn't a struggle but rather a simple bodily process actually on board with my intentions.

Let's take a look at how energy is used, stored, and burned in the body, so we can see how intermittent fasting unlocks weight loss in a healthy, natural, and ultimately effortless way!

WHAT HAPPENS WHEN YOU EAT

The human body is a pretty wondrous thing. All you have to do is eat! Systems beyond your control then break down the food and use what's needed for energy, growth, and repair, while also saving energy for future use. Unlike cars, which literally can't move when out of gas, your body is pretty capable of managing itself between meals. Pretty cool! Not surprisingly, your body also requires a *lot* of energy for its daily to-do list, and it's got two basic places to turn to for that: your last meal or your body fat. Let's zero in on the meal thing for a sec.

Though we like to isolate foods into single macronutrients ("Chicken is protein! Fruit is carbs!"), most foods actually contain protein, carbohydrates, fat, and occasionally alcohol, in varying amounts. The body doesn't store alcohol, which is used immediately for energy, and protein is preferentially used for growth and repair. That leaves us with carbohydrates and fat as potential fuel for both immediate use and long-term storage. I discussed all of this a bit in the "What?" part of this book, but here's another look at how the whole food process goes down.

When eaten, most carbohydrates are ultimately broken down into glucose, which becomes blood sugar. Excess blood sugar is toxic to the body, as it encourages glycation (a type of protein damage) and reactive oxygen species, which injure our cells' mitochondria. When the superhero pancreas senses a rise in blood sugar, it signals the release of the hormone insulin to shuttle the glucose out of the bloodstream and into your muscles and liver, where it can be stored as glycogen. But like any high-priced storage unit, your glycogen stores are limited, capable of storing around 15 grams of glycogen per pound of body weight.[1] While this suffices in a punctuated, whole-foods diet, minimizing constant food intake and carbohydrate consumption, it's often inadequate for our modern perpetual influx of sugary processed foods. So when the glycogen stores put up NO VACANCY signs, insulin escorts the glucose (along with the rest of your meal) to the backup storage unit: fat cells!

At the same time, insulin stops fat burning and encourages fat storage in general. This means if you eat constantly throughout the day (particularly insulin-spiking carbs), then you will likely be storing fat more than you are burning it. You'll also be limiting your *perceived* available energy. Ya see, when your body relies primarily on carb refills, it doesn't like to use body fat, despite having tons of it just waiting to be used! Instead, it lazily demands more food, making fat burning pretty difficult.

Unlike carbohydrates, which provide brief hits of short-term fuel and are restricted by limited glycogen stores, dietary fats function more like long-term fuel sources in the body. They do not, on their own, spike blood sugar and instigate the release of insulin. In the relative absence of carbohydrates, they become a preferred source of fuel in the body. That said, when fats are eaten with carbohydrates, they're pretty much just along for the ride, and are easily stored as fat.

You can think of this whole scenario like a bank. Our daily snacks and meals fill our limited "checking account," akin to our glycogen stores, with any extra funneled into our "savings account," akin to our fat stores. We can't access our savings account unless our checking account is empty—which rarely happens, since we constantly fill it up anytime we think it might be even *slightly* low. (We don't want to starve, now, do we?) This approach locks us *to* our checking account, and *out of* our savings account. We rely on temporary morsels ingested, rather than steady fat stores. Unable to access our abundant long-term energy, we become slaves to blood sugar swings and feelings of being "hangry," while putting an artificial ceiling on endurance.

WHAT HAPPENS WHEN YOU FAST

Now you may be thinking, *Gee, I wish I could just tell my body to burn my body fat instead of constant carbs!* Well, guess what! You can! And you don't really have to *do* anything—just *not do* something. If you can go about twelve hours without eating, your body will realize that mealtime doesn't seem to be an option anymore. While it may temporarily protest (perhaps too much, in your opinion), it will eventually #deal with the situation, and quite beautifully, I might add!

When you enter this "fasted" state (There! We said it!), the body gives up on using glucose and glycogen as the main source of fuel. It's basically like, "Well, since there's no energy coming in, we'd better prepare for the long haul!" and increases lipolysis—the breakdown of stored body fat into free fatty acids for energy.[2] And we're talking *tons* of energy. Between twelve and twenty-four hours after your last meal, the body typically liberates two to three hundred times *more* energy from fat stores than actually needed! This means the longer you run on body fat in the fasted state, the more energetic you can become: Talk about ultimate fat burning! In fact, the body will increasingly free up more fat stores for around seventy-two hours, at which point fatty acid levels in the bloodstream stabilize and plateau. (But that would be actual fasting, not *intermittent* fasting.)

Increased fatty acid oxidation also decreases glucose oxidation, as organs, muscles, and processes throughout the body begin to favor fat for fuel.[3] This means your fasting self simply needs less glucose from carbs! Yay! Fasting also regulates insulin levels and encourages insulin sensitivity, eradicating roller-coaster blood sugar levels and the associated energy dips and mood swings. As you finally access ample energy from stored body fat, hunger dissipates, since you're fueled from within![4]

KETONES

But wait . . . things get even better! In the fasted state, the body begins generating an alternative energy substrate known as *ketones*. Ketones can directly enter the cell mitochondria for fuel, unlike glucose, which requires an intermediate conversion step. They also generate more energy than glucose, with fewer toxic by-products, such as reactive oxygen species and free radicals. While 100 grams of glucose yields around 8.7 kilograms of ATP (a "currency" of intracellular energy), 100 grams of ketones create around 10.5 grams of ATP. Ketones are actually the preferred source of energy for the brain, and provide an array of benefits: They can protect neurons from degeneration; beneficially change gene expression; reduce inflammation; protect against metabolic diseases; and discourage Alzheimer's, epilepsy, and cancer.

The state in which the body begins using ketones as a primary source of energy is known as *ketosis* and can result from prolonged exercise, a low-carb diet, or fasting. (Surprise!) If you're uneasy with the idea of a "foreign" metabolic state, just know you likely routinely dip into ketosis at night: It's totally natural! To check your ketogenic state, you can order breath or urine analysis strips, which is how I became obsessed with the whole science-of-diet thing in the first place. After eons of vague protocols and questionable progress, I now had a test to corroborate my feelings of fat burning. Love you, ketones!

WHERE DO WE GO FROM HERE?

Okie dokie! Now that we've got a basic understanding of how intermittent fasting unlocks the fat-burning state, I say it's time to jump into the intense details of fat burning, as well as IF's astounding list of health benefits. While fat loss may be the immediate lure, the health benefits just may render you an IF fan for life. It's like marrying your high school crush! (Not that I have any personal experience in that matter, but stalking my Southern friends via Instagram gives me a pretty good idea.)

IF AND BODY COMPOSITION

In general, lipolysis (the fancy word for fat burning) is tightly controlled by various signaling molecules, the hypothalamus, and who knows what else. So despite your body having ample fat stores, fat burning can be lamentably difficult unless the body is #down on a hormonal level. This can make you feel powerless, in an "I have no money and am about to pass Park Place and Board-walk" type way. Thankfully, intermittent fasting initiates an epic metabolic state that actually encourages the body to plow through stubborn fat stores while maintaining muscle and discouraging weight gain. Let's take a closer look, shall we?

MORE WEIGHT LOSS

Intermittent fasting can produce greater weight loss than complementary dietary approaches . . . wait for it! . . . even when the *same* number of calories are consumed. A twelve-week study of thirty-two subjects found that an alternate-day fasting pattern yielded greater weight loss than a normal eating pattern, despite similar calorie intakes,[5] while a 2013 study found that dieting obese women who practiced IF twice a week lost substantially more weight than women practicing calorie restriction every day, despite overall similar calorie intakes.[6] Similarly, a 2011 review of seven intermittent fasting studies found that IF rivaled calorie restriction, providing significant weight-loss results in short amounts of time (two to three weeks), and increasing when extended for longer periods (eight to twelve weeks).[7]

HEALTHIER WEIGHT LOSS

Of course, weight loss is one thing; the *type* of weight loss is another. After all, dehydration can result in weight loss, as will losing an arm. But no one's selling a book called *Halt Hydration for a Hot Body!* or *Amputate Your Way Thin!* (At least, not that I'm aware of.) Thankfully, intermittent fasting targets the more unhealthy and inflammatory visceral fat stored around organs, in comparison to the more benign subcutaneous fat stored beneath the skin. And while typical calorie restriction tends to sacrifice muscle, studies show that intermittent fasting can actually *preserve* muscle. Check out "The IF Fitness Fanatic" section on page 180 for more on that!

STUBBORN FAT

You know those especially stubborn fat stores that won't budge, no matter what you seem to do? It's not all in your head! "Stubborn fat" is actually a very real thing. Ya see, fat cells are "guarded" by different receptors, which act like locks, and determine how easily the fat cells open. *Alpha-2* receptors in particular are quite difficult to open (think combination lock), while the *beta-2* versions are much easier to open (think your typical door). Various hormones and neurotransmitters called *catecholamines*, such as epinephrine and norepinephrine, serve as codes and keys.

Stubborn fat has a lot of alpha-2 receptors and not many beta-2 receptors. On the other hand, more "normal" fat stores have a lot of beta-2 receptors, and not many alpha-2 receptors. Women tend to have lots of alpha receptors on their hips, butt, and thighs, whereas men have more alpha receptors around their abs and midsection.[8]

Intermittent fasting does a few nifty things to help open tricky alpha receptors. For starters, when insulin is present, basically all fat stores are off-limits. Fasting lowers insulin, giving you a chance at tapping into fat cells in the first place! Second, fasting ramps up catecholamines in the system—those keys like epinephrine and norepinephrine that can open the pesky receptor locks. (Epinephrine also increases the metabolic rate in general, letting you grab more fat from the cells.) Third, fasting stimulates blood flow to deliver the catecholamines to the receptors. This is why stubborn fat pockets on your body may feel colder than places with little fat—due to the lack of blood flow. (It's also why "fat-burning" ab belts may actually help you burn more ab fat, by stimulating blood flow to the area.)

Of course, opening the alpha and beta doors is one thing; *burning* the fat inside is another. People who eat constantly often reach the "fat-burning state" with exercise, yet don't necessarily burn that much fat. When the body is accustomed to running on stored glucose from a recent meal, it "hits the wall" once glycogen stores are almost empty. Even though this is *prime* fat-burning time, you feel as though you *just can't do it*. But with fasting, the body has accepted fat burning, so there's no struggle in actually grabbing and burning the fat. You've got the green light!

FAT GAIN PROTECTION

Intermittent fasting also enhances nutrient partitioning, making you more likely to use food for fuel and repair, rather than shuttling it away as fat. A 2012 study found that mice that consumed a high-fat diet in an eight-hour window did not gain weight from excess calories, while mice that consumed the same amount of food and calories throughout the day *did*.[9] The study attributed this redirection of calories to changes in cellular signaling, fat-burning pathways, and liver and energy metabolism in the body.[10] Another study analyzing the effects of fasting on healthy, normal-weight men found that prolonged fasting increased fat oxidation once the men ate a normal meal again. In other words, intermittent fasting may cause you to burn more fat from what you eat than you would if you ate throughout the day!

IF HEALTH BENEFITS

Given that I personally started intermittent fasting for weight loss, I totally understand if this is your rationale! But while the weight *did* fly off, I soon noticed other changes: heightened energy, shining skin, improved mood . . . I stopped catching as many colds, and seemed to finally experience that elusive feeling of *resilience*. So when I sat down to research the mechanics of fasting, I wasn't surprised by the abundant literature on its health benefits, attributed to multiple biological mechanisms.[11] Let's explore these, shall we?

DIETARY RESTRICTION

Studies consistently link calorie restriction, especially when combined with a nutrient-rich diet, to longevity, insulin sensitivity, stress resistance, and disease prevention (including diabetes, heart disease, and cancer).[12] Similarly, intermittent fasting may acquire some of its benefits from (often unintentional) decreased food intake. IF often results in highly sustainable calorie restriction, due to the lack of hunger, meal satiation, and enhanced nutrition partitioning.

That said, intermittent fasting may yield metabolic benefits beyond calorie restriction. A 2003 rodent study found that alternate-day fasting protocols *with-*

out calorie restriction instigated greater blood sugar, insulin, and neuronal stress benefits than calorie restriction.[13] Similarly, a 2012 study found that intermittent fasting increased cellular stress resistance and protective stress genes more than calorie restriction alone.[14] Let's jump on this slightly *stressful* part, shall we?

THE BENEFITS (YES!) OF STRESS

When we think *stress*, we often think of the nail-biting, heart-pounding, nerve-racking type we've been told will kill us all. (Can I get some calming teas, mediation, and yoga over here?) This is chronic stress, which we'd like to avoid. But not all stress is bad, and perhaps even bad stress doesn't *have* to be bad. (For more on stress perception, check out Kelly McGonigal's *The Upside of Stress*, or Andrew Bernstein's *The Myth of Stress*.) But instead of embarking on a tangent about turning bad stress good, let's look at the "good" stress created by intermittent fasting.

In the good old days as hunter-gatherers, daily movement was necessary for securing food and shelter. As hunters, we'd intensely hunt in the fasted state to secure food. As gatherers, we'd do a lot of physical gathering to accumulate anything substantial. These environmental and physical stressors fostered a beneficial *hormetic* stress and adaptive resilience in our cells. Contrast this to today, as we work sedentary jobs and purchase ready-made meals, with a snack (or four) in between. While the mental stress is present, the physical stress . . . not so much. This lack of hormetic stress predisposes us toward diabetes, cancer, cardiovascular disease, and neurodegenerative ailments.

Intermittent fasting, however, activates stress-resistance pathways by temporarily stressing our cells.[15] This upregulates levels of neurotrophic factors and stress protein chaperones, which have protective mechanisms, instigating cell repair, optimizing functions, and rejuvenating the metabolism. Translation: IF is a beneficial stress that strengthens rather than weakens. Don't fear it—embrace it!

AUTOPHAGY

While "cleansing" may conjure images of green-juice fasts and beautiful people meditating by tranquil ponds, it manifests a bit differently on the cellular level!

When we cease eating for a substantial amount of time, the body begins recycling old, broken proteins for growth and repair, in a process called *autophagy*. Autophagy discourages the accumulation of toxins, which encourage frailty and cellular atrophy, slows the aging process, protects against age-related diseases, discourages neuron dysregulation, and even supports muscle mass.

It's like if you kept buying new clothes, despite having a closet *full* of old clothes. Say one day you ran out of money and couldn't buy new clothes. You'd be forced to go through your closet and make use of old clothes, and might even create new outfits from combinations of old clothes. In a similar manner, autophagy tackles the cluttered closet inside you, creating new cells in the process!

IF HEALTH BENEFITS

With fancy mechanisms such as caloric restriction, cellular stress pathways, and autophagy, it's no wonder intermittent fasting presents a shiny bundle of health gifts. Who needs Santa? (Ok, I do. It's fine.)

INFLAMMATION

Let us enter the murky waters of inflammation, simultaneous savior and slayer. On the one hand, acute inflammation can promote healing in times of physical distress, yet chronic inflammation run amok becomes a root cause of degenerative disease.

The eating process itself actually yields inflammation on some level, on a scale from slight to egregious. When we eat, we welcome in a lot of foreign (and occasionally downright toxic) stuff into our bodies: bacteria, problematic plant compounds such as salicylates and oxalates, *very* problematic plant proteins such as gluten and lectins, as well as the slew of toxins found in pesticides, conventionally raised animal fats, and processed foods. These compounds all hold the potential to instigate inflammatory responses and autoimmune conditions, while the prevalence of processed carbs and sugars in today's meals raise blood sugar and further boost inflammation.

A simple break from constant eating, however, can calm inflammation, enhanced by intermittent fasting's other anti-inflammatory mechanisms. A 2011 study, for example, found that fasting reduced inflammation in the neuroimmune system,[16] while two Ramadan studies found that daylight fasts reduced levels of the inflammatory biomarkers C-reactive protein, homocysteine, and interleukin-6.[17] More recently, a 2015 study revealed that ketones produced during fasting suppress inflammatory protein responses.[18]

On a purely anecdotal level, I find that intermittent fasting makes me feel like an anti-inflammation goddess. Whenever I feel inflammation's sneaky grasp (which tends to personally manifest in slight swelling or joint pain), I can easily remedy the situation with a nice bout of fasting!

LONGEVITY

Perhaps the fountain of youth lies not in some magic supplement but rather in a lifestyle practice. While the highly studied calorie restriction may increase life span, recent research indicates that intermittent fasting may do the same. In rodents, the effects are often dramatic: One study found that mice on fasting protocols lived around 83 percent longer than their normal-eating rodent friends![19] On the human side of things, a 2015 study spearheaded by Valter Longo, director of the USC Longevity Institute (fight on!), found that fasting-type diets in mice not only increased health and prolonged life span but even encouraged stem cell regeneration! A follow-up human study revealed similar beneficial effects on disease risk factors and longevity biomarkers.

While the exact mechanisms are unknown, fasting may lengthen life by affecting the rate of cellular aging, in part by decreasing oxidative stress. Yeast cells are up to one thousand times more protected against oxidative stress when fasted, while similar results have been found in mice.[20] In humans, a 2008 Ramadan study found that fasting protected body lipids from oxidative stress,[21] while a 2015 study revealed increased expression of the SIRT3 gene, an important factor in aging.[22] Other fasting effects at play may include down-regulated insulin and insulin-like peptides, increased insulin sensitivity, and better energy metabolism with fewer toxic by-products. Fasting also strengthens the immune system and wards off disease, as we'll discuss in a bit!

GUT HEALTH

My personal favorite IF health benefit is a gutsy matter! As discussed, the eating process itself is inherently inflammatory, though the extent of it depends on a myriad of factors, including the foods eaten, your immune system's personal calibration, and the status of your gut permeability. Periods of fasting instigate an anti-inflammatory state, allowing the gut lining to heal and seal and the immune system to calm down. It's no wonder studies find that fasting can reduce intestinal permeability, a.k.a. leaky gut![23]

For a further bit of inspiration, consider that the cells lining the small intestine boast the fastest turnover rate of *any* cells in our body, with some regenerating in as little as three to five days![24] This is insanely comforting. It means that even if your gut is in shambles, avoiding problematic foods while engaging in fasting may rapidly escalate healing! Our gut is primed for self-renewal, and IF catalyzes the process!

Many people also experience slowed intestinal movement, due to gut dysbiosis such as SIBO (small intestinal bacterial overgrowth) or nerve damage. This can result in food moving too slowly through the system and fermenting, leading to gas, bloating, and toxic bacterial by-products, which further exacerbates the problem. (For those with an overgrowth of archaebacteria associated with IBS-C, for example, the microbes produce methane from fermentation, which serves as a neurotransmitter further slowing intestinal mobility—yikes!)

Intermittent fasting, however, stimulates the migrating motor complex (MMC), the intestine's natural cleansing wave.[25] (It's what causes your tummy to grumble before a meal!) Activating the MMC helps keep things moving, discouraging buildup of food, toxins, and other residue. In fact, fasting has been shown to greatly benefit patients with IBS.[26] In a 2006 study, it improved seven out of ten IBS-associated problems, including stomach pain, diarrhea, and anxiety.

And lastly, while you'd think fasting would starve the gut microbiome, the opposite may be true! A 2015 study found that fasting can ultimately *increase* the beneficial variety of gut bacteria.[27] Fasting may starve pathogenic species, allowing the beneficial probiotic strains to get the upper hand. For people with gut dysbiosis (quite common today, thanks to antibiotics and the modern diet), less may be more, as an overabundance of eating (particularly of fermentable carbs) can exacerbate bacterial overgrowth.

So if you're struggling at all in the gut department, definitely try adding a bit of IF to your arsenal!

INSULIN AND DIABETES

If you were to walk into the control room of your body, you'd probably see a fancy-schmancy screen solely dedicated to your blood sugar levels, which must be in a very specific range for proper function. Too little blood sugar signifies insufficient energy, while too much blood sugar is toxic, meaning that potential death lies on either side of the spectrum!

Thankfully, both animal and human studies find that intermittent fasting regulates blood sugar and insulin levels, encouraging the body to preferentially burn fat rather than sugar as fuel, and discouraging insulin resistance. With less reliance on blood sugar comes fewer of the problems associated with blood sugar. One study found that intermittent fasting regulated blood sugar in diabetic rats to levels resembling those in nondiabetic rats, while multiple observational human studies associate fasting with lowered diabetes rates. Intermittent fasting may even regulate blood sugar on a genetic level, via the Forkhead box A gene. (Who comes up with these names?)

THE COMMON COLD AND IMMUNE SYSTEM

In grade school, getting sick was like a "get out of school free" card. Worries of perfect attendance aside, I treasured my mom's "stay home" decision, sinking back into bed instead of attending 7:15 a.m. roll call. In high school and early college years, sickness took on a new beauty: instant weight loss! Thankfully, such delights in infirmity have long since passed, and I welcome IF's cold prevention with open arms.

A lot of effort goes into food digestion. Just think about how tired you get after a big meal. Now consider that this energy expenditure happens after every meal, albeit on a smaller level. As discussed, eating also taxes the immune system, as it has to deal with ingested toxins, antinutrients, and invaders. Intermittent fasting can therefore redirect energy and immune resources normally spent on digestion toward other invaders, while also improving cell-mediated immunity and resistance.

Fasting further protects the immune system on a cellular level by discouraging inflammatory responses, reducing oxidative damage, and increasing stress resistance.[28] It also increases phagocytosis—the process by which white blood cells "eat" and expunge bacteria and other toxins. Recent findings even indicate that fasting may encourage the body to create *new* immune cells, by inhibiting genes that block stem cell rejuvenation![29] This means that IF holds the potential for generating new immune systems damaged by chemotherapy, or more common disorders such as autoimmune disease!

HEART DISEASE

As the leading killer in the United States, responsible for 25 percent of annual deaths, heart disease encompasses artery disease, heart attack, faulty heart valves, and heart failure. It usually arises from a buildup of plaque in the arteries, often from lifestyle and environmental factors, with risk factors including high blood pressure, cholesterol, and diabetes. Commonly prescribed heart disease preventions include not smoking, maintaining a healthy weight and diet, and exercising regularly. I'd like to cast a vote for intermittent fasting!

In both animal and human studies, intermittent fasting has been shown to reduce heart disease risk factors. IF can directly enhance cardiovascular function by increasing heart rate variability, helping the heart adapt to stress, building resilience to myocardial infarction and stroke, and affecting genes that regulate growth of heart muscle cells. IF also aids numerous other downstream factors supporting heart function, such as blood pressure, insulin, cholesterol, the inflammatory C-reactive protein, and neurotrophic factor signaling in the brain. It also increases adiponectin, a nifty little protein that regulates sugar and fat burning, protects blood vessel linings, and suppresses cellular aggravation from blood clotting.

CANCER

Cancer cells are essentially mutant cells that reproduce and wreak havoc on the body, forming tumors and destroying body tissue, while resisting the body's typical self-destruction systems. Rodent trials have found that intermittent fasting can reduce breast, prostate, and pancreatic cancers,[30] while human clinical trials show that IF reduces cancer risk and cell proliferation rates, reducing growth-factor hormones linked to cancer.[31] Fasting's beneficial effects can even work selectively on cancerous cells, encouraging growth of normal cells and protecting them from oxidative stress, while retarding growth of cancerous ones *without* shielding them from oxidative stress.[32] Pretty nifty!

Studies also suggest that cancer cells, due to their rogue mitochondrial nature, can only run efficiently on glucose, and are unable to sufficiently adapt to alternative energy substrates such as fatty acids and ketones.[33] The body's "normal" cells, on the other hand, are flexibly adept at utilizing these energy sources. As such, glucose-rich diets may predispose the body to cancer, while intermittent fasting, which minimizes glucose while upregulating fatty acids and ketones for energy, may starve cancer cells and kill tumors. Since energy generated from ketones requires less oxygen, fasting can further debilitate cancerous cells by reducing oxygen consumption and oxidative stress. This may be particularly relevant for brain cancer!

OTHER DISEASE STATES

Since intermittent fasting works on a foundational, holistic level, its therapeutic benefits go on and on! Fasting protocols may discourage liver disease, as the liver stores less fat during a fast. It may improve eyesight and treat eye disorders. (This is purely anecdotal, but when I began IF, my eyesight actually improved for the first time in my life!) Other maladies aided by fasting include spinal injury, brain lesions, kidney disease, and neurodegenerative ailments, such as stroke, Alzheimer's, Parkinson's disease, Huntington's disease, and dementia.

THE BRAIN

One could argue that the value of existence boils down to the brain, since you must be self-aware to perceive reality in the first place. Rocks' and plants' existence just can't hold a candle to consciousness! As such, I find it vastly rewarding to implement a dietary lifestyle that fosters an alert, meditate, reflective, and enjoyable state of being. What's the point of restrictive dietary protocols that seemingly boost body composition but render the dieter unhappy or lethargic? For the ultimate razor-sharp mind, look no further than intermittent fasting!

IF is highly therapeutic for the brain, discouraging inflammation and aging.[34] Ketones produced during the fasted state generate beneficial β-hydroxybutyrate (gotta love that fancy β!), protect neurons, slow neurological disease processes, and discourage excitotoxic and oxidative stress.[35] The lowered glucose levels may also discourage seizures, improve brain lesions, and aid mitochondria and cognitive function. Studies even show that IF can stimulate neural regeneration (a.k.a. new brain cells),[36] meaning your brain is never past the point of no return! If that's not uplifting, I don't know what is!

Fasting also keeps the brain "clean" by stimulating the aforementioned autophagy, as well as stimulating white blood cells called *macrophages*, which get their name from the Greek term for "big eaters." Macrophages go around the body "eating" unwanted and toxic particles, and become simultaneously more powerful and less inflammatory when you are fasting. A lack of this whole cleanup process, by the way, results in neural dysregulation and degeneration. So if ya feel like there's some brain gunk building up, a bit of IF might be just the thing you need!

MOOD

Studies show that meal patterns tend to influence mood in general, with fluctuating blood sugar notoriously fostering unpleasant tempers.[37] Since intermittent fasting promotes glycemic and insulin control, it eradicates feelings of being "hangry": that angry feeling you get when blood sugar drops and you don't want to talk to anyone because you *must eat something now.* A 2014 study even found that fluctuating blood sugar levels in nondiabetic adults were associated with anger, concluding that anger may be a risk factor for diabetes![38]

Fasting can also lift mood by raising levels of feel-good neurotransmitters such as norepinephrine and dopamine, modulating the nervous system, and regulating sleep. A 2014 study found that fasting correlated with decreased anxiety, social dysfunction, and insomnia,[39] while another found that it benefited self-esteem.[40] Other studies find that fasting mitigates depression, tension, and stress, while promoting a sense of peace.[41] It may do this in part by boosting brain-derived neurotrophic factor, in a similar mechanism to antidepressants. As one study put it, intermittent fasting improves vigor and "quality of life." Yep. That basically sums up this whole chapter!

IF PSYCHOLOGY

There's little point in any weight-loss protocol if it's too miserable to maintain. As concluded in a 2011 review, most weight-loss protocols bear minimal results, with weight regain common afterward.[42] Yet studies across the board[43] show that intermittent fasting actually promotes compliance! A 2009 trial, for example, found that adherence reached 86 percent during fasting days of controlled food, and actually increased to 89 percent during fasting days of self-selected food.[44] Another 2013 randomized controlled study found that IF adherence ranked at a stable 98 percent, while a 2013 IF review found similar compliance results compared to traditional diets.[45]

To understand how IF combats the circus of the mind, let's dive into the psychological side of things. These are not some sort of vague, feel-good changes in the land of lotus-eaters, but rather, very definite changes in the brain's neurochemistry that encourage effortless new habits.

WILLPOWER RESERVES

Willpower isn't some vague concept we prescribe as validation for completion (or lack thereof) of goals. On the contrary, willpower and self-control mandate ignoring animalistic drives that characterize the foundations of our being, such as the desire for food or sex. Studies suggest that our amount of willpower in a given day is a real thing, and it's *actually* limited. Every time you exercise a bit of willpower, you drain your reserves. That moment you don't hit the snooze button, don't snap at your coworker, or *do* go to the gym drains your willpower bucket.

Consider Roy Baumeister and Mark Muraven's famous "radish experiment," in which hungry students were presented with bowls of cookies and radishes in a room smelling of tantalizing, freshly baked goods. Some were told to only eat the cookies, others just the radishes. They were then given a geometric puzzle to finish, unaware it was actually impossible. Talk about cards stacked against you!

While the radish students easily gave up in less than ten minutes, the cookie students worked for almost double that amount of time, suggesting that the students who had "used up" some of their willpower in refusing the cookies had less leftover willpower to work on the puzzle. The radish students also reported feeling more tired and fatigued. A control group who bypassed the whole cookie/radish thing worked as long as the cookie group, so it wasn't like the cookies themselves magically boosted willpower.[46]

Over two hundred studies corroborate these findings. A 2007 *Psychological Science* study found that students who suppressed their emotions during upsetting movie clips performed worse on a follow-up, attention-demanding Stroop task than students who watched the movie without emotional suppression. (In the Stroop test, one must quickly identify the actual color of colored words. For example, the word "green" is written in a red font. It's trickier than it may sound!) Neural monitoring revealed that the students who exerted willpower exhibited a weakened brain monitoring system.

And if there's one thing that can overwhelmingly drain willpower reserves, it's dieting! When dieting, you must constantly refuse food while hungry (bye, willpower!), and constantly stop eating before full (bye, willpower!). No wonder another 2000 study found that students who had to refuse tempting snacks and/or control their emotional expressions to food stimuli lacked willpower in subsequent tasks.[47]

Intermittent fasting, however, requires *very little* willpower. Because fasting eradicates hunger, temptation during the fasting period flies away. It's like the equivalent of eating while sleeping or playing a sport: It's just not a thing! And when you do eat, you can eat abundantly and to satiety! Again, no tempting of willpower! (Of course, consuming nutritious whole foods when you eat will truly nourish your body and help you slay any resilient, lingering cravings!) Once you get through the first few days of metabolic and hormonal adjustment, IF frees up an insane amount of willpower for life, literally.

SELF-CONTROL AND BLOOD SUGAR

Any activity we do requires *actual* energy to power it, which just may include willpower and self-control! These "skills" may be some of the first things sacrificed in the face of a fuel shortage, given their relatively recent development (compared to, say, reproduction). In an extensive 2007 study, experimenters placed students in a variety of situations in which they did or did not exercise self-control, such as emotional suppression while watching a movie, or prejudice regulation while talking to someone of a different race. The researchers found that these activities actually lowered the participants' blood sugar levels, and they'd consistently perform poorer in follow-up self-control tests. A glucose drink administered between self-control tests, however, could reboot self-control. Another 2003 study found that dieters who faced peer-pressure Asch-type tests (imagine being asked to choose the obviously right answer on a test, when everyone else is oddly saying the wrong answer) ended up eating more than dieters who hadn't previously faced such draining decisions of conformity.[48]

With these findings, it's no surprise that a typical dieting scenario can diminish self-control. In a self-fulfilling prophecy, dieting requires self-control to resist food, which lowers blood sugar levels, which further depletes self-control. Talk about a dismal cycle! But does this mean that eating sugar is the cure? Not exactly. Doing so only constructs a blood sugar roller coaster. As noted in the first study discussed, "We do not intend to advocate consuming large quantities of sugar as an ideal strategy for improving self-control. Eating several candy bars, for instance, may give one a boost of energy and better self-control, but these benefits are likely to disappear when glucose levels eventually drop."

The key to blood sugar regulation for self-control is just that: *blood sugar regulation*. With intermittent fasting, the body relies on fatty acids rather than glucose as the primary source of fuel. A steady stream of energy, even when you're not eating, keeps the body fueled and ready to go, with consistent blood sugar levels. Happy blood sugar levels = happy self-control!

DECISION FATIGUE

You may be familiar with decision fatigue. It's that moment when you've made *so* many choices that you just enter a #whattheheckidontevencare moment. This often happens to me when I try on a million things in the dressing room for three hours, and then all of a sudden get this overwhelming, semi-panicky thought of *I give up! Buy everything and decide later!* (Thank goodness for return policies!)

Consider an extreme example of decision making: court cases. A 2010 study of 1,112 court hearings found that parole judges' rulings aligned with the time of day and meal patterns. At the start of a day and right after breaks, the judges would rule favorably 65 percent of the time. But at the end of a long session, like right before lunch or at the end of the day, favorable rulings fell to nearly zero.[49] The judges would hit decision fatigue and just be like, #guilty.

Decision fatigue is particularly relevant in the diet world. Eating throughout the day means you must choose when and what to eat constantly throughout the day. Such decisions add up quickly! *Should I eat breakfast? What should I eat for breakfast? Should I have a snack? Ok, I didn't have a snack, so now should I have a snack? What's for lunch? Should I be eating this? Should I have more? What's for dinner? Am I still hungry? Should I have dessert?* So. Many. Decisions.

Compare this to an intermittent fasting scenario, in which you make *very few* decisions. You decide what to eat in your eating window, and that's it! You don't even have to stress about the "decision" to stop eating, because you can eat until satiated. Bye-bye, decision fatigue!

HABITS

Up to an estimated 45 percent of our actions are habits,[50] which are *so* much more than some causally irresistible urge for déjà vu. Habits actually serve as shortcuts to enact seemingly necessary behaviors for survival with minimal effort, freeing up brain space for more pressing matters. This can lead to some uncanny activity, such as brushing our teeth in a zombie-like state, driving to work without thinking, and reaching for another handful of peanuts when we're not actually hungry.

How are habits created? When we first try a new action, we can't predict the process or outcome, so the sentient, decision-making part of the brain called the *prefrontal cortex* administers acute attention to everything along the way. If the new action yields a favorable outcome, we tend to repeat it. If we keep repeating it (and it keeps yielding a favorable outcome), then our prefrontal cortex is like, "This works! You got this! K bye!" and hands off the action to the basal ganglia, a part of the brain involved in patterns, memory, and movement. This means we no longer have to consciously *think* our way through routine actions. Just imagine how exhausting it would be if you had to intensely focus on getting dressed, driving to work, and eating a meal, like you'd never done it before? (Although such an experience of the world would be wondrous indeed!)

Now let's apply this to eating. Consider the history of your current go-to snack. (I'm looking at you, Cotton Candy grapes!) The first time you tried the snack, it was a new experience. You paid attention to the texture and flavor. You savored. Fast-forward a few days, and you just may have found yourself scarfing down the treat without a thought, barely remembering eating it in the first place as you reach for *just one more.*

As discussed in Charles Duhigg's *The Power of Habit*, the habit loop goes something like this:

1. **Cue:** An initial cue—such as time, place, emotions, people, or pre-ceding actions—sparks the habit chain, activating a habit "memory." *Example:* A nightly TV show comes on, and you crave a snack.

2. **Routine**: We enact the routine (what we perceive as the actual "habit") effortlessly and with little thought. *Example:* You walk to the fridge and eat the snack.

3. **Reward:** The habit loop yields a reward, which makes the whole thing #worthit. *Example:* Eating the snack gives you a shot of the feel-good neurotransmitter dopamine, stretches your stomach and/ or fulfills some mouth craving.

When a habit is something you intend to do, such as brushing your teeth or going to work, it's like an awesome life hack you didn't even have to research! But oftentimes habits trap us in unwanted behaviors: Think wolfing down excess sugar and calories, apocalypse-style. By the time a habit becomes a *bad* habit, it's ingrained in that memory-based basal ganglia, which is no easy thing to change. (If forgetting memories were easy, we'd probably have an easier time getting over our exes!) With intense habits, you can start doing things you know you shouldn't do, and don't even *want* to do, yet seemingly can't stop! Just consider that rodents habitually conditioned to push levers for food will keep pushing the levers when stuffed, or even when the food "reward" becomes toxic.[51]

Humans don't fare much better. A 2011 study conducted at the University of Southern California (fight on!) found that moviegoers willingly and readily consume stale movie popcorn out of habit. In the initial study, ninety-eight participants watched movie trailers in a movie theater. Half received fresh popcorn for the showing, while half unknowingly received week-old, stale popcorn. Though all the students claimed to prefer fresh popcorn (duh), it was their previous movie theater popcorn habits that determined how much they actually ate. Students with self-professed "weak" movie theater popcorn habits ate significantly less stale popcorn compared to fresh popcorn, while students who admitted having "strong" movie theater popcorn habits ended up eating the same amount of stale and fresh popcorn: around 63 percent!

When the researchers conducted the same experiment but with different environmental cues, things changed. When sixty students were given either fresh or stale popcorn before watching music videos in a campus meeting room, they *all* ate less stale popcorn. The students with "strong" movie theater popcorn habits now ate only *half* as much of the stale popcorn as fresh. Removing the movie theater cue short-circuited the habit loop, making eating more intentional. The experimenters next constructed popcorn boxes that "secretly" forced some students to eat with their nondominant hand, figuring this might break the habit routine by bringing attention to their eating, and encourage less stale-popcorn eating. It did just that.

Perhaps the most habitual thing we do, for better or worse, is eat. Studies suggest that overeating is highly habit driven, linked more to times and environmental cues associated with food consumption than to actual hunger.[52] In a society of perpetual food consumption, anything and everything can become a trigger to eat. TV Commercial? Eat something! Homework? Eat something! Sad? Eat something! Celebrity breakup? Eat something! Emoji? Eat something! And with dieting, you must constantly ignore cues to eat, and constantly refuse cues to keep eating when you do eat.

Intermittent fasting, however, frees you from this problem! By completely avoiding eating during a certain time window, rather than considering whether or not to engage, IF short-circuits habit cues all together. IF can also break your original dietary habits by slashing routine and reinviting intention. On your first day of IF, you will once again experience awareness in your eating pattern, welcoming back the prefrontal cortex and initiating the transition from old, controlling habits quick to betray to new habits quick to heal. You simply commit to the eating window, and the rest happens automatically, habit-style! Your eating habits become your best friend rather than your worst enemy!

INTENTION VERSUS DOING

Changing intentions is easy. How many times have you read an article or talked with a friend, and been like, "I'm doing it!" And then you just . . . didn't. Why? Because though changing intentions is easy, *executing* them is not.

This is perfectly summed up through the lens of *Star Wars*. As Yoda says, "Do. Or do not. There is no try." When I'd watch that scene as a youngster, I'd always raise an eyebrow and think, *Actually, Yoda, there* is *try. It's called trying.*

But now with intermittent fasting, it all makes sense! With IF, you either *are* eating or you *aren't* eating. It's "Eat. Or eat not. There is no try." If you try to not eat and you don't eat, then you did intermittent fasting! If you try to not eat and you *do* eat, then you didn't do intermittent fasting! "Try" doesn't even matter. You either do it or you don't!

I say this to be encouraging, not legalistic. Because with IF, you are *freed from intention*. You no longer have to *try* to restrict calories all day. You don't have to *try* to "be good" each and every time you eat. Instead, you commit to your eating and fasting windows, and the work is done! You just *do* it. I don't know about you, but I'm down for a lot less trying and a lot more doing!

HOW TO DO INTERMITTENT FASTING

Intermittent fasting is a dietary pattern of restricting the *hours* you eat each day, rather than the *amount of food* you eat. It's sort of like a coloring book. You pick a pattern, and then color it in with the meals of your choosing! You can color it however you like, as long as you stay in the lines. That's it! Your body will make the metabolic adjustments and do the rest of the work for you: No calorie counting, portion control, stressing, or coaxing required! Please go ahead and throw away your food diary, food scale, and any other nefarious memory of food regulation. (I would say donate them to charity, but why spread neurotic habits?) With intermittent fasting, you're either *not* eating, in which case it's simply not a thing, or you *are* eating, in which case it is *the thing*.

I suggest committing to one of the following outlined approaches when initially beginning IF. As you become more in tune with your body's natural fat-burning preferences, you can adjust and adopt whatever IF pattern best suits your lifestyle.

A FEW THINGS TO KEEP IN MIND WHEN BEGINNING YOUR IF JOURNEY

NO CALORIE COUNTING: This is huge! Please do not count calories in your eating time. Simply eat without restriction, and to satiety.

CELLULAR RHYTHMS: Your body's hormones and cells contain natural circadian rhythms, which respond to meal intake and timing. (The hormone ghrelin, for example, specifically adjusts to meal patterns, making you hungry at your normal mealtimes.) The more you repeat an IF pattern, the easier it will become, as your internal hunger cues sync to your new eating window.

ALWAYS AN OPTION: Unlike typical diet fiends, which mock you in a "Bet you can't do me!" type way, IF is like a close friend who's always got your back. You can always start IF, always do IF, and always adjust IF, whenever and however you please.

NO MISTAKES: If you "mess up" your IF pattern, you didn't really . . . you just did a different time window!

DAILY COMMITMENT: While the various IF patterns can be implemented on a more occasional basis, I recommend committing to a daily pattern in the beginning, to encourage your body to quickly make the necessary cellular and metabolic adaptions for fat burning, and catalyze your transition into the effortlessness of IF.

HYBRID FASTING: After you *do* accumulate a bit of IF under your belt (Yay!), feel free to experiment with more à la carte approaches down the line. You might fancy a longer fast here or there, an occasional calorie-restricted fast for boosted weight loss, a protein-restricted fast for enhanced autophagy, or even some days with no fasting. So many choices!

DON'T FREAK OUT: Remember, you can always break your fast if you need to! Sometimes just knowing you *can* break your fast can inspire you to *not* break your fast.

THE CLOCK APPROACH

WHAT?

In the Clock Approach to intermittent fasting, you choose the literal times each day during which you will eat and fast. This creates two time blocks on the clock—one of fasting and one of eating. You fast during the fasting times, and eat anytime during the eating times. For example, you may choose an eating time of 12:00 p.m. to 8:00 p.m. each day, with a fasting time of 8:00 p.m. to 12:00 p.m.

HOW?

- Decide on the number of hours you want to eat and fast per day in uninterrupted time blocks. You should ideally fast for a minimum of twelve hours. Many people find a sixteen-hour fast to be ideal. Of course, you can totally go twenty-four hours if you want!
- Assign these eating hours to a daily time block that fits best with your lifestyle. For example, if you choose a six-hour eating block, you could eat from 8:00 a.m. to 2:00 p.m., 12:00 p.m. to 6:00 p.m., 2:00 p.m. to 8:00 p.m., 4:00 p.m. to 10:00 p.m., and so on.

- Alternatively, you can choose the fasting time, from twelve to twenty-four hours, and assign it accordingly. For example, if you decide to fast for sixteen hours every day, you could fast from 5:00 p.m. to 9:00 a.m., 8:00 p.m. to 12:00 p.m., 10:00 p.m. to 2:00 p.m., and so on.

- I recommend making the eating times cover the meals you like. For example, you could eat from 7:00 a.m. to 2:00 p.m. if you love breakfast and lunch, or 12:00 p.m. to 8:00 p.m. if you love lunch and dinner. If you're just a dinner person (like me!), you could eat from, say, 5:00 p.m. to 9:00 p.m.

- In general, shorter time spent eating tends to yield faster weight loss, since you'll be fasting for longer.

- Stick to it! Follow your selected clock pattern each day, using the same times. Eat all meals during your selected eating time, and fast during your selected fasting time.

- You do not have to eat constantly during the eating time. You also don't have to start eating right at the beginning of the eating time, or eat right at the end. Simply eat when hungry *during* your allocated eating time.

WHY?

- The Clock Approach is clear and simple: Eat in your eating time, and fast in your fasting time. Stick to the clock, and watch the fat loss, health, and other benefits happen automagically!

- The Clock Approach can easily align with natural meal habits. You can choose a time that includes the main meals you like, be it breakfast, lunch, and/or dinner.

- When implemented every day, the Clock Approach is very habitual.

- There isn't much thinking or preparation involved. You simply fast during the fasting time and eat during the eating time, no questions asked! Fewer food choices = more willpower!

WHY NOT?

- Sometimes your chosen hours may not align with your schedule or a social function. (Remember you can always take a break from fasting or adjust your times if need be!)
- If you're the neurotic type, you might find yourself obsessing over the clock.

THOUGHTS?

I think a Clock Approach is a fantastic way to start intermittent fasting. It's very black-and-white, and removes all ambiguity. You simply stick to your fasting/eating times, and you're good to go!

THE WINDOW APPROACH

WHAT?

In the Window Approach to intermittent fasting, you create a daily fasting window, based on the minimum number of hours you want to fast. This is similar to the Clock Approach, though the windows each day may fluctuate and are not bound to certain times. Whenever a meal period ends, you essentially resolve to wait a minimum number of hours until you eat again.

HOW?

- Choose the minimum number of hours you want to fast each day, anywhere from twelve to twenty-four hours.
- When you finish eating on any given day, resolve to wait your minimum number of hours before eating again.
- For example, say you choose a sixteen-hour fast. If you finish dinner at 8:00 p.m., then you tell yourself not to eat again until at least 12:00 p.m. the next day. That next day, you might finish eating at 6:00 p.m., in which case you would wait until at least 10:00 a.m. the next morning to eat again. And if you continued to eat longer

that next day, say until 10:00 p.m., you would again not eat until 2:00 p.m. the next day. The key is simply maintaining the *minimum fasting hours*, regardless of the time on the clock.

WHY?

- The Window Approach allows for flexibility with eating, while ensuring minimum fasting hours.
- The Window Approach can create a more fluid and flexible approach to IF, with fewer feelings of being bound by the clock.

WHY NOT?

- Occasionally, your schedule or a social event may mandate eating again before your ideal fasting window has passed. If so, don't sweat it! You can always take a break from fasting on any given day. Plus, if you end up eating earlier than you like, you can always fast longer afterward!
- If you're the neurotic type, you might find yourself obsessing over your windows.

THOUGHTS?

I think a Window Approach is great for those who want to implement intermittent fasting without as many feelings of restraint on eating hours or thoughts of the clock. It also can create more fasting variety than the Clock Approach. You really just count your fasting hours, and you're good to go!

THE MEAL APPROACH

WHAT?

In the Meal Approach to intermittent fasting, you choose one or two meals to consume each day. You can snack in between the meals within the general eating window, but do not snack or eat beyond that, during the fasting window.

HOW?

Choose one of the following meal combinations to eat, and eat just those meals each day!

- Breakfast
- Breakfast and lunch
- Lunch
- Lunch and dinner
- Dinner
- Dinner and snacking till bed (that's me!)

WHY?

- The Meal Approach lets you eat your favorite meals!
- The Meal Approach may make you feel more "normal." For example, you could view it as "just skipping breakfast," or "having a late lunch and skipping dinner."
- The Meal Approach discourages any obsession surrounding the clock or time windows. If you choose lunch only, for example, you can have lunch whenever!
- If you choose one meal per day, it truly is a feast! It's great for those who tend to be big eaters rather than grazers.
- Choosing one meal per day frees up an insane amount of time.

WHY NOT?

- If you stick to the Meal Approach for the long term, you might have to come up with "excuses" for skipping breakfast, lunch, and/or dinner. For this reason, I recommend including dinner, which tends to be the most communal meal.
- If you can't sleep on an empty stomach, you won't want to skip dinner. On the flip side, if you can't sleep on a full stomach, you won't want to eat too late.
- You may be worried about skipping the "most important" meal of breakfast, or eating too much before bed. But have no fear! See "IF Fears" on page 122 for why that's not a problem.

THOUGHTS?

The Meal Approach is the intermittent fasting protocol I personally follow. I just eat dinner each night, with free snacking until bed. I find it wondrously liberating, as I gain time and productivity during the day, while looking forward to a massive, scrumptious feast each and every night. Viewing the fast as a meal mindset, rather than a time frame, allows me to eat dinner whenever I feel hungry and/or it's socially appropriate. And since dinner does tend to be the most social meal, I find this IF approach easily integrates into my social calendar. It has proven to be an effortless, effective lifestyle, which inspired the contents of this book!

OTHER FASTING INCARNATIONS

I strongly recommend you start intermittent fasting with one of the previously discussed approaches, which I have found work best for the lifestyle change, due to their habitual, nonrestricted nature. That said, fasting pops up in many other variants, so here are my thoughts for general informational purposes.

ALTERNATE-DAY FASTING (ADF)

This is a primary form of IF utilized in scientific trials. With ADF, you alternate "normal" eating days with fasting days. The fasting days are typically calorie-restricted (to around 25 to 85 percent of basal needs) to maximize fat loss, although fasting days with normal calorie intake can be utilized as well. Popularized forms of ADF include Michael Mosley's and Mimi Spencer's *The Fast Diet*, as well as Krista Varady's *The Every-Other-Day Diet*.

While I've never personally practiced ADF, I've definitely read about it for *hours* in the scientific literature. Across the board, studies show ADF approaches encourage adherence and maximize fat loss. That said, I don't recommend ADF in the beginning of your IF journey, as it's a bit complicated, less habitual, and typically requires calorie restriction, which I'm hoping you'll forget entirely. (Though it may happen naturally!) I also personally find that reverting to normal eating habits short-circuits IF adaptation.

BULLETPROOF™ FASTING

Bulletproof™ Intermittent Fasting is an IF method developed by Dave Asprey, author of *The Bulletproof Diet*. In this approach, you forgo breakfast and consume low-toxin coffee with butter or MCT oil in the morning. (Dave recommends his Bulletproof™ branded coffee, specifically created to be low in mold toxins, with his Brain Octane® oil.) You then break your fast with a high-fat, low-carb, and toxin-minimizing lunch or dinner, according to the suggested foods on his "Bulletproof Diet Roadmap."

On the one hand, this program can yield a good deal of energy and appetite suppression, combining the thermogenic effects of caffeine with a stable fat source for energy. On the other hand, there is a debate about whether drinking coffee with fat actually sustains or breaks the fast. Also, consuming massive amounts of fat in your fasting window may slow down your potential burning of body fat.

LEANGAINS

Leangains is a time-based IF protocol with a sixteen-hour fast and eight-hour eating period (16/8), tailored toward bodybuilders, developed by Martin Berkhan. The protocol implements careful use of branched-chain amino acids to support muscle mass, cycles macronutrients and calories, and features training and rest days.

PROTEIN FASTING

This involves more *what* you eat, rather than *when* you eat. With protein fasting, you drastically minimize protein intake in a given day, to encourage autophagy and the cellular renewal process.[53] (Autophagy is the process in which the body recycles old internal proteins for growth and repair. See "IF Health Benefits" on page 87 for more on that!) Of course, IF naturally stimulates autophagy during the fasted state anyway, but having a day here or there in which you further restrict protein intake in your eating window can ramp up the process considerably!

FASTING MIMICKING DIET (FMD)

Developed by Valter Longo at USC, the fasting mimicking diet is a short-term, very low-calorie, low-protein diet designed to nourish the body with micronutrients while still maintaining the cleansing and rejuvenating benefits of the completely fasted state—evident by similar glucose, ketone, and growth factor levels associated with longevity and stress resistance. The FMD purportedly allows for the therapeutic potential of an extended fast, without the deprivation and burden associated with fasting for multiple days on end. The official five-day protocol uses proprietary plant-based soups, bars, drinks, and snacks, as well as chamomile tea and a vitamin supplement.

LONGER FASTS

Longer fasts, as you may have surmised, involve fasting for more than one day, and are typically used for therapeutic healing processes of specific diseases, or under medical supervision for the severely overweight. While longer fasting definitely has its place, it is another beast entirely, and not something I prescribe in this book, or even encourage. Please discuss longer fasts with your doctor.

IF TIPS AND TRICKS

For maximum confidence in adopting your new intermittent fasting lifestyle (yay you!), I suggest reading all the sciencey parts of this book, to understand why *when* you eat will welcome a hunger-less state of fat burning and health. Knowledge is power! Beyond that, here are some concrete methods to help you easily transition to the IF life.

FEAST BEFORE

Don't start your first fasting day in a hungry mode. This will be fun for no one, trust me. While I don't recommend cheat days or bingeing, I see nothing wrong with a final "It's been real!" feast before your first fasting day. That way, you probably won't even be hungry for most of your first fast. Your body will then begin making the metabolic changes for fat-burning mode, so hunger won't even be a thing anyway! Plus, since you'll potentially be feasting every day anyway (depending on the length of your window), might as well get used to it!

STAY BUSY

Lying around in a melodramatically lethargic "I'm fasting" state will just make you more tired and hungry. Seriously. Start IF on a day with a full calendar. Rather than spending hours fantasizing about food and falling prey to boredom munchies, allow more pressing matters to demand your immediate attention. You can really only focus on one thing at any given moment, so might as well make it something productive! Physical activity also ramps up fat burning, catalyzing the transition into the fasted state and blasting through hunger. So get moving!

PLAN IT OUT

When you select your eating window for the first fasting day, plan out what you will eat during this time. You can go more freestyle after you've acclimated to IF, but a solid game plan is great in the beginning. If you're already a type A person, this should be easy. If you're not, just envision that OCD planner friend who gets nervous when people "branch out." ("Guys! We have to stick to the *plan*!") Create your plan and stick to it. Wiggle room just lets difficulties wiggle in.

TRACK YOUR PROGRESS

Many smartphone apps can help you chart your progress. Some are specifically geared toward fasting, while others provide more general motivation or target habits. Alternatively, you can go old-school and use a journal, or put happy stickers on a calendar to visually document successful IF days. (I recently ordered two hundred sparkly Lisa Frank stickers for the sole purpose of documenting my blog posts at MelanieAvalon.com—so gratifying!)

CAFFEINE

While I'm not saying you should become a caffeine junkie, this legal psychoactive drug undeniably promotes fat burning and energy expenditure, thrusting you into the fasted state and squelching appetite. Feel free to drink tea and coffee during the fast—just don't load them with cream and sugar. That said, if you find that caffeine keeps you awake at night, you might want to reconsider. Speaking of sleep . . .

SLEEP SMART

Not only is sleep simultaneously swell for your health *and* a fun time (lucid dreams anyone?), it also totally counts toward your fasting window! Try timing your sleep to create a "head start" in your fast. You could pick an evening window, and have a big early dinner. By the time you wake up the next day, you'll already have chipped away at a substantial portion of your fast! Oh hey, home stretch! Definitely don't begin your fasting adventures in a state of sleep deprivation, as this can increase hunger and diminish willpower.

FIND A FRIEND

Would Dorothy have made it to Oz without her friends? Debatable. Enlisting a pal (or three) to accompany you on your fasting adventure can work wonders. There's nothing like a friend's support when facing the fears of the unknown, especially if you feel like it's going to get darker before it gets lighter. Studies find that people in constant communication tend to mimic each other, leading to similar emotional and behavioral attributes,[54] so doing IF with a like-minded individual can amplify your own motivation and actions. Having an IF buddy also provides accountability for moments of doubt, and backup support for moments of social pressure. Perhaps best of all, an IF friend can provide reassurance that what you're doing isn't insane. (Or if it is, at least you'll go down together!) Can't find a friend? Try listening to "You Are Not Alone" from *Into The Woods* on repeat.

GO AT YOUR OWN PACE

While I advocate the cold-turkey, jump-all-in approach, if you are the type who requires some sort of warm-up, you can always ease into IF. Try skipping a meal here and there for starters, or slowly shorten your eating window.

TRY IT FOR A WEEK

Tell yourself, regardless of the outcome, you will try IF for just a week, which is significantly less daunting than a month or lifetime. Of course, if a week gets you hooked . . . well, it happens. When I first started intermittent fasting, I committed to a week. That was more than half a decade ago, and I haven't stopped!

EMBRACE THE "WHAT"

I cannot encourage you enough to embrace the "What?" portion of this book. Finding the best food choices for *you* can truly eradicate inflammation and stimulate vitality, while pairing wonderfully with IF! In fact, many people following whole-foods lifestyles easily fall into bouts of IF without even meaning to, while many IF-ers find they begin naturally gravitating toward whole foods. It all goes together!

IF FEARS

WILL INTERMITTENT FASTING DAMAGE MY METABOLISM?

Common dietary wisdom preaches that we must eat constantly to stoke our metabolic fire (at least 1,200 calories!), and if we go too long without eating (more than three hours!), our metabolism will automatically abandon us without a last look. We may fear doing irreversible damage or entering "starvation mode." In reality, the metabolism is not some rigid number of calories, like a lightbulb at a set wattage, but more like a fluctuating fire. The word metabolism even comes from the Greek word *metabolē*, meaning "change." To demystify it all, let's first establish what constitutes a person's daily metabolic rate, which includes the *basal metabolic rate* (BMR), *thermic effect of food*, and *physical activity energy expenditure* on a given day.

The BMR accounts for an estimated 60 percent of your metabolism, and refers to the amount of energy required to sustain all vital organs at rest. It's basically the amount of calories required to run your literal body if you did *nothing* for an entire day, in a calm, temperate environment. Your body will do *whatever it must* to generate this energy. Online calculators that ask for your height, weight, age, and gender calculate your general BMR. These formulas, however, do not account for body composition, and since muscle burns more calories than fat, two people could be the same height, weight, age, and gender, but have different BMRs.

The *thermic effect of food* refers to the amount of energy (calories) required for the digestion process, and is generally around 10 percent of calories consumed, meaning you can sort of write off some calories as lost to digestion. The type of food consumed affects this percentage. Fat provides a minimal thermic effect of 0 to 3 percent, carbohydrates provide around 5 to 10 percent, and the thermic effect of protein is a whopping 20 to 30 percent.

Physical activity energy expenditure refers to the calories burned through daily activity. This includes both conscious volitional activity (such as sports and exercise), as well as nonexercise activity thermogenesis (NEAT): all the movement you do in life that isn't "on purpose," such as fidgeting, walking from place to place, or even laughing. The hard-to-define NEAT can account for wildly varying metabolic rates, further convoluting the matter of metabolism.

Contrary to popular belief, BMR does *not* depend on meal frequency— researchers consistently find no overall metabolic adjustment to meal timing.[55] (As one study put it,[56] there is no metabolic difference "between nibbling and gorging.")[57] In fact, the metabolic rate can potentially *increase* while fasting! A 2000 study that analyzed the BMR of healthy lean individuals at various stages of fasting (between one and eighty-four hours) found that their BMR increased throughout the entire trial.[58]

Calorie restriction, *not intermittent fasting*, is what "slows down" a person's BMR and reduces the rate of weight loss. Your body does this as a protective mechanism, so you can keep on keepin' on at a lower calorie intake. That said, a lowered metabolic rate does not necessarily stop weight loss or fat burning, and your metabolism won't be stuck there forever. As long as the calorie intake is still below the number of calories required for that day, you'll likely still lose weight—just slower than if your metabolism *hadn't* adjusted for the deficit.

Consider a 2006 study on six months of calorie restriction in healthy, overweight humans: a control group on a maintenance diet, a 25 percent calorie-restricted group, a 25 percent calorie-restricted and exercise group (12.5 percent from calorie restriction, 12.5 percent from exercise), and a very low 890-calorie group.[59] While all the calorie-restricted patients experienced a decreased metabolic rate, they still all lost weight throughout the trial. At no point did weight loss stop. Also, the reduced metabolic rate occurred within three months, but didn't drop after that. This indicates that getting insufficient calories won't stop weight loss; rather, you'll simply burn less fat than if your BMR hadn't changed. (Of course, IF doesn't require calorie restriction anyway!)

Since BMR relies in part on a person's weight, it is possible for weight loss to plateau if you reach a lower weight requiring a lower BMR, and do not adjust accordingly. For example, say you restrict your diet to a rate that cannot sustain your present weight, but *could* sustain your body at a lower weight. Once your body reaches that lower weight, you would then need to further lower calories to continue weight loss. You didn't "damage" your metabolism; rather, the new, smaller version of you simply requires less of your metabolism.

That said, it's possible that fasting may "protect" one's BMR, even in the face of calorie restriction. The aforementioned 2006 study suggested that *energy deficit*, not calorie restriction specifically, is what lowers metabolism. Since fasting provides hormonal mechanisms for ample energy via fat and ketone metabolism, calorie restriction may be "safer" when fasting than when practiced throughout the day.

What about eating to speed up your metabolism? True, the body requires energy to process food, giving you a temporary "metabolic boost." This thermic effect, however, is a percentage based on the type and amount of food consumed, not the frequency. It doesn't matter if ten minutes or ten hours have passed since your last meal—the total thermic effect for the day will still be a percentage of the total number of calories consumed that day. For example, a study comparing two large meals with four small meals, containing the same number of overall calories, found no difference in their total thermic effect.[60] It's like if you went shopping all day and ended up with six outfits costing $180. Whether you bought them at different stores throughout the day or all at one store, the total cost would be the same. Of course, if you consume *more* calories in total with multiple meals compared to an IF window (which, speaking from experience, is easy to do), then you would indeed "burn more calories" via the thermic effect from eating more meals. However, you'd also be taking in more calories total, so it's a moot point.

WILL I GAIN ALL THE WEIGHT BACK IF I STOP FASTING?

A lower body weight correlates to a lower metabolism: If there's less of you, there's less energy needed to *sustain* you. A study of women who achieved stable weight loss through calorie restriction found they had "metabolic rates appropriate for their body sizes."[61] In other words, even if your metabolism settles at a lower point from weight loss, it won't be lower than it *should* be for the "new you." If you lose ten pounds, you may experience a lower metabolic rate compared to your formerly heavier self. While perhaps "permanent" at this new weight, the change is not irreversible. If you gain back the weight, you'll likely welcome back its correlated higher metabolism.

IS KETOSIS DANGEROUS?

Ketosis is a harmless, natural, and often beneficial state in which the body produces the energy substrate of ketones, at blood levels of around 0.5 to 3 millimoles per liter. People often confuse ketosis with ketoacidosis, which is typically an issue for diabetics, and occurs when a lack of feedback loops from a lack of insulin allows ketones to reach dangerous levels in the blood: around 15 to 25 millimoles per liter. This causes the blood's pH to become too acidic, leading to many potential problems. You don't have to worry about ketoacidosis when producing ketones, just like you don't have to worry about reaching toxic levels of vitamins. Unless you have a preexisting condition messing things up (which is why you should consult your doctor before you start fasting), the body regulates ketone and pH levels with dexterity.

WILL I GET ENOUGH NUTRIENTS WITH INTERMITTENT FASTING?

We tend to lump calories and nutrients into the common category of "food." A person is either eating enough or not eating enough—end of story. This does not account for the two critical subcategories of calories versus nutrients. *Calories* refer to the literal energy stored within food, while *nutrients* refer to specific building blocks required for optimal function, growth, and repair. You can take in too many calories while taking in too few nutrients. You can also take in too few calories while taking in ample nutrients. The former is highly common in modern society; the latter is much more rare. While starvation is a very serious issue that I do *not* take lightly, I'd wager that if you have the resources to read this book in the first place, you likely don't have to worry *too* much about getting enough calories. In any case, the ideal diet provides adequate calories *and* nutrients, granting the body the ingredients to thrive.

Perhaps most important, please know that intermittent fasting does not mandate calorie restriction, and the IF patterns discussed in this book can easily provide an abundance of calories. Your body is also quite intuitive: If you undereat calories at one meal, chances are you'll become hungrier at the next. IF teaches you to trust your body rather than fight it.

While this may be controversial, if you have to choose between calorie (not nutrient) restriction and calorie overconsumption, calorie restriction is likely healthier. While calorie overconsumption is linked to obesity, diabetes, heart disease, and many other conditions, calorie restriction is associated with disease prevention and longevity.[62]

Of course, getting enough calories is one thing. Getting enough *nutrients* is a different beast entirely. Although we have a tendency to slam our bodies with excess calories, we can still miss the nutrient train entirely. Proper nourishment involves the right *types* of food, more than the right *amount* of food. It is a composition issue, completely separate from meal timing. You could practice IF and consume junk food lacking adequate nutrition, or you could practice IF and consume nourishing food full of nutrients! You could also be simultaneously obese and malnourished, or underweight and nourished.

The path to adequate nutrition in your IF approach boils down to your food choices. I advocate embracing whole foods in abundance, rather than relying on "healthy" nutrient bars and/or pounding vitamins like candy. It's the whole "What?" part of *What When Wine*. Rest assured that nutrient intake is determined by one's overall twenty-four-hour consumption, rather than minute-to-minute activity. Simply focus on making the foods in your eating window healthy and nontoxic, and you'll grow more nourished by the day!

ISN'T BREAKFAST THE MOST IMPORTANT MEAL OF THE DAY?

Let's break down the word *breakfast*. Break. Fast. Yep, breakfast is the meal that breaks your fast. In that sense, I completely agree that breakfast is the most important meal! With IF, you're still eating breakfast—it just happens to be at a different time! But for reals, we're often told that breakfast is vital for health, and that skipping breakfast instigates weight gain, but is this the case?

To begin, flip to the footnotes of a study with the word "breakfast" in the title, and you'll likely find something to the effect of, "This review was commissioned and paid for by [insert cereal company here]." While this doesn't dismiss the findings, it does call for a discerning eye regarding the conclusions drawn from the data. In fact, a 2013 *American Journal of Clinical Nutrition* meta-analysis concluded that a majority of pro-breakfast studies feature biased interpretations, misleading language, improper citations, and inappropriate use of "causal" terminology.[63] To the last point, many studies linking breakfast to health and weight loss are observational and epistemological. Breakfast eaters tend to smoke less, drink less, eat more fiber and micronutrients, and be more physically active, so it may not be that breakfast itself controls weight, but rather that healthier people at healthier weights tend to eat breakfast.

Now for the more sciencey stuff! Breakfast is often assumed to be the most important meal because it fuels you for the day. This makes sense in a standard eating pattern relying on constant dietary intake for fuel. IF, however, switches your body into a fat-burning mode, squelching your reliance on constant meals. You already wake up in the fasted, fat-burning state each morning, so continuing your fast only further upregulates energy use, rendering the "breakfast for fuel" thing a nonissue.

Breakfast also supposedly keeps you from overeating later in the day, resulting in an overall calorie deficit. An opposing view, however, holds that skipping breakfast results in an overall *lower* calorie intake. So which is more likely?

I'll let the controlled, non-epistemological studies analyzing the relationship between breakfast, metabolism, and weight loss speak for themselves!

In a four-week 2014 study, researchers compared a high-fiber oat porridge breakfast, a nonfiber cornflakes cereal breakfast, and a skipped breakfast (fasting) in thirty-six healthy but overweight individuals. They found that, although the breakfast eaters felt fuller than the fasters, those who skipped breakfast lost significantly more weight than both breakfast groups. The study concluded that, while skipping breakfast may increase hunger, individuals are unlikely to eat enough later to make up for the missed meal, and eat fewer calories overall.[64]

In a six-week 2014 *American Journal of Clinical Nutrition* trial of thirty-three lean individuals, one group ate a breakfast of up to 700 calories within two hours of waking, while the other group didn't eat until after 12:00 pm. On the one hand, the breakfast eaters engaged in more light physical activity in the morning, and experienced diet-induced thermogenesis from digestion (which makes sense . . . since they were eating). But that was about it. No difference was found in the metabolic rate, appetite hormones (such as leptin and ghrelin), fasting glucose levels, or changes in body mass.[65] Breakfast and fasting also did not affect eating patterns later in the day: Once breakfast had passed, both groups consumed similar amounts of food and macronutrients. The breakfast group, however, *did* end up eating around 500 more calories in total during the day than the fasting group, significantly from sugar! The study concluded that skipping breakfast does not cause weight gain.

Two randomized crossover 2013 studies published in *Physiology and Behavior* also concluded that skipping breakfast does not encourage overeating.[66] In the first, twenty-four individuals alternated between a high-carb 335-calorie breakfast, a high-fiber 338 calorie breakfast, or they skipped breakfast. They next attended a buffet-style lunch, and their hunger and food intake was measured. The study found that, although those who had skipped breakfast were hungrier at the start of lunch, they ate no more than on the days they'd eaten breakfast, and, as a result, ended up eating fewer total calories than those who ate breakfast. Given these surprising results, the researchers wondered if the provided breakfast was too small to adequately affect lunch intake, or if the participants would end up eating more later in the day to make up for no breakfast.

So they did a second study, measuring food intake and hunger levels throughout the entire day of eighteen individuals who either ate a buffet breakfast or skipped breakfast. These participants ended up eating around 550 to 700 calories for breakfast. On these days, they felt less hungry and consumed fewer calories at lunch, by about 144 calories. But it ended there. Regardless of whether breakfast was eaten, hunger levels normalized by midafternoon, and breakfast's presence or absence bore no effect on hunger and calorie consumption after lunchtime. As a result, the participants ended up eating around 450 *fewer* calories when they skipped breakfast. The study concluded that skipping breakfast may be a good way to reduce overall calorie intake in some individuals.

Still on the fence? Here's a brief lowdown of several other studies:

- A 2011 study found that children who skip breakfast feel like they "could eat more" at lunch, but ultimately consume around the same amount, and end up consuming fewer calories in total for the day.[67]
- A sixteen-week 2014 study of 283 adults trying to lose weight in a free-living situation found no difference between eating or skipping breakfast.[68]
- In a two-week 2013 crossover study, men consumed either a 100-calorie or 700-calorie breakfast. While the men snacked more following the low-calorie breakfast, lunch intake was similar for both, and ultimately they consumed fewer calories when they ate a low-calorie, rather than high-calorie, breakfast. The high-calorie breakfast also reduced fat oxidation throughout the day.[69]
- A highly controlled 2001 study placed obese individuals in a pressurized chamber calorimeter, which calculates precisely how many calories its inhabitants burn by measuring the room's oxygen. The researchers found that skipping breakfast did not significantly affect metabolic rates or calories burned, though breakfast-skippers burned more calories at night than breakfast eaters. Eating throughout the day also resulted in more standing, potentially attributed to the participants getting up for the food (which I find a bit hilarious). The conclusion? Eating fewer meals or fasting does not encourage overconsumption.[70]

WILL EATING AT NIGHT MAKE ME GAIN WEIGHT?

On the flip side of the "eat early to lose weight" maxim, we've got the "eat late to gain weight" hypothesis . . . which turns out to be equally debatable.

From an evolutionary hunter-gatherer perspective, we scoured for food during the day and ate around the fire at night. Our natural cortisol rhythms support this, spiking in the morning to liberate energy stores for the fasted hunt for food. Studies on meal timing consistently show that total fat storage in a given day is not determined by *when* one eats but rather by the type and total amount consumed over twenty-four hours. A meal eaten at 9:00 a.m. requires the same amount of digestion and assimilation as a meal eaten at 9:00 p.m.

Beyond that, many of the studies linking night eating to weight gain involve night-shift workers or those with night-eating syndrome, or are epidemiological in nature, which can yield extraneous factors that independently contribute to weight gain, including skewed circadian rhythms, deteriorating sleep quality, insulin dysregulation, and potentially unhealthy diets or activity levels.[71] I'd also wager most night eaters *aren't* intermittent fasters, and so eat *more* in total per day by eating at night.

Studies that do look at "normal" eaters and late-night eating are far more heterogeneous, finding weight gain, no difference, or even weight loss. Most revelatory (but rare) are highly controlled metabolic-ward studies. One such study in 2007 of twelve obese women looked at the difference between 900 to 1,000 calories consumed either as five meals per day or confined to 9:00 to 11:00 a.m. or 6:00 to 8:00 p.m. It found no difference with regard to weight gain.

Other studies do find that night eating leads to weight gain and heightened morning insulin in obese women, but adding daily exercise obliterates these effects, instead yielding weight loss and muscle maintenance![72] This implies that perhaps it is not night eating that automatically causes problems but rather overall lifestyle patterns, such as sedentarism coupled with night food intake.

Depending on meal compositions, eating throughout the day *and* eating at night could perpetuate insulin, encouraging continual fat storge, but isolating insulin to a single release at night could yield the opposite effect. A 2012 study of seventy-eight obese police officers found that those who consumed most of their carbs (which spike insulin) at dinner rather than throughout the day lost more weight, experienced decreased cravings, and saw remarkable improvements in metabolic and hormonal factors.[73] This implies that insulin release at night may actually be beneficial if it is the only major insulin spike for the day. Plus, the police officers were still eating throughout the day and saw major benefits—imagine what would happen if they were completely suppressing daytime insulin with an IF approach!

The night-eating fear also assumes sleep to be a lazy state requiring little energy. On the contrary, a majority of metabolic and growth processes occur at night, with REM brain patterns similar to those of the awake brain. And despite a lack of physical activity, the nighttime basal metabolic rate is only reduced by around 15 percent, burning a similar number of calories as watching TV![74] Of course, what and when you eat can affect how well you sleep, and your body composition as a consequence. A controlled 2010 crossover study at the University of Chicago Sleep Research Laboratory found that sleeping less reduced weight loss by 55 percent, increased muscle loss by 60 percent, and spiked levels of the hunger hormone ghrelin.[75] You may sleep like a log after consuming a massive feast, or doing so might yield restless indigestion. I therefore encourage you to adopt an IF pattern that best suits your digestion and whisks you away to dreamland.

The takeaway? The whole late-night eating thing isn't so much about timing but rather about our accompanying habits, like how much we eat in total, spike insulin, or engage in physical activity. If you're eating throughout the day *and* heartily at night, it could spell trouble for your waistline. On the contrary, eating a night meal in an IF pattern controls food intake and insulin, while encouraging ample daytime fat burning, aligning with our natural rhythms to support a lean, healthy metabolic state.

IF Q&A

IF FOOD QUESTIONS

WHAT CAN I EAT IN THE EATING WINDOW?

What you consume in your eating window is entirely up to you! That said, why shoot yourself in the foot with your food choices when you could make *every* moment of your life rich in renewal? I wholeheartedly recommend an anti-inflammatory diet featuring whole foods that support health and encourage a fat-burning (rather than sugar-burning) state, as discussed in the "What?" section.

CAN I EAT UNHEALTHY FOODS OR BINGE DURING MY EATING WINDOW?

If you're transitioning from a standard American diet rich in processed foods, then continuing such eating in an IF pattern will still likely yield beneficial results by encouraging fat burning, decreasing inflammation, and minimizing damage done overall. However, the goal here is to ultimately free you from anything and everything that impedes your health, well-being, and success. So while you may start with just the "when" and not the "what," hopefully it shall be a stepping-stone to better food choices as well. I also don't encourage the "bingeing" terminology, which insinuates disordered eating. Instead, see IF as the opportunity to feast, if you so desire. (Which, yes, you totally can!)

CAN I CONSUME FRUITS OR VEGETABLES DURING MY FASTING WINDOW?

Consuming any food during the fasted state starts digestion and potentially releases insulin, breaking the fast, so commit to complete food abstinence during the fasting window. Snacks will simply keep hunger present and short-circuit metabolic adaptations for fat burning.

CAN I CONSUME FATS/MCT OIL DURING MY FASTING WINDOW?

If by "fasting" we simply mean maintaining a fat-burning state, then theoretically ingesting *pure* fat could possibly supplement this state, since fats do not affect insulin levels and do not immediately encourage fat storage. That said, consuming fat may influence related hormones and blunt growth hormone secretion, potentially discouraging muscle protection and fat burning. MCT oil, a ketogenic fat derived from coconut and palm oil, may be an exception, as it is directly shuttled to the liver for energy, rather than requiring digestion and filtration through the lymph system like other fats. Because it's all quite complicated, I advocate starting IF completely "dry" in the beginning. After you've got some fasting under your belt and know what the fasted state feels like, then you can experiment with MCT oil or other fats from there. In any case, ingesting fats will likely switch your source of fat burning from body fat to dietary fat, so you may want to do so when you've reached maintenance mode.

CAN I TAKE EXOGENOUS KETONES DURING THE FAST?

Exogenous ketones are an easily assimilated "pure" form of ketones—the alternative energy substrate generated during fasting. Studies suggest they can rapidly enhance the ketogenic state and provide therapeutic potential, including in regard to cancer. It's up to you if you want to experiment with exogenous ketones during the fast, either for enhanced energy, disease prevention, or to potentially catalyze your jump into the fasted state. If you do partake, look for pure forms without added fillers or flavors.

HOW MANY CALORIES BREAK A FAST?

The number of calories that break a fast is up for debate, and goes back to what we mean by fasting. I often hear 40 to 50 calories casually thrown around as some sort of upper limit, but I cannot for the life of me find any studies on the subject. In any case, the type of calories likely matter. A smidge of sugar or zero-calorie sweetener might break your fast by spiking insulin, while *perhaps* MCT oil doesn't. Small amounts of liquid calories, which do not spark mechanical digestion, might also be "safer," such as adding cream to one's coffee.

I advocate forgoing calories entirely during the fasted state: Why bother playing with temptation? Consider self-experimenting with things after you've got a substantial amount of IF under your belt. Keep in mind that if ingesting something instigates hunger, it's likely breaking your fast. And even if it doesn't increase appetite, it may minimize some of fasting's beneficial effects.

IF DRINK QUESTIONS

WHAT CAN I DRINK DURING MY FASTING WINDOW?

During your fast, you can consume noncaloric beverages such as water, tea, and coffee without sugar. Avoid artificial sweeteners, which can be inflammatory and toxic, and may negatively affect the gut microbiome, encouraging weight gain and other problems. If you *must* sweeten your drinks, try stevia. That said, most people find that forgoing the sweet taste is key for completely eradicating sugar cravings. As for coffee, you can add a tablespoon or so of half-and-half and/or cream in the beginning (if it doesn't cause hunger), but try to eventually adopt a black approach. It'll make things easier in the long run!

HOW MUCH WATER SHOULD I DRINK WHILE FASTING?

Drink when thirsty, and stop when full. You can use your urine as a gauge of hydration—it should be a nice pale lemonade color! (Note: Supplementing with the B vitamin riboflavin can turn your urine neon yellow.)

DOES DRINKING VEGETABLE OR FRUIT JUICE BREAK THE FAST?

Yes. Fruit and vegetable juices hit the system with a massive load of carbohydrates, halting the fat-burning state.

DOES DRINKING ALCOHOL BREAK THE FAST?

Alcohol does halt the fasted state, though it by itself is not easily stored as fat. Alcohol taken with a meal may also prolong digestion and slow the body's re-entrance into the fasted state. For more details, check out the "Wine?" section!

CAN I CONSUME ARTIFICIAL SWEETENERS DURING THE FAST?

I strongly urge you to forgo artificial sweeteners during the fast. Even if "technically" calorie-free, these sweeteners can sustain cravings, skew hunger signals, encourage overconsumption, and are highly correlated to weight gain! Most people find that once they slay the artificial sweetener demon, fasting becomes light-years easier. Check out "Fake Problems" on page 39 for more details.

IF PROTOCOL QUESTIONS

DOES IF REQUIRE CALORIE RESTRICTION TO LOSE WEIGHT?

One of the most awesome things about IF is no calorie restriction required! That said, if you do fancy some calorie restriction with IF (which can be pretty easy to do, for once), it can occur in a healthy, sustainable matter, yielding weight loss without hunger, muscle loss, misery, or rebound weight gain.

WILL IF MAKE ME OVEREAT?

A common fear is that temporarily restricting eating will make you ultimately eat way more than normal. Come mealtime, all hell will break loose as you stuff your face to oblivion. Yet IF may actually reduce appetite levels. In controlled studies, individuals do not typically "make up for" calories skipped at breakfast, and consume fewer overall calories for the day. And while a 2010 *Nutrition Journal* trial hypothesized that fasting patients would be hungrier and overeat on nonfasting days, they ended up eating 5 to 10 percent fewer than their baseline needs on these free days!

Furthermore, a 2013 study of 115 overweight women found that fasters spontaneously decreased their calorie intake and lost more weight than those poor souls implementing purposeful calorie restriction. Despite being instructed to eat a maintenance number of calories on their normal eating days, the fasters would eat around 600 calories fewer than they were "supposed to," mirroring the consumption of those on the calorie-restriction protocols.[76]

Finally, a 2011 analysis found that snacking tends to release insulin, decrease free fatty acids, and increase overall calorie intake.[77] Basically: The more you eat, the more you want to eat. Fasting, however, squelches appetite by ramping up lipolysis, stabilizing blood sugar, and modulating cellular circadian rhythms and hunger hormones, with supportive psychological changes to boot!

CAN I JUST SKIP LUNCH?

While you may be tempted to skip lunch for your IF protocol, eating in the morning *and* night eclipses the fasting period. You'll rarely go longer than twelve hours between meals, which is just when the fasting magic begins!

WHEN I'VE REACHED MY WEIGHT-LOSS GOAL, HOW WILL MY BODY KNOW TO MAINTAIN MY WEIGHT?

There's no need to stress about "teaching" your body to maintain its weight. Your body naturally favors homeostasis, and with healthy "what" and "when" choices, you'll likely stabilize at a weight perfect for your constitution! Don't revert to counting calories or portions: Simply eat intuitively to satiety!

HOW CAN I KEEP MY BODY GUESSING?

We don't need to purposely keep our body "guessing." As you regain meta- bolic harmony, you'll likely find that you desire different amounts of food and macronutrients each day. Some days I eat a lot, some days less. Some days more carbs, other days more fat. I don't do it on purpose—it just *happens*. You can also always play around with your windows, throwing in a longer or shorter fast here or there! Ultimately, IF should be a stress-free lifestyle that ebbs and flows like the tide, not some sort of fake, controlled, perfect pool, Disney World–style. (Though I totes love Disney!)

WHEN DOES THE FASTED STATE START?

The fasted *state* is technically different from the fasting *window*. While the fast- ing window begins the second you stop eating, you're not in the fasted state yet, since your tummy is full of food! Studies suggest that the actual fasted state begins around twelve hours after one's last meal, though this is easily affected by the type and amount of food consumed, digestion time, and numerous other fac- tors. In any case, you can just monitor your fasting window overall, rather than the fasted state per se. The fasting window starts when you put down that fork, and should last a minimum of twelve hours, up to around twenty-four hours.

WHAT IF I START IF AND DON'T LOSE WEIGHT, OR GAIN WEIGHT?

Some people find that when beginning IF, they don't immediately lose weight, or even temporarily gain weight. If such is your predicament, don't panic! The body can do a lot of wonky things with hormones and water retention when we radically shift our diet. Stick it out for a couple of weeks, and your body should eventually come around! Since IF encourages fat loss and supports muscle, which weighs more than fat, you also may experience substantial changes in body composition, but not weight loss per se. Go by how you feel and how your clothes fit, rather than what the scale says! (I thought we threw those away?)

CAN I DO LONGER FASTS?

In the IF protocols discussed in this book, the fasting windows do not exceed twenty-four hours; a meal is consumed each and every day. Though you can certainly do longer fasts, this is different from IF as discussed in this book. (I've actually never fasted beyond a day. True story.) Please engage in any longer fasts with caution, and, as with any fast, consult your doctor accordingly.

SPECIAL IF SCENARIOS

WHO SHOULDN'T FAST?

Fasting is safe for most people. If there were significant health problems from fasting, we wouldn't have been safely doing it, not to mention *healing* from it, for thousands of years. We'd also probably die between meals. (Too extreme of an assumption?) That said, I do not recommend fasting for children, pregnant women, or for those severely underweight.

CAN I DO IF WHEN I'M SICK?

Who doesn't know the slight panic from that tickle in the back of the throat, as you feverishly chug vitamin-C cocktails like it's your twenty-first birthday? When you succumb to the nasty visitor, you lie in bed, secretly grateful for the excuse to skip work and binge-watch *Game of Thrones* or *Real Housewives*. Though colds used to be a common thing for me, just a part of life in a "Sorry 'bout it!" type way, they are now much more rare thanks to IF. But what if you do find yourself with a case of the sniffles? Should you eat it off or fast it off?

You'd think we'd become hungry when sick. After all, what better time for extra energy and nutrients than when you're fighting a foreign invader, right? Yet in the immediate response to microbial invaders, cell-signaling proteins called *cytokines* act on the central nervous system to *decrease* appetite, which is likely a sign that food restriction can somehow fight pathogens.[78] In fact, force-feeding sick lab animals decreases survival time and increases death rates. In one study, 5 percent of mice that hadn't eaten for three days died of an induced bacterial infection,[79] while 95 percent of mice who *had* eaten died within twenty-four hours.[80] And despite often severe reductions in white blood cells, studies even show that anorexia can lower rates of infection.[81]

Perhaps it goes back to the saying "Starve a fever, feed a cold," which may involve the two types of immune helper cells predominantly at play. Eating may upregulate *T1 cells* to fight viruses (which typically manifest as a cold), while fasting may upregulate *T2 cells* to fight bacteria (which typically cause a fever). Fasting while sick also may reserve energy otherwise spent searching for food, reduce nutrient resource availability for pathogens, enhance immune function of macrophages, minimize inflammatory effects of the acute-phase response, and encourage apoptosis, or cell suicide of infected cells.[82]

But while a temporary bit of fasting when sick may be beneficial, it might not be appropriate in all scenarios. The T1-to-T2 ratio response developed in prehistoric times of more bacterial infections and fewer viral infections. While we've got the upper hand on bacteria today (through a potential overuse of antibiotics), viruses and cancers have become ever more resilient and sneaky. They may hijack the system by inducing a psychological lack of hunger, at a time when eating (along with sleep and hydration) would be in one's best interest. And while short bits of fasting may help fight infections in the beginning stages, prolonged fasting may ultimately delay recovery by inducing nutrient deficiencies and susceptibility to further infection.

So if ever there was a time to practice intuitive eating, it's when you're sick! At such a time, don't feel pressured to eat or not eat. Don't stick to any specific "window." Forget IF, and do what your body tells you to do. If you're not hungry and just want to sleep—do that! If you're hungry—eat food! While I advocate always eating healthy, immune-boosting substances (oh hey, Paleo!), this is especially important when under the weather. In fact, maybe we should always consume the foods we would feed a struggling body? #Foodforthought.

CAN I DO IF WITH BLOOD SUGAR ISSUES?

In Kingdom Glycemia, the moody tyrant King Blood Sugar reigns over pitiful peasants plagued by a myriad of conditions. Those with hyperglycemia experience bouts of excess blood sugar, often with diabetes and weight gain. Those with hypoglycemia face low blood sugar's grip of dizziness, tiredness, and fainting spells. Those with reactive hypoglycemia suffer sharp blood sugar drops after meals, with shakiness and ravenous hunger, despite having just eaten.

If you identify with one of these, have no fear! Since IF encourages the body to rely less on blood sugar and more on fatty acids and ketones, it may help manage blood sugar problems and welcome glycemic control. I suggest combining a low-carb, whole-foods diet with a small fasting window to start, increasing as you feel comfortable. You can also try adding some MCT oil or exogenous ketones during the fast to further mitigate blood sugar swings. IF just may be your ticket out of Kingdom Glycemia!

(Please do not take my suggestions as medical advice, and know that medications can also interfere with your blood sugar levels. Please discuss any dietary changes with your doctor.)

WHAT SHOULD I DO IF I FEEL COLD DURING FASTING?

You shouldn't feel uncomfortably cold while fasting, though I've personally become a colder person (in body, not spirit!) since losing body fat from IF. If fat does one thing, it can keep ya warm! If IF does make you a little chilly, make sure you're eating enough in your fasting window, as unintentional undereating may or may not cause issues for you personally. To combat cold, consider eating more, fasting less, or eating thermogenic foods such as coconut oil. If you can't seem to fix your inner thermostat, consider getting your thyroid checked.

IF I FEEL FAINT OR SHAKY, SHOULD I STOP FASTING?

It depends. When you begin IF, your body may protest with feelings of lethargy. As you become fat-adapted, and your body learns how to #deal, such weakness should pass. Shaky feelings when you're already comfortable with fasting, however, may indicate an underlying issue. Ensure that you're eating enough in your window, and consider monitoring blood sugar levels. Always feel free to stop fasting, and discuss things with a medical professional if necessary.

WHAT IF I NEED TO TAKE MEDICATION WITH FOOD DURING THE FAST?

Always take your medication as prescribed. If that's in the morning with food during your fast, then that's in the morning with food during your fast. Don't worry—it will be ok! Try to find something that minimally affects your blood sugar levels and insulin, such as low-protein, low-carb, high-fat stuff. You could try a smidge of butter, or something more normal, such as some avocado or heavy cream. As long as you take the medication with a very minimal amount of food, I wouldn't sweat it. You'll be back in the fasted state pronto!

WINE?

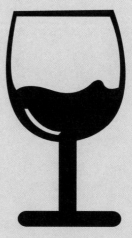

ALCOHOL AND FAT BURNING

While the "Wine" of *What When Wine* may seem a bit self-explanatory, there's a lot going on in that glass or Solo cup. For definition #itscomplicated, look no further than alcohol! After all, drinking promises the good times of released inhibitions, followed by physical and emotional regrets if one engages *too* fully. It's undeniably correlated to health benefits and longevity, yet can be toxic in excess. Popular thought holds that alcohol promotes weight gain, yet the studies (spoiler alert!) show almost the opposite. And if all that weren't enough, government and religious worldviews further convolute matters.

I suggest approaching this topic with an open but scrutinizing mind as we analyze the situation through and through. (If wine is going to play a supporting role in our diet, you better believe we're gonna know who we cast!) We'll start with the metabolism of alcohol and its relationship to fat burning, then examine alcohol's relationship to health and longevity, and finally jump hardcore into wine specifically. (Just what *is* resveratrol?) We'll wrap things up by addressing a few lingering questions. (Curious if alcohol is Paleo? The answer may surprise you!) So sit back, pour yourself a glass, and pore over these next few chapters! Cheers!

ALCOHOL AND FAT BURNING

Conventional wisdom says you can't drink if you *really* want to lose weight. And at first glance, alcohol *does* brim with the potential to inflict damage upon our waistlines. It contains 7.1 calories per gram, second only to fat's 9 calories per gram, with studies showing that we don't tend to eat less to "make up for" these calories.[1] In fact, we often eat *more*, as alcohol may be the least satiating macronutrient,[2] and can enhance food reward via GABA, opioid, or dopamine receptors.[3] Alcohol also minimizes fat oxidation when consumed, at least in the short term.

But before you're like, "OMG, I can never drink again," here comes the twist ending, M. Night Shyamalan–style: Clinical and epidemiological studies typically find that light to moderate alcohol intake correlates not only with healthy weights, but actually with *weight loss*.[4] Perhaps even more shocking, some studies suggest that *not* drinking favors weight gain.[5] A 2010 analysis of almost ten thousand people found that, despite *increasing* total daily calories, alcohol consumption was related to *decreased* body weight. These effects may be particularly potent in women, as girls who drink tend to weigh less than girls who don't drink, while women who drink heavily tend to have less subcutaneous fat.

WHAT'S GOING ON HERE?

It would seem that calories from alcohol do not act like "normal" calories. In clinical trials, substituting alcohol calories for carbohydrate calories typically leads to weight loss, while calories consumed in excess from alcohol don't necessarily result in weight gain. In one study, hospitalized alcoholics gained *no* weight when 1,800 calories in the form of alcohol was added to their standard diet.[6] In another, substituting 50 percent of patients' daily calories with alcohol yielded weight loss. And while adding 2,000 calories of chocolate to a patient's diet steadily increased weight (shocker), adding 2,000 calories of alcohol negligibly affected weight.

Theories about the alcohol paradox range from its thermogenic nature (estimated to be between 10 and 30 percent), a resulting increase in the basal metabolic rate (around 5 percent), or a "wasting" of alcohol calories. Additionally, when alcohol is consumed in super high amounts, the body upregulates the inefficient microsomal ethanol-oxidizing system (MEOS) to break it down, which requires a lot of calorie burning.[7] As such, it'd be difficult (perhaps impossible) to gain weight on an alcohol-only diet. (But please don't do that!)

Alcohol's weight-sparing effect may also involve long-term metabolic changes or reductions in food intake, despite any increases in a single meal. Alcohol can notably reduce ghrelin levels in the body—a hormone that stimulates hunger. And unlike carbohydrates, alcohol does not induce fat-storing enzymes and seemingly bears no overall effect on fat storage, despite the fact that it temporarily "turns off" fat burning.[8] On the flip side, alcohol does stimulate proteins that can encourage fat burning, increase insulin sensitivity, and discourage the accumulation of unhealthy visceral fat.[9]

ALCOHOL METABOLISM

When we drink, alcohol initially undergoes first pass metabolism, in which the alcohol dehydrogenase (ADH) enzyme converts it into a compound called acetaldehyde. This occurs a smidge in the stomach lining, then primarily in the liver. How fast alcohol actually reaches the liver (via the portal vein) involves how much alcohol and food is ingested. Alcohol hits the liver faster when consumed on an empty stomach, whereas food can slow its absorption. Either way, the alcohol *will* ultimately be dealt with, so you can't actually block absorption with food. (Flashback to the first time I drank in college, in which my dearest friend Kylie prescribed running to the late-night drive-through, because we *needed* carbs to "soak up the alcohol"!) That said, food *can* increase alcohol processing in the stomach, reducing the amount delivered to the liver, which can adequately handle around one drink per hour.[10] If the amount of alcohol absorbed is too great, the liver begins releasing the alcohol into the bloodstream, so the rest of the body can deal with it. The alcohol then concentrates in the body's water and raises blood alcohol content (BAC).

Ultimately, around 90 to 98 percent of alcohol is oxidized, rather than stored. We have no established "holding place" for alcohol in the body; the body burns alcohol preferentially over protein, fats, and carbs. Alcohol cannot be directly converted to glucose, and conversion to fatty acid is neither simple nor practical. Worst-case scenario, around 10 percent of alcohol could possibly be converted to fat, although this is unlikely. It's sort of like being given coupon cash that you can only spend at a particular store, rather than actual money you can save for later.

WINE WEIGHT BENEFITS

If you *really* want to up your body-composition alcohol odds, raise a glass of wine! The polyphenols found in wine (which we'll look at in detail in the next chapter!) can actually act as "antidiabetic agents,"[11] by regulating blood sugar, affecting glucose absorption in the gut, blocking beta cells channels to lower insulin release,[12] and modulating genes to improve insulin sensitivity.[13] The polyphenol piceatannol, for example, has been shown to slow fat cell growth and inhibit baby fat cells from growing in the first place, possibly by affecting insulin and gene signaling. Similarly, wine's anthocyanins can inhibit body fat,[14] while its ellagic acid may discourage the formation and growth of fat cells, and support fat burning in the liver![15]

Or consider the polyphenol resveratrol. This famed wine compound has been shown to activate proteins that encourage the formation of brown fat—a highly thermogenic fat that actually helps you burn more stubborn "white" fat.[16] Resveratrol may also serve as a sort of mock exercise! In a 2011 study, scientists were trying to find a way to prevent atrophy and bone mineral density loss in astronauts.[17] They simulated the sedentary effects of zero gravity by hanging rats by their hind legs (poor little guys!), and found that those rats who were fed resveratrol were protected from muscle loss and insulin resistance. Another 2012 study found that resveratrol supplementation enhanced the beneficial effects of exercise and increased endurance rates in rats, providing benefits similar to endurance training.[18] So having a glass of red wine *may* slightly make up for not hitting the gym! (Please see "The Tipsy Elephants in the Room" on page 162 for a further discussion about debates surrounding resveratrol supplementation.)

ALCOHOL WEIGHT GAIN

All that said, alcohol-related weight gain is still a thing. While alcohol itself does not easily become body fat, whatever you eat or drink *with* the alcohol can surely show up on the proverbial scale. (Not that we support scales around here!) Many cocktails are insulin-spiking, calorie-laden sugary concoctions, and loosened inhibitions or mere expectations associating alcohol with food consumption may further encourage feasting on weight-promoting goodies. (I shudder to think about all the times my college friends and I hit up Denny's for pancakes, or Jack in the Box for a large bucket of curly fries, circa 3:00 a.m., because it's just *what you do* after partaking in cheap drinks, beer pong, and existential life contemplations at the weekly film frat party. Shout-out to DKA!)

Studies also suggest that weight gain from drinking can stem from a person's naturally impulsive tendencies, rather than from the actual alcohol per se.[19] This means that if you're more likely to go overboard with drinking, you may be more likely to go overboard with eating. Of course, a Paleo and/or IF approach can help restore normal eating behavior, and nip binge tendencies in the bud!

The takeaway? Sensible drinking as a part of a healthy diet and lifestyle can readily support a lean figure. The body *is* capable of handling alcohol in appropriate amounts, and may even benefit from it—just please use good judgment! Unlike grains and other goodies, you *can* have your drink and drink it too!

LONGEVITY AND ANTIOXIDANTS AND POLYPHENOLS, OH MY!

ALCOHOL AND HEALTH

Okay, so alcohol does not automatically instigate weight gain, but does drinking actually provide health benefits? Therein lies the question.

Correlational studies often find that, surprisingly enough, those who drink moderately tend to live longer than people who drink heavily or not at all.[20] According to a 2014 analysis, the maximum amount of daily alcohol that may support boosted life span likely falls somewhere around 20 grams—the equivalent of around one and a half glasses of wine. It also suggests that you may need to drink around 72 grams of alcohol per day (around five glasses of wine) to "equal" the mortality risk of not drinking, and around 89 grams (over six glasses of wine) to "hurt" your longevity odds. Worst-case scenario, avoiding drinking likely won't magically extend your life. A 2016 meta-analysis of eighty-seven studies encompassing 3,998,626 people and 367,103 recorded deaths found that, while moderate drinking of alcohol did not consistently seem to reduce mortality rates across the board, neither did abstaining.

Daily light to moderate drinking may serve as a beneficial hormetic stress, causing the body to adapt and grow, while providing just the right amount of oxidative stress to help break down inflammatory fatty acids. Epidemiological studies also consistently correlate moderate alcohol consumption to reduced risk of cardiovascular disease, perhaps due to ethanol's effects on endothelial function,[21] blood pressure,[22] blood profiles,[23] and insulin sensitivity.[24] Alcohol consumption also favors healthy cholesterol ratios (raising "good" HDL and lowering "bad" LDL cholesterol),[25] and is associated with decreased risk of stroke.[26]

Of course, more controlled trials are desired, and these findings are often hotly debated. (See "The Tipsy Elephants in the Room" on page 162 for more on that!) Alcohol's health benefits may also be influenced by timing, genetic factors (such as if you're a slow or fast alcohol metabolizer), environmental factors (which can green-light various genetic and immune reactions), as well as correlational lifestyle factors. I'm definitely *not* prescribing alcohol to live longer (I'm quite an anti-prescription girl myself); rather, I think these findings indicate that a moderate amount of drinking may do more good than harm. Channel your inner Goldilocks: Not too little, and not too much!

WINE AND LONGEVITY

Time to discuss the spirit of the matter! While alcohol alone may play a key role in health, wine really ramps up longevity benefits, due to the numerous polyphenols found within grapes.[27] (Spoiler alert: It's not just resveratrol!) The polyphenol-alcohol combination may be key in rendering wine a "functional food" with health-enhancing, disease-preventing potential. Before we jump into the specifics, let's look at the whole "antioxidant" concept, so when I'm like, "This compound is an antioxidant!" we'll totally be on the same page.

THE ROLE OF ANTIOXIDANTS

The supplement industry loves to obsessively commercialize the latest health trend, which may leave you a little incredulous about the whole "antioxidant" thing. ("Try this *magical* antioxidant compound only found in a bean located at 3.4653° S, 62.2159° W of the Brazilian rainforest, and never age again!")

That said, antioxidants are actually legit . . . just please don't think they're best attained via a pill.

Here's how it goes down. Your body is sort of like a war zone, where invaders such as reactive oxidative species and free radicals inflict oxidative damage on your cell membranes. While free radicals often come from environmental toxins, they're also common in processed foods, as natural by-products of cellular energy generation, and are even generated in the body's own attack system.

Now, before you freak at the idea of an R-rated battle shattering your innards, please know that we're equipped to deal with free radicals via *antioxidants*, produced in the body and present in food. Antioxidants neutralize free radicals and help repair damaged cells. Yay! As long as the balance between free radicals and antioxidants is all good, then we're all good! Unfortunately, our modern environment typically yields a free radical mess and a state of oxidative stress, in which continual wear and tear on the body's cells, membranes, and DNA invites aging and disease,[28] while hindering our ability to heal.[29]

Embracing an antioxidant-rich diet can really give the body a leg up in the battle. And what's chock-full of polyphenolic antioxidant compounds? Oh *hi*, red wine! Better yet, many polyphenols can actually function as *both* antioxidants against free radicals and as oxidants against cancerous cells, and can cross the blood-brain barrier to protect the cerebral region! A 2007 randomized controlled crossover study found that red wine reduced markers of oxidative stress across the board. Forty subjects alternated two weeks of drinking about two glasses of red wine per night, with two weeks of no wine. The researchers found that red wine significantly increased total antioxidant status, and significantly decreased the toxic oxidation by-product malondialdehyde.[30]

Now that we've got antioxidants under our belt (hopefully literally!), let's take a closer look at those specific polyphenols, so you'll be able to throw out fancy-sounding words to wine naysayers!

POLYPHENOLS

Scientists have identified over ten thousand polyphenols, which provide fruits, veggies, and other plants with their vibrant colors, and affect the flavor, aroma, and bitterness of plant-derived food and beverages.[31] While it may seem like they exist to provide sciencey reasons for eating your fruits and veggies like your mother told you, polyphenols actually serve a fascinating purpose as a defense mechanisms in plants.[32] Since they can't exactly run away from danger, plants release polyphenols in response to infection, stress, and damage, to ward off pests, bacteria, and fungi, and even to combat UV light exposure. This defensive nature creates potent antioxidant power when we ingest polyphenols, which can scavenge free radicals and cancerous cells, support the immune system, and encourage cellular regeneration! Better yet, polyphenols often target malicious cells and invaders while sparing healthy cells, and do not tend to become toxic, even at high amounts.[33]

Grapes are one of the fruits highest in polyphenols, and "injuring" them in the wine-making process creates a beverage even *more* concentrated with polyphenols. The wine maturation process also often occurs in oak, which can further increase polyphenol content. These polyphenols contribute to the sensory experience of wine (like aromas and mouthfeel), as well as to wine's outstanding health benefits. Though it varies, a typical glass of red contains around 125 milligrams of polyphenols, while white clocks in at a much lower 15 milligrams (though it still ranks in the top one hundred polyphenol-rich foods). For the highest polyphenol content, turn to the widely popular Cabernet Sauvignon, or the more obscure Refosco from Italy.

In addition to the widely popular polyphenol resveratrol, there are *hundreds* of other polyphenolic compounds, all with potential health benefits! Let's look at the main ones, to see how they affect not only the glass of wine in your hand, but your body's well-being as well!

FLAVONOIDS

Flavonoids constitute approximately 60 percent of all plant polyphenols, and potentially greater than 85 percent of those in wine. Residing primarily in the grape skin and seed, they're particularly abundant in red wine, which gets its color from fermentation in contact with the skin and seeds.

Flavonoids are potent little health-promoting beasts, with anti-inflammatory, antibacterial, antiallergic, and antioxidant powers. In addition to scavenging free radicals, they can influence enzymes involved in oxidative stress and bind to dangerous metals. They hold a particular affinity for cells around our vital organs, and are highly anticarcinogenic, instigating apoptosis (programmed cell death) of cancerous cells at all stages, and often superseding conventional cancer therapy. They also tend to act selectively on cancer cells, while sparing normal cells. Talk about a win-win situation!

Quercetin

Quercetin is a primary flavonoid in the human diet with potent antioxidant and antiaging powers. It can fight free radicals, activate antioxidant enzymes, discourage fatty acid oxidation, and support glutathione production.[34] It also may lower blood pressure and discourage obesity, and it is one of the most studied polyphenols to combat cancer.[35]

Quercetin is also *highly* anti-inflammatory.[36] Like many common nonsteroidal anti-inflammatory drugs (NSAIDs), quercetin inhibits the inflammation-green-lighting COX-2 enzyme. But while NSAIDs can reduce pain, they also injure the gut in the process, encouraging intestinal gut permeability, bleeding, and ulcers![37] Quercetin, however, actually *reduces* intestinal inflammation, supporting the intestinal lining and protecting from NSAID-induced injury.[38]

While most people eat and drink an estimated 5 to 40 milligrams of quercetin per day, consuming quercetin-rich vegetables, fruits, and beverages can increase this by tenfold. Wine is particularly rich in quercetin, and its synergetic alcohol effect may actually enhance quercetin's absorption in the body. The varietal Sangiovese has tested particularly high in the compound, so try some Chianti next time you're craving some quercetin!

Catechins

Catechins contribute up to 60 percent of the polyphenols in the grape seed. They give wine its dry, mouth-puckering sensation and add bitterness and structure. As potent antioxidants, catechins can inhibit inflammatory protein transcription factors and cytokines throughout the body's tissues, particularly those damaged from aging or degenerative disease. Catechins also boast anticancer, antibacterial, and antifatigue properties, and can discourage weight gain![39]

Anthocyanins

Anthocyanin comes from Greek words meaning "blue flower," which is an appropriate nomenclature, since these flavonoids provide many fruits and veggies with their vibrant red, blue, and purple hues, and are responsible for red and rosé wines' crimson colors.[40] With over six hundred types identified, anthocyanins can protect DNA,[41] regulate hormones and the immune system, strengthen cell membranes,[42] and discourage the development of diabetes, heart disease, and cancer.[43] Anthocyanins also have some funsie features, such as upregulating night vision (flashback to night-vision goggles from childhood!), enhancing memory, and upregulating brain and motor abilities. Oh hey, body upgrades!

NON-FLAVONOIDS

On the flip side of the flavonoids are the . . . wait for it! . . . non-flavonoids, which pack their own health punch.

Phenolic Acids

Phenolic acids provide wine with astringency, bitterness, and some characteristics associated with oak aging. These antioxidative, anti-inflammatory, antimicrobial compounds include gallic acid, caffeic acid, and ellagic acid, and are particularly combative against cancer cells, while sparing healthy cells.

Stilbenoids

Chance are you've heard of the most famous stilbenoid: resveratrol. Studied to an almost overwhelming extent, you can totally drop the word "resveratrol" in casual conversation without blank stares, and pick it up in commercialized form in your local supplement aisle. Studies show that resveratrol can regulate genes, proteins, enzymes, hormones (particularly estrogen), insulin, and calcium levels in cells, to encourage a state of homeostasis.[44] Resveratrol also influences apoptosis and inflammation (discouraging or encouraging them when they best suit the body) and may protect against atherosclerosis, diabetes, cardiovascular disease, and many types of cancers. And as a girl who has sworn off pain pills, I love that resveratrol can reduce both acute and chronic pain,[45] while encouraging cellular tissue repair.[46]

If you're drawn to the allure of youth, resveratrol has also got you covered! As revealed in a 2003 Harvard study and its 2013 follow-up, resveratrol can activate aging-related proteins called *sirtuins*, which affect DNA restoration, apoptosis, inflammation, and metabolism, and are a proposed mechanism for the longevity benefits of calorie restriction.[47] But why restrict calories when you can potentially have some wine instead?

While resveratrol may be all the rage, let's not forget its stilbenoid cousins living in the shadow! Pterostilbene is structurally similar to resveratrol, but likely more bioavailable, thanks to its fat-attaching tendency.[48] It also may provide more antioxidant and antiaging potential than resveratrol, while encouraging healthy circulation, cardiovascular health, and cancer protection. Or consider one of my personal favorites, piceatannol, which can actually stop fat cells from forming and growing, and may be more powerful for COX-2 inhibition pain relief than resveratrol.

TANNINS

Yay for another sort of familiar word in a sea of sciencey nomenclature! The various polyphenols in red wine can combine to form tannins, which contribute to wine's mouthfeel by creating a drying sensation (irony of the liquid medium aside). Tannins also lend hints of bitterness for complexity. While you may associate tannins with nebulous descriptions, à la "silky expressive tannins," there's actually a pretty cool reason for why tannins do what they do.

The word *tannin* comes from the tanning process of turning animal hides into leather, thanks to their drying power. This goes back to the whole plant defense mechanism thing. Tannins can attach to the proteins of invader fungus, bacteria, and other microbes, as well as the digestive proteins of animals that might eat the plant. And guess what! A primary function of *our* saliva is to attach to compounds like these, so they can't bind to our digestive enzymes.[49]

So wine's "drying" sensation comes from tannins attaching to your spit! (This is also why some wines are surprisingly not vegan, as proteins such as casein, egg whites, or gelatin are often added in the "fining" process of wine-making to bind the tannins, reducing bitterness and/or astringency.)

This also means tannins can be a bit sticky, no pun intended. Unlike other polyphenols, which tend to exhibit no side effects even in very large concentrations, tannins' protein-attaching, antimicrobial power may be a bit *too* potent. That said, the small amount of tannins found naturally in wine may provide all the bark without the bite . . . or just the right amount of bite, synergistically interacting with other polyphenols to yield antioxidant, antimicrobial, anti-inflammatory, anticancer powers.

Though it varies widely, red wine averages around 80 milligrams of tannins per glass, from around 50 milligrams in light Pinot Noirs to around 100 milligrams in high-tannic reds, such as Nebbiolo or Petit Verdot.[50] Older vintages also feature more tannins, which continue to form with age, as do barrel-aged wines, since the oak lends its own tannins, while "softening" the preexisting ones.

A WINE-FUELED
ROUTE TO OZ

Now that we've got a perspective on wine's polyphenol powerhouse, you hopefully understand how the beverage can enhance many aspects of our biology. So embrace your inner Dorothy as we go on a wine-fueled journey!

WINE AND THE BRAIN

If only the Scarecrow knew the time spent lamenting his lack of brain might have been better served drinking a nice Merlot! (Plus, it probably would've made the whole stuck-to-a-stick-in-the-middle-of-a-field thing more bearable.) As it turns out, wine may be just the thing for providing a cognitive boost!

Studies have shown that moderate alcohol consumption correlates to enhanced brainpower, including mental processing rates, motor skills, memory, recognition, and both short- and long-term memory.[51] Alcohol in general also may protect the brain and discourage degenerative diseases such as dementia and Parkinson's by regulating cholesterol, boosting blood platelets, and improving insulin sensitivity.[52] A well-controlled three-year 2011 German study of more than three thousand elderly participants found that 29 percent fewer of those who had one to three alcoholic drinks per day developed dementia than those who did not drink, and 42 percent fewer of those people developed Alzheimer's.[53] Similarly, a 2001 Italian study of over fifteen thousand people found that moderate daily alcohol consumption (fewer than 40 grams for women and fewer than 80 grams for men) correlated to reduced risk of cognitive dysfunction.[54]

Of course, that's just alcohol in general. The polyphenols in wine, which are particularly capable of crossing the blood-brain barrier, may further boost brain benefits by mitigating inflammation, boosting antioxidants, and relaxing blood vessels.[55] The highly bioavailable anthocyanidins can enhance function and memory, while resveratrol activates "longevity" sirtuins, which may discourage neuronal loss.[56] Resveratrol has also been shown to increase blood flow in the brain, which may support cognition.[57] In a small 2014 pilot study, researchers found that resveratrol-enhanced wine boosted performance in elderly patients given tasks that demanded extra brainpower.[58] Research also indicates that wine may protect the brain via the gut. A 2017 study found that metabolites produced from wine compounds by gut bacteria can discourage neurodegenerative disease by protecting neurons from stress![59]

What about the more "subjective" states of mind, a.k.a. mood? While I in no way advocate relying on alcohol as a coping mechanism, studies find that moderate alcohol use can reduce tension, anxiety, and the stress hormone cortisol, and may actually aid recovery from stressful situations. Granted, this may involve the *expectation* of a glass of wine easing our woes, but the actual effects are definite—placebo effect or not!

A 2014 randomized control trial looked at alcohol's effect on mood when consumed with a meal.[60] The participants drank three glasses of sparkling white wine, unknowingly with or without alcohol, in rooms with either a pleasant or unpleasant ambiance, achieved via music, light, cleanliness, and either happy or sad film scenes from *Bambi* and *The Lion King*. (Cracks. Me. Up.) Though alcohol did not substantially increase mood when one was already happy, it *did* increase mood in an unpleasant ambiance. So, a nice glass of wine with dinner may be the key to pulling you out of a funk.

Studies have also found that the proper amount of alcohol consumption may actually discourage rates of depression. The previously discussed German trial found that alcohol intake correlated to decreased rates of depression, as well as dementia. And a 2013 study that followed over five thousand individuals at high risk for depression over seven years found that, while heavy drinking correlated to higher rates of depression, moderate wine intake (up to around one glass of wine per day) seemingly reduced depression.[61]

To reiterate, drinking wine occasionally and sensibly to *enhance* one's life is different from relying on wine to *deal with* one's life. (If we hang out, choose the cute wineglass in my cupboard that says CELEBRATE! rather than the one that says CAN'T ADULT TODAY.) But if we can benefit both physically *and* mentally from wine consumption—including dealing with the huge downer of Mufasa's death—then I'm all for it! Who's with me?

WINE AND THE HEART

Turns out the Tin Man could have potentially benefited from a nice Cabernet, as an exhausting list of correlational and controlled studies find that moderate alcohol consumption consistently benefits heart health biomarkers and is associated with decreased risk of cardiovascular disease.[62]

Red wine loves our heart in many ways: It can scavenge free radicals, reduce blood pressure and blood clots, support the arteries, increase "good" HDL cholesterol, lower "bad" LDL cholesterol, regulate insulin and blood glucose levels, and discourage hardening of the arteries, all while priming blood vessels for optimal function.[63] The fact that de-alcoholized red wine has been shown to protect the heart indicates that these cardio-protective components likely involve the polyphenolic compounds we discussed!

In a 2015 long-term randomized trial, 224 diabetic nondrinkers drank a glass of mineral water, red wine, or white wine with dinner for two years, while following an unrestricted Mediterranean diet. The researchers found that, compared to the other beverages, red wine correlated to reduced cardiometabolic risks and enhanced lipid factors, potentially due to a synergy between its alcohol and polyphenol content.[64] So please put down that bowl of "heart-healthy" cereal, and have a drink instead, to your heart's (actual) content!

WINE AND (SEXY) COURAGE

Ok, so maybe it goes without saying that a glass of liquid courage could have motivated the Cowardly Lion. But I'm not even gonna go that route. Instead, let's look at how wine can actually boost sex appeal . . . and thus confidence. (Is this a stretch in the metaphor? I'm just going with it.)

Wine itself is often considered sort of sexy. After all, what other drink can you totally indulge in while maintaining a semblance of class, and notably *not* end up schammered. (And, not gonna lie, if a guy says his favorite drink is Tempranillo or Carménère, I'm just like . . . *potential.*) But did you know that wine's aphrodisiac nature may be rooted in legit chemistry?

Yep, some red wine may *literally* increase the attractiveness factor. The spicy earth and musk aromas of the smooth, luscious Pinot Noir mimic the male pheromone androstenone. When the olfactory bulb in your nose detects these scents, it can mistake it for this mating chemical. This can effectively green-light your sex drive . . . before you even consciously realize it! (Though maybe that's more of a con than a pro? Debatable.)

THE DESTINATION

Like Dorothy awakening to reality, I hope that you now grasp the clear science of red wine, rather than some hazy, vague idea of "health benefits." (Though the benefits were there all along!) Of course, while some wine consumption may be great for your health, it's *even better* when combined with a healthy diet and lifestyle, rich in whole foods, social connections, vibrant movement, and the joy of life. May you use wine to *enhance* your life, not escape from it, and know that happiness is in your own backyard!

THE TIPSY ELEPHANTS IN THE ROOM

Now that we're raising a proverbial (literal?) toast to our health, I suppose we should address any similarly raised eyebrows. But is red wine *Paleo*? What about *toxins*?? Causation versus correlation!! Let's take a deep breath, a sip of wine (I know I just did!), and look at these one by one.

IS ALCOHOL PALEO?

Might as well start with the biggie! For starters, I remind you that Paleo is not so much a rigid list of predetermined "right" and "wrong" foods, but rather an informed template of which foods are compatible with our bodies from a genetic and biological perspective. While a historical approach can help clarify this, it is not the be-all and end-all.

When it comes to wine, we *do* harbor specific genetic adaptions to process alcohol. While it is unlikely that our Paleolithic ancestors had the time and means to distill a potato into vodka or sugarcane into rum, early primates likely lapped up fermented fruit sugars as early as eighty million years ago. Then things got real . . .

Our ability to process alcohol involves the ADH4 alcohol dehydrogenase enzyme, found in the tongue, throat, and GI tract of primates. A ground-breaking 2014 study discovered that a key mutation around ten million years ago made the gene around forty times more effective, likely because primates at that time shifted to a ground-based environment, and began eating fallen, fermented fruit rather than the fresh, virgin fruit found in trees.[65] The alcohol enzyme ensured a safe fuel source, so tipsy monkeys weren't casually parading about in the dangers of the wild. This alcohol gene may even be why humans enjoy alcohol, which we associate with energy and nutrient-rich fruit.

Though the amount of alcohol naturally present in fruit varies widely, a Panama study found that alcohol concentrations average around 0.6 to 0.9 percent in ripe palm fruit, and 4.5 to 8.1 percent in super-ripe fruit.[66] As such, a monkey dining all day on ripe palm fruit would likely take in more total daily alcohol (relative to body composition) than a human who drinks a glass of wine with dinner. That said, dining throughout the day on fruit with low amounts of alcohol differs from drinking higher concentrations of alcohol in wine, in more punctuated amounts (or #shots! style). It's possible that when we began isolating alcohol into pure form about nine thousand years ago, we began brewing trouble. (Sort of like when we began refining grains and sugar!) Our enzymatic system simply may not have adapted to tolerate chronic or punctuated alcohol in larger amounts.

Beyond evaluations of historical alcohol enzymes, I raise a larger question: Can wine inhabit a place in our diet compatible with our constitution, and contributing to health and vibrancy? I believe the answer is a resounding *Yes!* Unlike the more recently produced liquors, wine is a whole-foods drink with beneficial compounds. We've been consuming it for thousands of years, and wine and beer containers have even been found from Stone Age times!

That said, many (if not most) wines contain a variety of unsavory components added for color, flavor, consistency, and profitability. (Thank you, government regulations, for keeping such nefarious additives hidden!) I'm talking things such as animal proteins, gums, folic acids, chalk, and even the colorizer "Mega Purple." (Google it!) We've also got the many pesticides, fungicides, and herbicides sprayed on the grapes, which consistently rank high in pesticides according to the Environmental Working Group. For this reason, I encourage you to favor wineries using sustainable, organic, and even biodynamic production methods. (Check out DryFarmWines.com/melanieavalon for my favorite resource for natural, clean wine!) Studies have also found that organic grapes feature higher levels of polyphenols, and resveratrol specifically.[67]

WHAT ABOUT TOXINS?

Excessive alcohol intake can undoubtedly encourage problems, including increased reactive oxygen species, endothelial dysregulation, cirrhosis, and cardiovascular disease, despite alcohol's heart protection benefits. Some studies also indicate that drinking wine may increase the risk of breast cancer (though these are debated, with a myriad of factors likely involved.) And don't worry—I'm not gonna make the argument that red wine is good for your liver.

That said, the connection between alcohol consumption and liver disease is less clear than one may imagine. According to a 2011 panel conducted by the U.S. government's National Institute on Alcohol Abuse and Alcoholism, only a small percent of people who drink heavily develop liver disease, and little clinical evidence has even linked moderate drinking to liver disease.[68] Problems arise in part due to classification. Even though liver problems commonly develop from diets high in refined fat and sugar (particularly soft drinks), the simple parameter of whether one *does* or *does not* drink is often used to classify the type of liver disease as either alcoholic (ALD) or nonalcoholic (NAFLD). ("Do you drink? Then you have ALD! Do you not drink? Must be NAFLD!") So many cases of "alcoholic" liver disease may actually be nonalcoholic liver disease primarily resulting from other dietary factors.

Despite the fact that we've been consuming alcohol for thousands of years, liver disease is now particularly on the rise. A 2006 study found that 10 percent of children (who presumably aren't drinking) have NAFLD, even though young people tend to harbor more robust livers. I point this out *not* to downplay any damaging effects of alcohol, but rather to draw awareness to the importance of overall diet and lifestyle choices. If we establish alcohol as the sole source of liver trouble, we risk ignoring the many other potential burdens on our liver, including obesity, diets rich in processed and refined foods, and toxic environments (such as chemical and mold exposure).

If you minimize dietary and environmental toxic burdens, then moderate alcohol consumption should be fine. On the other hand, if your liver is already burdened with a toxic onslaught, then you probably don't want to run to wine for health. In any case, an overwhelming excess of *anything*, be it food or drink, is best avoided. While I don't believe we should make alcohol the scapegoat for liver disease, that doesn't grant you a free pass to go wild like it's your twenty-first birthday. Use good judgment to love your liver and life!

HOW MUCH CAN I DRINK?

I recommend consuming alcohol in moderation, with careful attention to avoid binge drinking. Many factors influence the "right" amount of drinking. Gender is a biggie.[69] Men seem to handle alcohol better than women in the short term . . . if by "handle" we mean feel and appear less intoxicated. This may be due to the fact that men tend to be leaner than women, with higher bodily water content. Since alcohol concentrates in the body's water, less body water for ladies leads to a quicker onset of higher blood alcohol concentrations (BAC).

The fact that women become intoxicated sooner than men (and consequently are more likely to experience negative health outcomes if they *do* indulge) may serve to discourage overconsumption of alcohol in order to protect an unborn baby from toxins. Despite significant differences in body weight, women's livers tend to be similar in size to men's, further indicating that they're wired to process toxins.[70] As a final note, the more rapid rise in the female BAC may impair cognitive function (such as short-term memory) more steeply than in men, meaning ladies *are* more likely to black out.

That said, since men take longer to experience higher BACs, they're more likely to develop related problems in the long term. Epidemiological data consistently reveals that, compared to women, men are more likely to drink to excess,[71] experience legal and personal ramifications, develop liver disease, and become alcoholics.[72] So regardless of whether you're a lightweight or heavy-weight, the takeaway is the same: Don't go crazy, people!

Genetics also may play a key role. Variations in genes that affect alcohol-processing enzymes can influence alcohol metabolism, tolerance, side effects, damage, and addiction.[73] On chromosome 15, for example, CHRNA5 may influence one's reaction to alcohol, as measured by body movements and "high" feelings.[74] And genetic variations in the PNPLA3 gene, involved in proteins for the metabolism of fats, have been linked to increased fatty liver and inflammation, with some studies suggesting it may be the primary predictor for the likelihood of developing alcoholic cirrhosis.[75] Other potential genes correlated with alcoholic troubles include CYP2E1, NCAN, GCKR, LYPLAL1, SAMM50, and more. Since this is starting to feel like alphabet soup, I'm going to stop now.

Other additional factors may influence alcohol-consumption reactions. Obesity, diets high in processed and refined foods, old age, and ethnicity (such as Asian and Latino) may increase liver risks. Situational factors can also play a prominent role, such as drinking on an empty versus full stomach, a person's mindset, or the time of day.

For practicality, keep a few things in mind: The liver can process approximately one standard drink per hour; pure alcoholic spirits and/or mixing different types tends to do more liver damage (step away from the Long Island Iced Tea!); and chronic heavy drinking is likely worse than occasional binge drinking. In other words, the dose makes the poison (and health benefits!), and sensible, slow wine intake is likely best.

CAN I EAT GRAPES INSTEAD OF WINE FOR THE HEALTH BENEFITS?

Sort of . . . but not so much. Alcohol independently contributes health benefits, particularly for the heart. And you'll get more polyphenol bang for your buck (with less sugar!) via the vino, since alcohol increases levels of wine's polyphenols, and the alcohol/polyphenol synergy supports wine's advantages.

The vinification process also ramps up wine's health potential. Polyphenols reside largely in grape skins and seeds, and are activated when the grape is threatened. Macerating the grapes to create wine renders them more potent and bioavailable than if you just ate a grape! The oak-aging process further instills wine with valuable compounds.

CAN I TAKE SUPPLEMENTS FOR WINE'S BENEFITS?

If you're tempted to choose supplements such as encapsulated resveratrol for wine's treasures, I encourage you to reevaluate this itinerary. For starters, let's be blunt: It's much more *fun* to drink wine than to take a pill. While you may not see the allure in munching on some grass-fed liver for vitamins, I'd wager wine is a *smidge* more appealing for polyphenols.

Consuming polyphenols in whole form also trumps a stripped-down pill, since wine's *hundreds* of compounds work synergistically, with no single one determining total anti-inflammatory or antioxidant potential. This is partly due to the fact that plants naturally contain many protective compounds to ensure that attackers (such as bacteria and viruses) do not become resistant. Studies have found that the interaction of various polyphenols found in the grape seed and skin is key for preventing blood clots, and multiple polyphenols more effectively combat cancer than an isolated compound.[76] We also have no idea just how many of these interacting compounds exist. We used to think there were eighteen different stilbenoids, for example; then, in 2013, researchers discovered a whopping twenty-three *more* when they analyzed red wine samples.

Critics of the wine-health hypothesis also point to the large amounts of polyphenols used in many studies. ("You'd have to drink a gallon of wine to reap the benefits!") True, while in vitro and rodent studies often do use relatively large amounts of isolated compounds, it is because they seek to identify the root mechanism by which the polyphenols reap the benefits experienced by average wine drinkers, who are presumably *not* ingesting wine by the gallon. Studies also suggest that the biological makeup of various polyphenols influences their bioavailability more than the amount. Think quality, not quantity!

Supplementing with isolated wine compounds may even do more harm than good. Slamming your system with pure antioxidants may downregulate your own production of them, and highly concentrated forms of isolated polyphenols have been shown to encourage cancer, rather than prevent it. Consuming antioxidants in whole food or drink form, on the other hand, vastly reduces risk of toxicity. Extracted polyphenols are also prone to oxidation, and many supplements contain problematic additives. I cannot advocate enough that you get your polyphenols from fruits, veggies, and wine, rather than a pill—no matter how tempting the commercial copy or discount may be!

DOES WHITE WINE HAVE HEALTH BENEFITS?

What if you're the type of person who naturally gravitates to Sauvignon Blanc or Pinot Grigio? Or maybe you're just #over the red wine teeth stains? Can you still reap wine's health benefits?

A majority of wine's health-enhancing compounds come from the grape skin and seeds, which play a starring role in red wine fermentation, a supporting role in rosé wine fermentation, and never even got an audition for white wine fermentation. As such, red wines may contain around ten times more polyphenols than white wine. That said, given all the studies that look at alcohol and longevity, rather than wine specifically, there's definitely some benefit to white. Some non-flavonoid polyphenols also notably reside in the grape pulp, and studies have found value in white wine consumption specifically, including positive influences on inflammation (such as decreased C-reactive protein), metabolic factors, and insulin regulation.

So while you may not reap all the potential benefits that you'd get from red wine, feel free to raise a glass of Chardonnay or Pinot Grigio to health as well!

THE BATTLE OF THE SEXES

Though women may need to maintain more awareness of calories and nutrients for hormonal and reproductive health, that doesn't mean that intermittent fasting should be feared or avoided by us ladies! I've thrived for years on IF, and find it an excellent tool for health and well-being, when properly implemented. That said, men and women just aren't the same creatures, so let's take a look at how biological sex differences affect fat burning and fasting, before addressing women and IF specifically.

FAT USAGE IN MEN VERSUS WOMEN

While intermittent fasting boosts fat burning in both sexes, male and female bodies typically utilize dietary and body fat in different ways, resulting in stereotypically different physiques. It all goes back to one simple concept: babies.

Ya see, a girl's body intrinsically anticipates supporting another living being inside itself for nine months—an anabolic state that *doubles* energy requirements. No big deal. As such, the female body can be a *bit* jealous of its fat reserves. During pregnancy, fat use and storage ramps up considerably. After the first ten weeks, the amount of fat in the blood is 20 percent more than in a nonpregnant woman, and can continue to climb to 300 percent. By the seventh month of pregnancy, women gain an average 7.3 pounds of body fat, supplying around 30,000 calories of energy!

The body knows how much body fat it needs to bear a child, and can temporarily adjust fertility accordingly, which is why low body weights can affect menstrual cycles. During pregnancy, the body will do whatever it must to ensure adequate fat reserves, including downregulating metabolism, adjusting how it uses nutrients, and even extracting more calories from food than normal. (So much for "a calorie is a calorie"!)

Because of the whole presumed-future-baby thing, women typically display a higher body fat percentage than men. They also tend to store more fat for the long term in the butt and thighs, while men store more (in a less healthy manner) in the midsection and abs. In fact, a woman's thigh fat is specifically reserved for pregnancy to nurture the infant, which explains why this fat can be extremely difficult for women to burn. Women also fare better with short-term fat storage, and are more likely to store fat in the more easily usable subcutaneous tissue beneath the skin, whereas men are more likely to store it in visceral tissue around the organs, which is more hazardous to health.

Women are also wired for fat-fueled fasting and exercise, experiencing higher rates of fat burning (including from the muscles) than men, who favor more glucose. The ladies also experience more sympathetic activity (such as epinephrine and norepinephrine) while exercising than men, increasing alertness.

The game changes after menopause, when the whole pregnancy idea isn't so plausible, and women begin storing more abdominal fat like men. Obesity also levels the playing field, with obese men and women featuring more homogeneous fat storage. (It would seem that fat stored unhealthily in excess is granted license to go everywhere.) Lean men and women, however, tend to release similar amounts of fat from their abs and lower body.

I hope all this encourages ladies *not* to begrudge their body's love of fat, which is highly context specific and supports the life and energy of both mother and (potentially future!) child.

SHOULD WOMEN FAST?

Time for the elephant in the room! While a female's fat use efficiency would seemingly suit an IF protocol, a girl's body can understandably become a bit panicky with fat reserves, since pregnancy when malnourished could mean not enough fuel to sustain both mom and baby. That said, a woman's state of fertility involves various hormones and nutrient levels, of which intermittent fasting may or may not play a part. Let's take a closer look at the studies on fasting females, and then I'll make recommendations for how women may maximize IF benefits while minimizing any potentially negative effects.

RODENT TRIALS

A few trials have analyzed the gender differences of various restrictive dietary protocols in male and female rats. Two six-month studies—one in 2007[1] and a follow-up in 2008[2]—implemented novel diets in our Mickey and Minnie friends: 40 percent calorie restriction, 20 percent calorie restriction, alternate-day IF, and a high fat/high glucose diet (HFHG). Except for the HFHG group, all were calorie restricted. Both studies assumed that varying levels of dietary restriction would affect males and females differently, due to different reproductive roles and energy requirements. I'll spare you the computer manualesque details, but here are the basic findings.

The 2007 study begins by pointing out that lab animals that are provided constant access to food tend to overeat, suffer more disease, and die sooner than those on calorie-restricted or fasting diets. The study's actual results were all over the map, with *most* of the protocols affecting *most* hormones and neurotransmitters one way or another (including the HFHG diet, which yielded pretty unfavorable results overall). The researchers found that IF enhanced cognitive activity in females much more than in males, resulting in substantially fewer errors and faster maze completion on their part. (Whenever I think of rat mazes, I think of the *Wonder Years* episode where big brother Wayne vacuums up Kevin's rat. Anyone?) IF also elevated brain-derived neurotrophic factor (BDNF)—which encourages growth of new neurons in the central nervous system and positively affects memory, learning, and higher thinking—in the plasma (but not hippocampus) of the females. The study also found that both calorie restriction and IF increased adrenal size in the females, but not in male rats, indicating that they were pumping out more related hormones. Yet despite their increased activity, IF decreased circulating ghrelin levels—the "hunger" hormone—in the females, but not males, meaning they were likely less hungry, despite the calorie restriction. Oh hey!

On the downside, the IF protocol affected female, but not male, fertility. While too few or too many calories bore no effect on the male rodents' testicular weight, it decreased female ovary size. (Interestingly, the HFHG diet also decreased ovary size.) That said, while 20 percent calorie restriction, IF, and HFHG instigated menstrual cycle fluctuations in some of the females, only the severe 40 percent calorie-restricted diet actually *stopped* it. In other words, if you fiddle with the number of calories in a female rat's diet—either decreasing or adding them—you'll likely fiddle with the pattern of her cycle as well.

In the end, the researchers concluded that female rats are more sensitive to calorie intake, due in part to energy requirements for reproduction, and that heightened performance in times of fluctuating energy availability helps them better compete for food.

The 2008 follow-up study shifted focus to the hypothalamus: the "central governor" in the body, in charge of appetite, energy levels, metabolism, and a whole bunch of other stuff! In this trial, the researchers found that the energy-restricted diets, including IF, increased the size of the females' hippocampi considerably more than in the males, with IF upregulating sixty pathways and, again, leading to better performance in maze tests. The IF diet also upregulated genes involving cellular energy regulation, oxidative stress resistance, cell survival, and the breakdown of old proteins in the females specifically. That said, the IF protocol increased daytime activity of the females, but not the males. Before you're like, "Yay! Productivity!" . . . rats are actually nocturnal, so this implies that IF might not be ideal for female circadian rhythms.

Perhaps most notably, female rats were more sensitive to the specific level of calorie restriction, whereas males displayed a more general response. To anthropomorphize this: Only when calorie intakes reached extremely low or high amounts were the boy rats casually like, "Oh hey . . . stress. Let's maybe do something about that?" Yet, even *slight* shifts in calories resulted in the females being like, "Oh my goodness! We are experiencing X amount of stress at this moment! We should precisely adjust our genes and hormones to ensure both we and our future offspring survive this stressful time!"

Sound familiar?

The researchers concluded that female rodents are highly in tune with degrees of calorie restriction, and react accordingly, becoming more alert and active to ensure energy for fertility. They also noted that the female brain cells deal better with metabolic and oxidative stressors than males.

In other words, female rodents react more intensely to restrictive diets, including IF in this case, for better and worse. While a bit of restriction upregulates brain and physical activity, it may increase stress biomarkers. Taken to the extreme, it may pause the reproductive cycle, since pregnancy requires substantial energy. In contrast, a male's brief reproductive role means he can afford to be horny 24/7. (In fact, a male's fertility may be preserved during calorie-restricted states, so he can keep the line going despite nutritional hardships.)

HUMAN TRIALS

Time to move up the food chain! Unfortunately, human studies on fasting females are a bit sparse. Most studies look at females in relation to stressors in general (such as calorie restriction and exercise) rather than fasting. These often find that such stressors indeed affect hormones and menstrual cycles. However, since they often involve inadequate calorie intake, it is uncertain if the implications extend to an IF protocol providing *adequate* calories and nutrition.

IF-specific studies looking at basic health biomarkers between the genders are often conflicting, without addressing whether fasting is detrimental to women specifically. For example, some studies find that IF majorly benefits fasting glucose in women,[3] while others find it statistically insignificant.[4] One study found that alternate-day fasting protocols (ADF) reduced insulin post-meal for men but not women, while another found ADF did zilch for men's insulin. Another found that ADF lowered glucose, insulin, free fatty acid, and

LDL cholesterol more in women than men. These wildly varying results make it difficult to pinpoint anything specific regarding IF's hormonal effects, and I'd wager a person's baseline health, genetics, and lifestyle may play a pivotal role.

As for the more reproductive-specific studies, a 1994 study of women on three-day (aka *not* intermittent) fasts found that, despite significant weight loss, fasting bore no effects on reproductive hormones, including immune luteinizing hormone, follicle-stimulating hormone, oestradiol, and progesterone.[5] More recently (and applicably), a 2013 study of fifteen overweight women found that an IF protocol alternating eat-all-you-want days with severely calorie-restricted days led to decreased body weight, waist circumference, blood pressure, and cholesterol, and did not affect menstrual cycles.[6]

We can also turn to studies on Ramadan—a Muslim religious fast of complete food and drink abstinence during daylight hours—for more findings. On the plus side, these fasts do not mandate calorie restriction during the eating window, making them similar to the protocols in this book. On the downside, they forbid hydration during the fasting window.

For starters, a 2010 Ramadan study specifically analyzing fasting and menstrual cycles found no significant negative effects.[7] Another 2013 Ramadan study looked at forty women with polycystic ovary syndrome (PCOS)—the most prevalent endocrine disturbance in females, which yields metabolic, reproductive, and psychological problems. Because a proposed mechanism for PCOS is a shutdown of the reproductive system due to increased nervous system activity, the study aimed to investigate fasting's effects on nervous system factors such as cortisol, catecholamines, and sex hormones. In contrast to the rodent studies, where fasting upregulated nervous system activity, the Ramadan study found that fasting proved therapeutic for the PCOS women, decreasing levels of the stress hormones cortisol and noradrenaline. In the same vein, a 2002 study found that fasting benefited ovulatory issues in women with PCOS.[8]

As for the aforementioned stress hormone cortisol, a 2007 metabolic-ward study on meal patterns in women found that, compared to eating throughout the day, IF produced no differences in salivary cortisol.[9] Studies also suggest that light exposure, rather than food intake, may be the primary factor regulating cortisol rhythms.

Ironically, even if dietary restriction "pauses" the menstrual cycle, it may potentially extend fertility, possibly by preserving female eggs. Mice put on ADF protocols experience menstrual cycles later in life than mice who eat normally. And Dutch women who suffered starvation during World War II ultimately experienced no change in fertility (despite fluctuations during the war), and in fact bore children who were, in turn, more fertile.

THE TAKEAWAY?

Reviewing the literature can be downright confounding. One minute IF seems detrimental to reproductive health, the next it's a saving grace. In any case—and I believe this is key—most studies that find fasting to increase stress are those in which women were subject to some sort of dietary restriction, whereas IF as discussed in this book does *not* require calorie restriction and is designed to provide ample energy intake. Fertility also may be influenced more by the amount of baseline body fat a girl's got, rather than immediate food intake. It's quite probable that *actual* starvation most affects a girl's cycle, rather than fasting.

On the flip side, intermittent fasting can also attenuate many health problems and metabolic issues that typically upset reproductive cycles. Excess weight is connected to a host of fertility issues, and even small amounts of weight loss can significantly improve reproduction. That, coupled with IF's metabolic benefits, make it potentially beneficial for enhancing reproductive health.

I believe diet should support a fertile gal, and intermittent fasting can definitely instigate a healthy shift in metabolism, hormones, and body composition. I also believe IF will be most beneficial when viewed as a healthy hormetic stress, rather than a taxing chronic stress. While a girl's cycle may initially fluctuate on an IF protocol, it should not automatically result in long-term menstrual irregularities, especially when consuming adequate calories and nutrients in the eating window. That said, fasting is not one-size-fits-all. If you do IF and your body reaches a weight that it "views" as inadequate for childbearing, or if your unique hypothalamus interprets fasting as particularly stressful, you may experience negative effects such as, but not limited to, restlessness and irregular cycles.

TIPS AND TRICKS FOR FEMALE FASTERS

If you *do* experience seemingly stress-related effects from intermittent fasting—such as fatigue, depressed mood, or menstrual irregularities—consider the following adjustments:

- Make sure you're consuming enough calories in your eating window. Since IF lets you eat a ton and still lose weight, why *not* go big?
- Perhaps more important than calories, make sure you are getting adequate *nutrition*. Favor whole, natural foods, while minimizing or (better yet) eliminating grains, sugar, and processed foods.
- While intermittent fasting and low-carb can be two peas in a pod, some women's bodies may desire more carbs. Consider adding these in healthy forms, such as in fruits, tubers, and/or sweet potatoes.
- On the flip side, if you're eating higher carb and lower fat, you may want to consider upping your fat intake.
- This may or may not be applicable, depending on the length of your window, but you can try consuming lower-carb meals during the day, and higher-carb meals at night, to support natural cortisol, insulin, and adrenal rhythms. In any case, having some carbs before bedtime may just whisk you away to dreamland!
- Don't do IF in a time of poor nutrition, lack of sleep, and/or immense stress, *unless* it honestly makes you feel less stressed. Perception matters. If you're implementing IF while following a healthy, nutritious diet, and view your fast as *strengthening*, I believe it will greatly benefit your body. If, however, you view your fast as dangerous, then repercussions are more likely to arise. I wholeheartedly recommend reading Kelly McGonigal's *The Upside of Stress*.
- Consider cutting back on the fasting a bit. You might try IF once or twice per week, rather than every day. You can also shorten your fasting window or lengthen your eating window.
- Consider adding MCT oil to your morning tea or coffee, à la Dave Asprey's Bulletproof™ Intermittent Fasting Protocol (see page 116).

Ingesting fat without protein or calories may keep your body in a "fasted" state and encourage ketosis and autophagy, while potentially minimizing stressful effects.

- Pay close attention to overall adrenal, hormonal, and thyroid health. If you don't feel well, ask your doctor to run adrenal and thyroid tests. Be mindful of your body, and how certain foods and eating patterns *make you feel.*

- Address your chronic stress levels via therapeutic outlets, such as mindfulness, meditation, and social support. Try to maintain natural circadian rhythms, with bright lights during the day, and minimal lights and technology at night. I personally wear blue-light-blocking goggles at night, and use f.lux on my computer to do the same. It's pretty life changing! Check out MelanieAvalon.com for more on this!

- Above all else, know that your body is doing what it does to *protect* you and your future. Practice IF out of a keen interest to improve your health, in a state of love. Be kind to yourself, and embrace fasting as nourishment, rather than fear. Keep in mind that the IF protocol that best served you yesterday may not be the same one that best serves you today or tomorrow. Listen to your body, and adjust accordingly. Intuition and mindset are key.

THE IF FITNESS FANATIC

D o you #heart the gym? Greet the day with a run through the country-side? Compose your life soundtrack to the hypnotic beats of a treadmill? Does lifting weights lift the weight off your shoulders? Maybe you're married to CrossFit, or instead favor a more casual workout relationship of sweat-drenched one-afternoon stands? In any case, if physical activity for fat burning and body composition fuels your fire, this section is for you!

THE FITNESS FANATIC IF BENEFITS

FAT BURNING

Studies consistently find that fasted exercise significantly increases fat oxidation, meaning you'll burn *more* fat during your gym efforts with the same (or even less) amount of effort.[10] Enough said.

ENDURANCE

Ever hit the wall? It's like one moment you could traverse the entire country Lewis and Clark–style, and then all of a sudden you can't move another muscle? While it may seem like you simply "ran out of energy" . . . you didn't. You just *thought* you did.

Typical nonfasted exercise is primarily fueled by glucose (sugar from carbohydrates) and its stored form of glycogen in the muscles and liver. While glucose serves as an easily accessible fuel source during exercise, it can actually *inhibit* fat burning. When your body has abundant glucose reserves from its last meal, it resists tapping into fat stores. In the ultimate irony, we store substantial energy via fat to traverse hundreds of miles, yet are restrained by our limited glycogen stores, which we can deplete in a single exercise session.

When relying on glucose, our body will "hit the wall" when it runs out. When this happens, the brain stops physical activity in its tracks, like the police shutting down a college party. In fact, you'll likely "hit the wall" *before* complete glycogen depletion, as the brain slows ya down in anticipation of running out! It's like leaving the party when you hear the sirens coming, even though the police aren't even there yet! To avoid hitting the wall, athletes often turn to sugar-filled sport drinks or energy gels to provide hits of glucose.

By sparing glycogen, lowering insulin levels, regulating blood sugar, and raising stimulatory neurotransmitters such as epinephrine, fasted training bypasses the whole glucose issue, jumping straight into fat stores, and near-limitless energy! It's like graduating from a weekly allowance to becoming a financially stable adult. Oh hey, self-reliant sustainability! One clinical trial found that rats that fasted for twenty-four hours ran longer than rats in the fed state, even when their blood sugar dropped *below* that of the fed rats: Their proverbial wall was gone![11] Human studies find similar results, with fasted exercise boosting performance by increasing fatty acids and ketones for energy.

The endurance benefits also extend to the muscles. A 2011 study found that fasted training encouraged the breakdown of fats within muscle for energy, while another found that fasted training increased muscle proteins involved in glucose regulation by 28 percent.[12] Speaking of muscle . . .

MUSCLE PROTECTION

Numerous studies find IF protects muscle. Fasting increases insulin sensitivity and enhances nutrient partitioning, conditioning the body to efficiently use protein for muscle synthesis. It also upregulates ketone production, which reduces muscle catabolism, and promotes autophagy—the recycling of old and damaged proteins for growth and repair, which is *required* to maintain muscle mass.

IF may even protect muscle in the catabolic state of calorie restriction. A 2011 review of eighteen studies examined the effects of calorie restriction practiced in either typical eating patterns or IF eating patterns.[13] It found that, compared to "normal" calorie restriction, intermittent fasting seemed to encourage the preservation of muscle mass. Similarly, a 2013 study found that overweight woman who dieted for three months lost weight from fat rather than muscle when fasting, while normal calorie restriction yielded more muscle loss.[14]

What's better than muscle protection? Muscular *enhancement*! Research conducted by the Intermountain Medical Center found that IF can increase human growth hormone (HGH), which is key for muscle growth.[15] Fasting for twenty-four hours resulted in HGH increases by 2,000 percent in men and 1,300 percent in women! Other studies indicate that IF can enhance activity of the muscle-building protein kinase mTOR, increase enzymes that prime muscles for regrowth upon refeeding, and encourage genes for protein synthesis.

THE FITNESS FANATIC IF Q&A

WHAT IS THE BEST IF APPROACH FOR THE FITNESS FANATIC?

The Fitness Fanatic may appreciate the schedule-friendly, time-based Clock Approach, allowing you to pencil in your IF and exercise windows, scheduling the latter at the most efficient fat-burning time of your fast. Or you could try a Meal Approach and implement your workouts before your lunch and/or dinner.

WHEN SHOULD I WORK OUT DURING THE FAST?

I recommend working out when it best aligns with your (admittedly subjective) fasting "zone." Some people find that working out earlier in the window catalyzes their transition into the daily fasted state, while others prefer the enhanced fat oxidation and potential for *really* tapping into stubborn fat when working out later in the fast. If you find that working out makes you hungry afterward, you might want to work out later in your fasting window, and closer to your eating window. Play around to see what works for you!

DO I NEED TO EAT RIGHT AFTER EXERCISE?

While conventional wisdom mandates food consumption immediately post-workout to refill muscle glycogen and ensure adequate protein synthesis, this may not be necessary. Since fasted exercise is primarily fueled by fat rather than glycogen, it requires less (if any) "refilling" post-exercise. According to the 2014 *Journal of International Society of Sports Nutrition*, adequate glycogen refilling can occur at any point within twenty-four hours of a workout.

As for protein, studies show that muscle synthesis can also occur over a twenty-four-hour spectrum, even after fasted workouts. A 2000 study found that females who ate adequate protein throughout the day experienced identical nitrogen levels and protein synthesis as those who consumed all of the protein within one meal,[16] while a 2007 trial in middle-aged men and women found similar results in muscle retention when comparing one versus three meals.[17] Translation: As long as you consume adequate protein within your daily eating window, you should be good! According to the official Recommended Dietary Allowance (RDA), that means around 0.36 grams per pound of body weight per day for the average person. Strength training individuals may bump that up to an estimated 0.5 to 1 gram per pound of body weight. (That said, I suggest acquiring your protein by eating nutritious whole foods to satiety, without necessarily counting anything.) In fact, daily protein restriction during your fast can even benefit muscle preservation, since consuming protein shuts off the previously discussed autophagy.

Of course, if you want to schedule your fast so you work out and then eat, go for it! But don't sweat it (pun intended) if you work out earlier in the day and don't eat until later.

WILL FASTED EXERCISE MAKE ME OVEREAT?

Ya know that moment when you're feeling pretty confident about your gym efforts, only to get home and be slammed with a wave of "OMG let me eat all the things!" A bit of fasted exercise can help with that too! A 2013 University of Illinois study found that, while fasted exercisers were just as likely to exercise for the same amount and intensity as fed exercisers, only fasted exercise reduced uncontrolled, emotional food consumption post-workout.[18]

Even if you *do* "overeat," fasted exercise may mitigate the damage. A 2010 study looked at healthy males who ate 30 percent more calories than needed per day (amounting to 1,000 calories or more!) for six weeks.[19] Some did carb-fueled aerobic training, some did fasted aerobic training, and some didn't train at all. Unlike the carb-fueled trainers and nontrainers, the fasted trainers gained no significant weight, even when engaging in the same amount of exercise and consuming the same number of excess calories!

SHOULD I SUPPLEMENT WITH CAFFEINE?

Controlled studies find that caffeine—the most consumed psychoactive drug—upregulates metabolism and fat burning, increases endurance, and lowers rates of perceived exertion. In other words, it can make you burn *more* fat, while making it seem *less* hard to do so. Double win. Caffeine's fat-burning effects may even remain after the actual substance has left your body. A 1995 study found that caffeine ingestion continued to increase fat burning by 10 to 29 percent the next day. And habitual caffeine likely doesn't downregulate its fat-blasting potential, as one study found that endurance exercisers experienced no difference in fat burning when ingesting caffeine habitually, compared to a four-day withdrawal period.

More caffeine, however, is not necessarily better. In a 2012 study, though caffeine improved performance in cyclists, doubling the dose conferred no further benefits.[20] Studies also indicate that caffeine's thermic effects may be more potent for lean individuals than for obese individuals. I take this as a sign that caffeine might be a smart fuel for blasting those last bits of fat, rather than initiating the beginning of a weight-loss journey.

In any case, having some caffeine preworkout can likely benefit performance and body composition, but if you find it overstimulates you or encourages insomnia, you might want to reevaluate or lower your dose.

SHOULD I TAKE BRANCHED-CHAIN AMINO ACIDS DURING MY FASTING WINDOW?

Some IF-ers argue that branched-chain amino acid (BCAA) supplements may minimize muscle loss and support an anabolic state. Yet IF naturally preserves muscle, and taking BCAAs during a fast may encourage insulin release or shut-off autophagy. For these reasons, coupled with my preference for whole foods over supplements, I don't consume BCAAs. But feel free to experiment and see how you react. And if you're worried about muscle loss, simply believing you are protecting your muscles with BCAAs could be beneficial. Oh hey, placebo effect!

HOW MUCH SHOULD I EAT IN THE EATING WINDOW?

While fitness aficionados may fervently log calories and macronutrients to the decimal, I advocate a much more intuitive approach: Eat the (whole) foods you crave, to satiety. If you do unintentionally undereat, you'll likely find yourself hungrier come your next eating window. I also do *not* advocate processed workout "foods," as such concoctions can fiddle with natural satiety signals. After all, we've been consuming whole foods for thousands of years (with a lot more physical activity, historically speaking), with nary a workout shake in sight!

A FINAL WORD OF CAUTION

While fasted exercise can catalyze fat burning, support muscle mass, and provide a number of health benefits as discussed, I encourage you not to go overboard. Please moderate your exercise, and do not overtax your body. Punctuated fasted gym sessions a few times per week is not the same as engaging in exhausting hours of cardio and CrossFit each and every day. Know that more is not always better, and take comfort in the fact that fasted exercise will make your workouts more efficient, so less can truly be more! Please allow for adequate recovery time, supported by rest (yay!) and nutritious food (yum!). If you experience signs of overtraining—such as a fluctuating heart rate, insomnia, continued joint pain or soreness, or chronic fatigue—please slow down. After all, exercise should ultimately make you stronger, not weaker!

THE IF WORKAHOLIC

D o you swim in the turbulent ocean of professionalism, with dreams of deadlines, deals, and meetings? Would you rather climb ladders than play Chutes and Ladders? Maybe you're the desk-job type, swimming in proposals and spreadsheets, or perhaps you turn a profit from more creative endeavors. In any case, if to-do lists, coffees, and #productivity stamp your identity, this section is for you!

THE WORKAHOLIC IF BENEFITS

ALERTNESS

Because most weight-loss protocols mandate energy restriction without adequate nutrition, and because 20 percent of daily energy goes toward the brain, it's no surprise that common diets—with the exception of fleeting highs from diet pills and caffeine—dull brainpower. Intermittent fasting, on the other hand, amplifies alertness, yielding a hyperaware state of laser-beam focus as sharp as your PowerPoint.

Studies show that excessive food intake dampens cognitive function. (Can

I get a food coma over here?) IF, however, upgrades the mind by changing the brain's primary fuel source. While the brain typically runs on glucose influenced by wavering blood sugar levels, it functions *better* on fatty acids and ketones. Fasting also upregulates stimulatory neurotransmitters such as epinephrine and norepinephrine, and supports alert cognition, learning, and memory. In fact, upregulation of the central nervous system may be a reason for the seemingly contradictory finding of occasional *increased* resting energy expenditure while fasting. Translation: Fasting may make your brain *so* wired that it literally burns more calories!

STRESS REDUCTION

With its array of traffic commutes, deadlines, and bosses, career stress can quickly turn chronic. Thankfully, the fasted state can help cultivate a healthy stress response. In a 2013 study, heart rate variability tests indicated better norepinephrine stress responses and improved autonomic nervous systems when fasting,[21] while a 2015 study found that IF decreased the stress hormones cortisol and noradrenaline in women.[22] Other studies show that fasting protects the brain from excitotoxic stress, possibly due to changed glutamate and GABA ratios.

FLEXIBILITY AND FREEDOM

Intermittent fasting perfectly suits busy, fluctuating schedules, cutting the proverbial chains of snacking, eating, and the clock. With IF, you don't have to worry about scarfing down breakfast, planning meals, or hunting for snacks to keep you going—especially when you can't leave the desk!

With IF, you simply no longer fear *having* to eat in order to function. Instead, you'll find yourself laughing in the face of former food temptations, as you easily complete your job tasks without worries about energy dips and appetite. You can adapt to whatever is thrown your way like it's not even a thing. While other people may be slaves to coffees, lunches, and snacks, you can power through like the boss you are (or will be!).

COMBAT THE EFFECTS OF SEDENTARISM

Perpetual physical inactivity is connected to a host of health problems, including weight gain, cardiovascular disease, and oxidative stress. And if there's one thing worse than sitting all day, it's sitting and eating all day. Thankfully, IF can address these dilemmas, relieving oxidative stress and serving as a beneficial hormetic stress similar to exercise.

THE WORKAHOLIC IF Q&A

WHAT IS THE BEST IF APPROACH FOR THE WORKAHOLIC?

A Clock Approach is great for the Workaholic, who likely runs by the clock anyway! You can simply pencil in your eating times right alongside your other daily tasks! Alternatively, a dinner-only Meal Approach may perfectly suit the nine-to-five desk job: Think epic unbroken energy at the office, avoidance of cafeteria temptations, and a delicious feast upon return to your humble (or perhaps not so humble?) abode!

HOW DO I DEAL WITH SUSPICION OR PRESSURE FROM COWORKERS?

Unfortunately, I can't promise you won't temporarily become the subject of workplace gossip, as coworkers raise eyebrows under piercing fluorescent lights. "Well-meaning" work buddies may swear they'll break your fasting habits, passionately presenting home-baked goodies as well as detailed descriptions of the commissary's current offerings.

If such is your workplace situation, I encourage you to have faith. If you remain steadfast in your choices, the obsession shall eventually pass. People can be threatened by change, but routine and time breaks all novelty. When you face hurdles from your coworkers, feel free to explain your personal choice in however much detail you wish, and then go about your business. You've got better things to deal with! Check out the "Social Guide" on page 202 for more tips and tricks!

THE IF SUPERMOM

Are you battling diapers and temper tantrums? Waking up at 6:00 a.m. for bright yellow buses? Living a life defined by carpools and oddly difficult questions about algebra and U.S. history? Perhaps you're struggling to burn a bit of that lingering pregnancy weight gain? In any case, if you're currently raising the next generation (for which I thank you!), this section is for you.

THE SUPERMOM IF BENEFITS

MORE ENERGY

While your child may desire a pony or rocket ship for Christmas, perhaps you'd settle for just a smidge more energy? No need to turn to Santa for that! Adopting an intermittent fasting lifestyle rapidly instigates fat-burning, insulin-regulating metabolic changes that increase energy and decrease fatigue. You'll likely find you now have the motivation to do #allthethings, from dragging your kids out of bed in the wee hours of the morning, to helping construct a messy miniature volcano for the science fair, to driving back to the school to deliver the book they left on the counter.

BETTER MOOD

As if pregnancy didn't screw with your hormones enough, raising your kid(s) may be further taxing your humor, loving them aside! Many moms have told me the best thing about IF is their uplifted mood. By stabilizing blood sugar levels and regulating neurotransmitters, IF can banish irritability, lend more patience, discourage fights, quiet raised voices, and help temper temper tantrums. Plus, a happy mood can be infectious, which can cultivate a warm spirit in the household!

MORE TIME

Who has time? As a mother, you may find the clock ticks a bit too fast as you scramble to take care of not only yourself but the needs of your family. Intermittent fasting has a tendency to free up time you didn't realize you had. Even if you spend the same amount of time actually eating, you nevertheless gain an immense amount of time in not stopping and starting your life three to ten times per day to eat. (Feeding another human being is time-consuming enough!) Just think about how much time you stand to gain in the mornings by simply skipping breakfast!

MORE MONEY

Stressed by grocery bills? IF has totally got you covered! Even though you may be eating the same amount of food as before, you'll nevertheless likely save a wad of cash with an IF pattern as you forgo snacks and mindless munchies. You may even find you personally require *less* food overall, since IF discourages overeating and teaches your body to become more efficient with fuel.

In the bigger picture, IF has a tendency to keep you healthy, which can mean substantially less money spent on health care costs. From simple cold medications to more expensive medical procedures, this can really add up!

HEALTHY EATING

IF eradicates cravings for toxic and addictive foods, making you more in tune with your body. You'll likely find it easier to create an atmosphere of wholesome food choices, and lead by example for your family. This newfound clarity could arguably be the best benefit for the health and wellness of the entire household!

Speaking of healthy eating, money, and time, check out the "Recipes" on page 269 for delicious Paleo-style meals, the "Shopping Guide" on page 240 for money-saving tips, and the "Cooking Guide" on page 246 for time-saving, healthy cooking methods great for the whole family!

SNACK/HUNGER PERSPECTIVE

The growing rate of obesity among today's children is, quite frankly, alarming. Data collected in 2014 revealed that more than a third of children are overweight, and more than one-fifth are obese.[23] Seemingly gone are the days of active children working up appetites between meals; they've been replaced by sedentary kids scrolling on iPads and shoving constant snacks into their mouths.

In adopting an IF protocol and understanding the science of energy regulation and hunger cues in the body, you'll likely gain a new perspective on snacks and hunger. While, of course, children should *not* be fasting, you may realize they don't need to be chowing down every second either, and will be just fine (if not *healthier*) if they eat when hungry and don't when not. You'll be absolved from feeling the need to force-feed dinners, or, on the contrary, worrying about having adequate snacks as you run out the door. Perhaps your new perspective shall renew the eating patterns of former generations, which featured concentrated, wholesome meals, yet typically fostered less excess weight and degenerative disease.

POST-PREGNANCY WEIGHT LOSS

Fat gain during pregnancy wondrously supported the growth of your future child. That said, perhaps you'd like to bid farewell to some of it, after all's said and done? Just like you teamed up with your body to produce your child (congrats!), a great way to shed body fat after birth and breastfeeding is also by teaming with your body. Your body was super controlling with body fat while pregnant, and it's still super controlling after giving birth. To blast away body fat, you need to create a constant fat-burning mode coupled with ample nutrition, in tune with your body's preferences. Oh hey, intermittent fasting!

THE SUPERMOM IF Q&A

WHAT IS THE BEST IF APPROACH FOR THE SUPERMOM?

For the Supermom, I strongly encourage an IF approach that includes a communal meal, such as dinner. A routine meal together is key for family bonding, and I believe family life should take precedence over diet any day!

HOW DO I MEAL PREP WHEN FASTING?

If you're an IF Supermom newbie, I suggest prepping meals during your eating window to avoid cravings. You can also plan meals in advance to save time, and to ensure that you don't forget about the other meals for your family. (IF can banish appetite *so* effectively that you can forget other people eat on a more steady schedule!) Consider having nutritious whole foods such as fruits and veggies available for your kids in the fridge, rather than "easy" processed snacks in the pantry.

CAN I PRACTICE IF WHILE PREGNANT?

During pregnancy, your body requires substantial energy and nutrition (which I hope you satisfy via whole foods). Do not place IF restrictions on your body while pregnant or when nursing. But once your child has graduated from breastfeeding, full speed ahead!

HOW SHOULD I DISCUSS IF WITH MY CHILDREN?

This one is huge. Your child may become suspicious of your eating habits if you're not partaking in the meals you fix for them. I am never a fan of lying to or misleading children, but I also don't want impressionable young minds burdened with ideas of "diets" (even though IF isn't a "diet"!). It is up to you to decide how to best approach the IF topic with your children.

If your children are quite young or not very invested in your eating habits, you can simply tell them you're not hungry, or are eating later (both are true!). If your children are older or more inquisitive, you might choose to engage in an honest dialogue with them about your fasting practices, emphasizing they are for health purposes, *not* weight loss. Make it very clear that fasting is not appropriate for growing children, who should eat when hungry. That said, you can discuss the difference between hunger and cravings, and assure them they don't need to eat if they're not hungry either!

Ultimately, I encourage you to foster a wholesome approach to food in your household, embracing it as a nourishing path to vitality rather than viewing it through the lens of restriction or weight loss. Emphasize the importance of loving our bodies, not loathing or fearing them. Depending on your child's age and temperament, you also may wish to engage in an honest dialogue about eating disorders and disordered eating. In any case, I do believe that a mother who practices healthy food choices, which may include fasting, provides a better example for children than a "dieting" mom constantly logging calories and food intake, trying to lose another pound.

Also consider establishing a food "morality" clause, in which food is neither "good" nor "bad." Branding food itself with ethics can encourage obsession and invite an unnecessary psychological component that is hard to let go of down the road. Let your children know that some foods are more nutritious than others, and certain foods may make certain people not feel good. I encourage you to make it very clear *why* you choose to eat the foods you do, rather than relying on easy, vague labels of "It's healthy!" or "It's bad for you!"

THE IF SOCIAL BUTTERFLY

Are you the life of the party? Do you thrive on social soirees? Are you energized, rather than drained, from a gathering of people in a single location, accompanied by the sound of loud music? Do you categorize wine-filled nights as "networking"? If so, this section is for you!

THE SOCIAL BUTTERFLY IF BENEFITS

SOCIAL FUNCTIONING

Though you may already be pretty comfortable when out on the town, a bit of IF can nevertheless ramp up your confidence. Studies have found that fasting increases mental markers of social functioning and self-esteem and decreases anxiety. It can also benefit mood and cultivate a positive mindset, which can further enhance your social outings!

FOOD ENJOYMENT

From restaurant dates to potluck suppers, social gatherings often involve food. Assuming it's in your eating window, intermittent fasting allows you to actually embrace these meals without worries of calorie counting or portion control. You no longer stress about what you will (or will not) eat at that family get-together or reunion with friends. You can look like someone who'd order the salad but instead chow down on a juicy rib eye. So. Much. Freedom.

AVOID FOOD TEMPTATION

On the flip side, when social events *do* occur in your fasting window, IF's psychological effects grant you pristine willpower and self-control to resist temptations. The only real difficulty comes from dealing with other people, who can get a little freaked out by fasting. For that, I refer you to the "Social Guide" on page 202.

DRINKING

With IF, you can totally indulge in your share of drinks with friends and coworkers, with minimal (if any) negative effects to your waistline. Though drinking can easily support a healthy lifestyle and even lower body weight, IF nevertheless instigates damage control by shortening the time for loosened inhibitions, discouraging oxidative stress, and ensuring a detox period. You'll also likely save money, as IF can quickly turn you into a lightweight. To that point, I strongly encourage you to go slow when drinking in an IF protocol, embracing moderation and good judgment! For all the details on alcohol, check out the "Wine?" section on page 143!

THE SOCIAL BUTTERFLY IF Q&A

WHAT IS THE BEST IF APPROACH FOR THE SOCIAL BUTTERFLY?

I suggest a Meal or Window Approach for the Social Butterfly, so you don't have to worry about specific times on the clock for social functions. You might like to include dinner, which tends to be the most social meal. Suggest tea or coffee in lieu of breakfast and/or lunch.

CAN I DRINK WHILE PRACTICING IF?

As discussed in the "Wine?" section, alcohol itself does *not* easily contribute to weight gain, and can actually regulate or even lower insulin. You can definitely consume alcohol as you please during your eating window—just know that alcohol breaks the fast, and alcohol consumed with a meal may prolong digestion and slow the body's re-entrance into the fasted state. In any case, IF definitely liberates spirits, since you can drink and lose weight! Yay! Of course, try not to go crazy, and keep in mind that fasting can lower tolerance.

WHY DOES FASTING AFFECT MY BREATH?

As a social lover, you may be super aware of your breath. Some people do experience "keto breath" when fasting, described as everything from dog hair to acetone. The latter is likely most appropriate, as ketosis, or even excess protein in the diet, can increase by-products such as acetone. Fasting can also encourage detoxification in the gut (Yay!), the smelly effects of which may escape through your tongue (Boo!).

While you can turn to mints and gum for bad breath attacks, these may break the fasting Zen and encourage cravings in some people. I recommend experimenting with natural homemade breath fresheners made of purified water and peppermint oil. You can also supplement with chlorophyll, parsley, and cloves for internal deodorizing.

HOW DO I DEAL WITH SOCIAL PRESSURE?

Check out the "Social Guide" on page 202 for all the tips and tricks on this!

THE IF TRAVELER

Are you a globetrotter? Would you have been BFF with Christopher Columbus? Do road trips, airport lines, and signs in foreign languages incite thrills rather than stress? Can you recite the flight attendant monologues by heart? Do you feel most at home when not at home? In any case, if wanderlust is in your blood, or a vacation rides on the horizon, this section is for you!

THE TRAVELER IF BENEFITS

EASIER ROAD TRIPS

IF perfectly complements cross-country road trips. You don't have to worry about tracking down healthy snacks at gas stations or finding suitable restaurants near the exit. Bathroom trips also become way less of a worry. And if you break down on the side of the road . . . at least you won't starve!

UPGRADED AIRPLANE TRAVEL

Intermittent fasting extinguishes travel annoyances such as finding suitable airport food, or, even worse, air*plane* food. With IF, you don't have to worry about going hungry or bringing healthy snacks that may or may not make it past the TSA. You'll also experience newfound willpower in resisting the in-flight peanuts and/or biscotti cookies, which, let's face it, aren't that good anyway. With IF, all you need is some water, and you'll be just dandy! Airport travel may actually become a time of detox (or at least status quo) rather than a toxin-fueled journey! Plus, you can eat *more* deliciousness when you arrive at your destination!

FINDING FOOD

IF obliterates the difficulties of scavenging for suitable food when staying at your less-than-five-star hotel. No longer will you be a slave to gift shops, room service, and the exuberantly overpriced minifridge. Simply eat your main meals when out and about, and you're good to go! And since IF intensifies food taste, perception, and awareness, you'll get more pleasure and appreciation from your exotic meals (which, depending on the exchange rate, may cost a pretty penny!).

FIX JET LAG

Jet lag isn't just some casual excuse for feeling less than #onpoint when arriving in a new city. Rather, it's a psychological phenomenon involving the body's internal biological clock in the hypothalamus, which regulates mood, appetite, and energy, among other things. When we experience changes in a day's timing beyond one hour, our internal clock sort of struggles, and we may experience fatigue, insomnia, lethargy, mood changes, nausea, and irritability.

Since meal patterns influence our biological clock, IF can be used to reset it in new time zones, mitigating or even eradicating jet lag! A 2002 study involving 186 personnel in the National Guard found that those who implemented fasting were 7.5 times less likely to experience jet lag on the initial flight, and 16.2 times less likely on the return![24]

STOP VACATION WEIGHT GAIN

With IF, vacation weight gain can become a thing of the past! If you maintain your IF protocol while traveling, you can still eat *all the things*, with minimum collateral damage to your awesome body. And since vacation typically boosts dopamine, sociability, happiness, sleep, and often physical activity, it can even become a time to effortlessly *lose* weight. Who would have thunk?

GUT PROTECTION

This one is *huge*. Traveling abroad can introduce your gut to exotic substances and bacteria. If you struggle at all with IBS, you likely know the stress of worrying about your body's reaction to foods, *especially* foreign foods. IF allows the gut ample time to clear out and reset itself, while building stellar gut walls. Though you may not be able to completely squelch stomach issues when traveling, IF can definitely minimize reactions and deal with the aftermath, should any unfortunate events arise.

THE TRAVELER IF Q&A

WHAT IS THE BEST IF APPROACH FOR THE TRAVELER?

With changing time zones and unpredictable mealtimes, I think a Meal Approach is best for the IF Traveler. Choose which meals you consume, and when traveling, stick to them, according to the new time zone.

HOW DO I ADJUST IF FOR CHANGING TIME ZONES?

I find I can use IF to easily reset my sleep schedule: When I eat dinner, my body knows it's sleep time! To adjust to a new time zone, go by the new time zone you're in, rather than the time zone you were in. I recommend fasting prior to and during travel, and then eating your next typical meal that arises in sync with the new time zone. So if you're typically an evening eater, wait to eat an evening meal at the new location. If you're an earlier eater, wait for breakfast or lunch the next day.

SHOULD I STOP IF ON VACATION?

This one is totally up to you. If you're going on a short vacation, feel free to pause IF entirely. That said, the longer you do IF, the more you'll realize you likely feel better when practicing it, and consequently will have a *more* enjoyable vacation if you maintain some sort of IF protocol, even if it's a more lax one. You might try, for example, lengthening your eating window.

If you do implement IF on vacation, you can actually indulge in #allthethings, with minimal (dare I say no?) weight gain! But even if you don't stick to IF on vacay, you can rest assured knowing it awaits you upon your return, to quickly banish any vacation weight gain! (Of course, if you're going on a month-long vacation, I definitely recommend sticking to your IF protocol.)

SOCIAL GUIDE

You'd think the hardest thing about Paleo or intermittent fasting would be the whole "not eating certain things" thing, or just the straight-up "not eating" thing. As it turns out, those things are kinda a breeze. Once you begin eating nourishing whole foods and/or falling into the groove of fasting, your hunger levels, hormones, and circadian rhythms sync accordingly. Appetite vanishes in the presence of newfound energy, and the whole "eating thing" shifts from an obsessive gluttony for food ("Guys! Let's eat *all the things*!") to a pleasurable behavior that nourishes life's activities. ("Guys! Let's *fuel* ourselves!") So just what *is* the hardest part about these dietary changes?

Other people.

Or allow me to rephrase.

Dealing with *your* reactions to *other people's* reactions.

I cannot tell you how many times I've faced accusations of unhealthiness, obsessiveness, and/or eating disorders, thanks to my food choices and fasting habits. In fact, a primary reason I wrote the original *What When Wine Diet* was to concoct a scientific arsenal for such accusatory moments. In this chapter, we'll first take a look at the psychological underpinnings for people's #freakouts, so we can avoid making our own judgment about others' judgment. Acceptance for the win! We'll wrap things up with some tips and tricks for rocking social settings while following a Paleo/IF lifestyle.

THE CHANGE

When you first adopt a new dietary protocol, it can be this cool thing you're "trying." People can put up with others "trying" things because they assume they're, well, just trying. As in, "It's a phase." Perhaps this is why friends and family were mostly silent when I undertook a myriad of ineffective and weird diets, from obsessive calorie counting to diet cookies, as they figured each would pass in time. But then I started low-carb . . . and didn't stop. Next I adopted intermittent fasting . . . and didn't stop. (I planned to do IF for a single week, and half a decade later I can count the number of times I've broken my fast.) Finally I adopted Paleo, and—like the changes before—it became pretty permanent.

And then it becomes a *thing*.

Because now you're not the person who's *trying* a new diet—you're the person who *has* a new diet. And even though you might try your very hardest to *not* bother other people, you *will* bother other people. Politely declining food becomes a terrible insult. Sincere statements of no hunger become insidious excuses masking ulterior motives. I've spent a good amount of time contemplating how to *not* offend people with what I'm *not* eating, which, to be frank, is quite a silly concept indeed!

There's also an odd double standard at play. While a vast number of health issues in our present society are linked to excess weight, engaging in weight-loss measures, is somehow socially acceptable to critique. While we may silently judge gluttony, we can vocally reprimand abstinence. When you practice IF, you may find that friends, family, and strangers alike will adamantly try to thwart your plan, employing everything from passive-aggressive remarks to vendetta-driven monologues. Criticizers may easily say, "You can just have one bite!" or "You're taking this too seriously!" or "You're ruining the fun!" to an intermittent faster, yet would likely pause before saying, "Maybe you shouldn't have one more bite!" or "You're not taking this seriously enough!" or "You're having too much fun!" to someone else.

I don't point this out to demonize overeating, which is the *furthest* thing from my intentions. It's a wonder we don't all eat ourselves to death, given the present food situation! I'm simply highlighting the construction of societal judgments, which rest on illogical foundations, in the hopes that you might not stress about them, and even stop thinking about them entirely.

I GET IT

Before I get carried away with the "People are crazy" banter, I must remember that I once sat on the other side of the proverbial dinner table. A typical standard American diet lacklusterly fueled the first two decades of my life. I ate breakfast, lunch, and dinner, with snacks in between, devouring prepackaged brownies with sparkling cosmic sprinkles and whatever lured me from the vending machine. (Does anyone *actually* eat the Moon Pies?)

While I maintained a "normal" weight, I nevertheless suffered from an acute case of toned-body envy. In grade school, one of my best friends happened to be, in my opinion, a beautiful athletic goddess. As we'd vacation in Sanibel each summer, she'd follow a strict diet in preparation for soccer camp. I'd order gluttonous restaurant dishes, and she'd stick to Caesar salads with chicken. Always Caesar salads with chicken. And I would just get ever so slightly . . . annoyed. My interior monologue would go something like this: *Why can't she eat normal food like the rest of us? She's missing out on the experience. She's ruining the fun.*

I now realize the faulty logic of these thoughts, which held that the amount of "fun" to be had depended on what another person put into her mouth. This reasoning rested on bricks of self-consciousness, envy, and personal insecurities: Since I *knew* deep down that pigging out on teriyaki cheese quesadillas and red velvet cake wasn't good for me, any third-party abstinence seemingly drew attention to my actions. In reality, my friend did nothing to draw attention to anything, except politely decline my dessert offerings.

If we were all truly content with our personal choices, we would likely look at each other's actions with joy, indifference, sadness, or simply see beyond them completely. Instead, we fixate on ourselves, foster resentment, and sacrifice kindred fellowship at the altar of protective scrutiny.

IDENTIFYING THE REASON

Understanding intentions is key for discouraging fear or resentment. After many years of careful food choices, intermittent fasting, and much contemplation, I've gathered what I believe to be the main reasons people #freakout about IF (which tends to be the most incendiary diet change), listed on a sliding scale from sincere (re: *your* well-being) to selfish (re: *their* personal insecurities). With these in mind, you can put yourself in another's shoes, and decide how to appropriately respond when faced with backlash.

HEALTH CONCERNS

Since intermittent fasting radically departs from common dietary wisdom, it can understandably appear to be detrimental. It's hard to blame a person for being concerned about your health. Heck, before my fasting days, I thought I was unhealthy when I skipped a single meal; I would have been downright worried if any friend did so *routinely.*

The good news? Health concerns can be satisfactorily alleviated if the doubter is open to hearing you out. In reading this book, you should be armed with knowledge for why IF is not only safe but *healthy.* While I don't recommend trumpeting biological mechanisms and supportive studies if no one is asking ("Guys! Let me tell you *all* about this new study in the *New England Journal of Medicine*!), feel free to briefly explain the science behind your protocol when appropriate. (Or gift them a copy of this book! #shamelessplug)

APPEARANCE CONCERNS

You know the cliché of popping up at a high school reunion in some radically changed body? While potentially shocking, such drastic changes are easily attributed to the vast amount of time allowing for such a transformation. Or take yo-yo dieting, in which people fluctuate around a given 10 pounds or so, and small wins are easily congratulated. In both cases, body changes—both big and small—are typically accepted (despite any jealousy or skepticism hiding behind the outward "praise").

IF, however, can make you lose weight *fast*, with substantial body recomposition to boot. Such quick, drastic changes can make people genuinely uncomfortable when they're used to a different you. They may fear you're "disappearing," or reckon that only unhealthy measures could yield such effects. Your physical shift may also unconsciously register as a threat to your current relationship, as you are seemingly becoming someone else (if only physically).

Unless you're willing to gain weight to grant the comfort of familiarity, there's not much you can do about these fears. I recommend simply sticking it out until your new look becomes the norm, and they come around. If people can get over the constant Facebook platform changes and iPhone OS updates, they can adapt to your new body as well!

SOCIAL CONCERNS

Sometimes concerns come not from what others personally think but rather from what they think *other* people will think. Your friend may be bothered by the idea of bringing you to a social event involving food. Your mother may be worried you will offend your grandmother by not eating her refrigerator cake. This can be tricky to combat, as you yourself may agree with the logic.

I recommend evaluating each situation on a case-by-case basis, keeping in mind that everyone is entitled to his or her own choices. You definitely shouldn't have to eat anything you don't want to, nor should anyone else. Act as you see fit: If you want to engage in a social eating event—do it! If you don't want to break your fast—don't! I definitely encourage you not to break your fast or eat something toxic to your body out of worry that others are worried about others' worries; that's a really long chain of questionable reasoning! (Plus, my grandmother ended up being *super* supportive of my dietary habits, claiming they were the way "things used to be.")

SELF-CONSCIOUS CONCERNS

Perhaps the most common cause of diet backlash stems from insecurities. As discussed, when you adhere to a diet protocol, it can seemingly shine a spotlight on another person's *own* dietary habits, for better or worse. Although you may harbor *no* intention of making someone feel bad, you will, inevitably, make him or her feel bad. By *not* eating the cake, it may make the other person more aware that they *are* eating the cake. Rather than deal with their own cake eating, they may find it easier to squelch the issue entirely by attempting to drag you back to status quo. ("Oh, come on, one slice won't kill you!")

I suggest you stand your ground, provide reasoning for your choices when appropriate, and move on from there. Say it was career rather than diet related. Being successful can stir up jealously in others, but would you stop pursuing your goals just to make them feel better? Keep on keepin' on, and perhaps one day they will see you as an inspiration rather than a threat.

IF SOCIAL TIPS AND TRICKS

While we may not be able to remove the interpersonal roadblocks surrounding IF, we can at least navigate around them! Use these tips and tricks to exit communal events unscathed, with both your eating habits and friendships intact!

SAY NO NICELY AND CONCISELY

When offered food in your fasting window, politely decline with minimal explanation. While you may be tempted to spout out a carefully prepared "Science of Fasting" lecture, complete with footnote studies, consider using short and sweet phrases instead:

- "I'm good, thanks!" (Because you *are.*)
- "I'm not hungry, thanks!" (Because you *aren't.*)
- "I'll get some in a little bit!" (Substitute an outright refusal with noncommittal procrastination.)

- "I already ate, thanks!" (I love this one. It's technically 100 percent true: You *did* already eat. It just happened to be a while ago.)

AVOID ATTENTION

Don't draw unnecessary attention to your eating patterns. Just don't. While you may want to parade around and be like, "Guys! I'm intermittent fasting and it's changing my life and I'm losing weight and #allthethings!" it's probably best to refrain. When not eating at a party, do not be like, "Hey! I'm intermittent fasting and not eating!" Just do your thing. Talk to people. (Isn't that the point of a social gathering anyway?) Laying low is the name of the game. You'd be shocked what you can get away with by just holding a cup of water. Remember, people are often far more aware of themselves than of others. Also, do NOT bring your own food to a social event, unless it's a potluck. Very. Bad. Idea.

HAVE A GO-TO EXPLANATION

For those times when discussing IF is inevitable, have a succinct, prepared explanation that quickly combines personal and scientific reasoning for why you have chosen an IF lifestyle. Consider mixing and matching these pointers:

- **Personal reasoning**: "I do IF because it gives me energy, kills my appetite, and lets me eat all I want, all while losing weight."
- **Timeline for legitimacy**: "I've been doing IF for a month!"
- **Science of fat burning**: "When fasting, the body releases stored body fat for energy, supporting metabolism and activity."
- **Health benefits**: "Studies show that fasting may increase longevity, boost immune function, and prevent many diseases."
- **Something "sciencey" sounding**: "Fasting promotes autophagy, which is the recycling of old, broken-down proteins in the body. Fasting upregulates neurotransmitters and catecholamines in the body, which creates an alert, energetic state."

PRIORITIZE HEALTH

Since most concerns surrounding fasting involve its seemingly "dangerous" nature, it can be helpful to emphasize IF's health benefits rather than weight loss. Become BFF with the "IF Health Benefits" chapter on page 87!

INFLUENCE THE PLANS

If you can, weigh in on plans, encourage activities that align with your eating window, or that avoid the issue altogether.

- **Breakfast/brunch/lunch alternatives**: Tea/coffee, hiking, beach/pool, yoga, shopping, manicures, Pinterest craft day, etc.
- **Dinner alternatives**: Movies, theater, comedy clubs, bowling, game night, escape rooms, etc.

DON'T BE DEFENSIVE

Becoming argumentative or defensive regarding your fasting habit will only fan the flames. Let a quiet peace surround you. Know why you practice IF, without feeling the need to explain yourself to anyone. It's your body, your life, and your choices! Let any arising hostility come from someone else, not you. If you do sense negative energy, accept it and move on, rather than fixating on it or letting it bring you down. Channel an accepting, resolute mentality!

STAY POSITIVE

If you find yourself in a situation where you must explain yourself, err on the side of positivity. It's hard to doubt someone who genuinely proclaims, "This lifestyle makes me feel great!" with radiating energy. A sense of humor can work wonders as well. Infuse your testimony with smiles and laughter!

SPEAK IN THE FIRST PERSON

When discussing IF with others, focus on how it makes *you* feel, rather than how it can make *them* feel. For example, instead of saying, "It can make you run on fat!" say, "It makes my body run great on fat!" The key is to make it all about something that works for *you* personally, so other people don't feel like you're imposing your lifestyle on them, or insinuating that *they* need to change.

FIND A DIET BUDDY

Studies have found that having a buddy in a weight loss plan substantially ramps up the amount of weight loss, as long as one of you is successful! (Translation: Success breeds success!) Enlisting a friend to join you on your IF journey can be excellent for motivation and for sticking to the plan, and with more communal success comes more "evidence" of the legitimacy of your lifestyle. Having a friend on board can also transform you from feeling like an ostracized outcast to a secret team hacking the system.

EMPHASIZE YOUR LOVE OF FOOD

Fasting may worry friends and family who believe you are unnecessarily and unhealthily restricting yourself. To alleviate such concerns, parade your love of mealtime. When I discuss IF, I emphasize how it lets me eat *all I want*, because I *love* eating. I also point out that I never fast more than a day, because I adore my nightly feast and can't sleep on an empty stomach. Which I can't.

STICK IT OUT

Each time you stand your ground, you'll gain more confidence that you can *continue* to stand your ground. The longer you practice IF, the more impressive testimony you'll have. When you've only done IF for a few days, it can seem faddish and unsustainable—but stick it out! As you rack up the days, months, and even years, the sustainability of your protocol will speak for itself.

DO YOU

Appreciating, helping, and loving other people does not equate sacrificing your well-being for other people. How can we be truly happy if we place our own value only in the opinions of others? Confidence must come from within. Your life is your life, and you are entitled to follow the dietary approach that best suits your health and happiness. You gotta do you!

MINDSETS

Our reality is conceived in our mind. Use these mind hacks to change your perception so you can effortlessly adopt a new "what" and "when"!

CHOOSE CHOICE

Doing something you didn't seemingly choose to do, or that is outside of your control, can deplete mental resources and darken the finish line. On the contrary, feelings of choice encourage feelings of self-empowerment, serving as psychological fuel for goal completion. So view all dietary decisions as a choice! No one is forbidding you to eat, or conversely, making you eat. You are simply eating what *you* want to eat, when *you* want to eat it! If you want to eat all Paleo whole foods, you totally can! If you want to have something more Neolithic, you also totally can! If you want to break your fast early, you totally can! If you want to fast longer, again, you totally can! Everything is in your control and your power. You are not a slave to diet; rather, your diet is a beautiful pattern of eating that serves *you*.

DON'T VERSUS CAN'T

Say "I don't" instead of "I can't." For example, say "I don't eat grains" rather than "I can't eat grains," or "I don't eat breakfast" rather than "I can't eat breakfast." Studies show this trick can literally make actions easier to do, by increasing feelings of self-empowerment rather than invoking a third-party restriction. When participants in a 2012 study said "I don't," 64 percent later willingly chose a "healthy" snack over a candy bar. But when participants said "I can't," only 39 percent chose the healthy snack. In a follow-up study, 80 percent of women who said "I don't" completed their health-related goals, compared to only 10 percent of women who said "I can't."

BEND TIME

Our linguistic phrasing can affect our perceptions of time. Try these simple adjustments to make your fast seem short and your feast seem long!

- **Anytime versus only**: Say, "I eat *anytime* between 2:00 and 8:00," rather than, "I eat *only* between 2:00 and 8:00."
- **Number of hours versus specific time**: Say, "I eat *in* two hours!" rather than, "I eat *at* 7:00 p.m."
- **Imply little time versus a lot of time**: When fasting, say, "Only five hours *until* I eat!" instead of "I *still* have five hours until I eat." When eating, say, "I *still* have five hours to eat!" instead of "I *only* have five hours to eat!"

JUST SAY NO

A 2007 study found that "vigilant monitoring" was great for slashing unwanted habits.[25] Literally telling yourself, "Don't do that!" may be more effective than avoiding the temptation or distracting yourself. In other words, totally feel free to just be like, *"Stop."* This also means completely forgoing food groups (Paleo-style!) or meals (IF-style!) may be more effective for habit control than simple "dieting."

NO DEPRIVATION!

Typical weight-loss diets discourage dwelling on food, since a satisfying meal-time is off the proverbial (and literal) plate. Yet studies find that deprivation easily leads to exacerbation and plain ol' giving up. (Though I'm guessing you didn't need a study to know that!) Thankfully, this is rarely a problem with Paleo, which doesn't require restriction or calorie counting, or intermittent fasting, which lets you eat bountifully each and every day! Log that thought away for any nervous fasting moments, as you remember that the yummy, abundant food shall soon come!

STRESS PERCEPTION

Fasting is a hormetic or "good" stress, which conditions the body to resist future stress. But even if it weren't a good stress, studies show that stress perception matters. Thinking a stress is bad can make it have more damaging effects on the body, while thinking a stress is good may not only deter negative effects but actually strengthen the body. Embrace your fasting window as a beneficial, hormetic stress to encourage resilience and success!

THE POWER OF ROUTINE

Repetition creates patterns in the brain. This means each time you successfully "fulfill" your chosen dietary protocol, you're making it *that much easier* next time! See each successful Paleo meal or IF day as another brushstroke forming a beautiful dietary painting, one you can soon hang on your wall and casually be like, "Oh yeah, I bought this self-portrait of me the Paleo, intermittent faster, ya know . . ."

LEARNING EXPERIMENT

Studies find that achieving goals is easier when viewed as a learning experiment rather than a performance test, so don't see Paleo or IF as a pass-or-fail exam.

Instead, see them as a new experience, which will show you how a different meal approach *feels*. Rather than thinking, "I will do this right, otherwise it was pointless," think, "I will do this, and then I will know how it feels."

IMAGINATION

Obliterating cravings via imagination harkens all the way back to my lamentable days of *actual* calorie restriction. While munching on bland 100-calorie Frankenfoods, I'd envision myself in my epically dieted body, evoking the grace of Grace Kelly at some fancy-schmancy party, waltzing with a dashing gentleman to the envy of onlookers. Such fantasies tended to nip cravings in the bud! And apparently it's not just me. A 2005 study found that dieters who imagined being on vacation experienced fewer subsequent food cravings throughout the day, compared to dieters who imagined their favorite food.[26] And there's a reason for this. It's a survival thing. We're basically wired to indulge in what feels good *now*.

Ya see, back in our hunter-gatherer days, it didn't make sense to value the future over the present, since the future was uncertain. So even though we may *know* that eating something crappy will make us feel crappy later, our brains are programmed to ignore that. To hack this, you can utilize "episodic future thinking," in which you vividly imagine yourself in the future. This encourages your brain to perceive the future as more immediate, and thus weigh its importance more heavily. Studies show that episodic future thinking can reduce food temptations by around 30 percent!

A person's vision of his or her future self can also shape his or her current self-perception and actions. Those who imagine a certain future are more likely to literally believe it will transpire, and they attain their goals as a consequence. So embrace the law of attraction, since imagining your way to the proverbial finish line just might help you reach the *actual* finish line!

FIND A HIGHER CAUSE

Identifying a reason outside of yourself for *why* you want to make a lifestyle change makes it more likely you'll stick to that lifestyle change. Studies show that doing things for external causes, especially other people, heightens self-control. You could consider starting Paleo or IF not entirely for yourself, but also to inspire others to make lifestyle changes. You could do it for your parents, spouse, friends, and/or future children. You could do it for God, or out of respect for your own health and body. While I discourage you from feeling pressured to do things for others, some selfless purpose can solidify a lifestyle-change commitment, while potentially encouraging others along the way! Everybody wins!

JUST #COMMIT

Resolute commitment fosters more drive and motivation than a lukewarm "Well, maybe . . ." by shifting focus to empowering goal attainment, rather than personal impediments. Studies find that strong intentions are more often realized than weak intentions, while specific and challenging goals lead to better performance. So choose your specific dietary plan, make it as challenging as you want, and just do it! You got this!

MAXIMIZED FAT BURNING

Like starting a round of Mario Kart with a perfectly timed rocket boost, implementing a Paleo and/or IF approach puts you leagues ahead in the fat-burning game. But why stop there? After adopting your new "what" and/or "when" for a few weeks to establish a baseline, extremists can use these tips and tricks to maximize fat burning!

ADJUST YOUR MACROS

I firmly believe that no single carb/fat/protein percentage works ideally for everyone. (After all, 1 + 7 = 8, but so does 4 + 4!) That said, feel free to play around with different macros. Sometimes switching things up—even if just temporarily—with a bit of keto here, or some higher-carb there, can shake things up a bit.

ADJUST YOUR FOOD INTAKE

Don't freak out! I'm not about to unsay everything I've said about not counting calories, and I do not support a restrictive mindset by any means. I do, however, believe you can engage in healthy dietary energy restriction while implementing IF, particularly if you have lots of fat to lose. Studies consistently link calorie restriction with decreased oxidative stress and aging, reduced inflammation, and increased longevity. If you've got the fat to burn and want to fiddle with eating less, I say go for it! Just make sure you're getting adequate nutrition via healthy, Paleo whole foods. Plus, a "calorie-restricted" diet while intermittent fasting may not even be calorie-restricted from your body's perspective, since IF assures ample fuel from fat stores!

ADJUST YOUR WINDOWS

Your IF windows are totally flexible, and you can always fast longer or shorten your eating window. The longer you fast, the more fat you burn! I personally never eat until I'm actually hungry, even if it's my "normal" eating time.

HIIT

To really blast away fat via fasted exercise, try a bit of High Intensity Interval Training (HIIT). It's sort of like a hot, temporary fling granting an epic body, with minimal time or emotional pain investment required. HIIT is a form of cardiovascular exercise in which you alternate short, intense, maximum-effort sprints for around fifteen to thirty seconds, with slower recovery periods for around thirty seconds to two minutes. Unlike hours of cardio, a typical HIIT session lasts anywhere from four to thirty minutes. Studies suggest a mere half hour of HIIT three times per week may yield the same physical improvements as an entire hour of normal cardio five times per week!

HIIT supports both aerobic and anaerobic fitness, for all types of people: men and women, trained and nontrained, diabetic and nondiabetic. It's great for insulin sensitivity, blood sugar stabilization, and cardiovascular health, with even very small amounts significantly increasing heart rate. HIIT also increases VO2 max—which involves the body's use of oxygen for energy—much better than endurance training. In fact, studies suggest HIIT might be the *only* way for trained athletes who have stabilized at a certain level of fitness to substantially improve these endurance exercise factors.

HIIT *really* shines in the fat-burning arena! In the best of both worlds, HIIT uniquely chips away at glucose stores activated by short, intense movement, while also tapping into body fat typically used in longer, steady-state activity. It upregulates catecholamines such as epinephrine and norepinephrine to unlock fat cells throughout the body, including from subcutaneous fat, stubborn fat, and abdominal fat. And HIIT discourages skinny fat syndrome by supporting muscle, rendering them both glycolytic (sugar burning) *and* oxidative (fat burning), while also jacking up growth hormones, which encourage muscle growth and recovery.

But we're not done yet! Even after the sweat from your HIIT fling has dried, the afterburn lingers on! Catecholamines released during an HIIT session remain elevated for a substantial amount of time, stimulating the body to continue burning fat post-exercise, no conscious effort required! The body also burns fat post-HIIT as it works to remove excess lactic acid, resynthesize glycogen, and rebuild muscle oxygen stores for an estimated sixteen to twenty-four hours *after* an HIIT session! This means you may easily burn more from a brief HIIT session than from a longer endurance session, with less effort to boot!

As a cherry on top, HIIT actually *reduces* appetite post-workout, possibly by the release of an anorectic peptide called corticotropin-releasing factor. So bid farewell to the ravenous *"Eat all the things"* monster, which may have undone your workout attempts of old.

HOW TO DO HIIT

Please keep in mind that HIIT is meant to be short in duration, and should not be extended beyond thirty minutes or so. If you're new to HIIT, please start gradually, and increase only as you feel comfortable. (Do not jump right to the highest speed that your machine allows—not a good idea!) Make sure to stay hydrated, and monitor yourself post-workout for adequate recovery. If you experience muscle loss or injury, fatigue, or an overall decrease in energy, please scale back on the HIIT, or discontinue it entirely. So with that disclaimer (gotta keep things real!), try one of the following simple HIIT protocols, once or twice per week:

The Structured Approach

1. Warm up for three to five minutes.
2. Intense period—run/elliptical/whatever *intensely* at your max effort for fifteen seconds to one minute.
3. Recovery period—walk/jog/whatever *slowly* or *moderately* for fifteen seconds to two minutes.
4. Alternate the intense period and recovery period until you reach your time block goal, between four and thirty minutes total.

That's pretty much it! While studies indicate that a two-to-one ratio of workout time to recovery period may work best, you can play around with the ratios. Find what works for you!

The Four-Minute Quickie

Only got a little bit of time? Try alternating twenty seconds of intense activity with ten seconds of recovery. Do this eight times. Four minutes down, and you're done!

The Musical Approach

In this more laissez-fair approach to HIIT, turn on an upbeat pop song. Simply walk/sway during the verses, and sprint/jump/dance during the chorus! Repeat as desired!

GOLDEN HOUR

If you choose to engage in any movement, such as traditional exercise, HIIT, or more functional activities (hiking, cleaning, dancing, etc.), consider doing so in the "golden hour" near the end of your fast. This is when any physical activity will most likely tap into particularly stubborn fat stores. (After all, you don't really go to your last resort until it's your last resort.)

If you want to take a more casual approach, begin a ritual of ending your fast with some sort of pre-meal, ten-minute victory dance. Jump around for pure joy to the tune of {insert favorite song here} before your feast, and watch the pounds melt away!

COLD THERMOGENESIS

I'm a big fan of fat burning that just sort of happens, in a "Who, me?" type way. You simply create the situation, and all the cellular work is done for you! Cold thermogenesis is just that. It occurs when you subject your body to cold temperatures, which responds by generating heat to keep you warm. Not only does cold thermogenesis boost the metabolism, it notably tackles brown adipose tissue: a type of body fat specifically reserved for heat production. You're not gonna easily burn this stuff unless things get a little chilly! That said, cold thermogenesis is actually of the *nonshivering* sort: The *more* you increase consistent cold exposure, the *less* you end up shivering, and the warmer you feel! So embrace your inner Elsa to let that fat go!

Better yet, cold thermogenesis comes with an array of health benefits! It can promote anti-inflammatory metabolic changes, reduce oxidative stress, support healthy cellular mitochondria, boost the immune system, and combat feelings of fatigue.

FUNCTIONAL EXERCISE

Truth be told, I believe we have done *movement* a bit of a disservice in labeling it as "exercise," like it's some quota to be filled. Rather than simply supporting our ability to rejoice in physical activity, our modern perspective brands movement with negative connotations, in a "No pain, No gain!" type way. We believe we must commit to a certain number of sweaty gym hours to atone for sedentary and dietary sins.

Before IF, I both loathed and loved my gym excursions. The first thirty minutes would be spent in a dread-filled, weary attempt to feel energized and enter "fat-burning mode." By the time I reached this elusive zone (which *did* feel pretty good if actually attained), I typically had to wrap things up. The whole experience would leave me with minimal fat burning and a seemingly warranted appetite to devour everything in sight. Needless to say: not very effective. Strength training was equally suspect. While I avoided carrying heavy things in "real life" and saw lifting objects as a chore, I'd march to the gym and painfully strain against apathetic machines to make myself "stronger." Silly me!

IF changes the exercise game by welcoming fat-burning mode *all the time*, so everything you do becomes "exercise." You don't need to "do" cardio to burn fat, because you're *always* burning fat. You can exercise less, while making it mean more. You also may begin viewing daily physical activity with newfound joy, as such activity is fueled by generous fat stores, rather than greedy glycogen and the sum of your last meal. Rather than go to the gym, I now simply embrace the wondrous movement of life, and am in much better shape for it! (Of course, if the gym is your thing, do your thing!)

NEAT

NEAT refers to all of the subconscious movement we do as a daily part of life, such as fidgeting, cooking, pacing, dancing, fighting, and laughing. NEAT's energy-burning potential is so vast that a person can burn up to 2,000 calories per day just from NEAT alone. Such. A. Fan. Since IF puts you into a perpetual fat-burning mode, body fat will automatically fuel any NEAT activity, which quickly adds up! NEAT also does not register as abnormal physical exertion in the body, and thus discourages a rebound response to conserve calories. (You typically don't get a raging appetite from laughing for hours with your friends.) Basically, IF plus NEAT allows you to burn more fat without ramifications: You don't sweat the small or big stuff, while kinda sweating *all the stuff.*

HOW TO MAXIMIZE NEAT

- Pace while talking on the phone.
- Sit up straight. (You can wear an ab or posture belt to keep yourself aware of this.)
- Park in the farthest spot from your destination. Not only will you rack up NEAT points, you'll also never worry about parking again. Double win.
- Offer to open doors and carry things for people. Not only will you burn more NEAT calories and build more muscle, but people will also think you're a super nice person. Again, double win.
- Use a grocery basket rather than a cart.
- Embrace housecleaning as NEAT expenditure. Rock that vacuum for all it's worth!

- Listen to upbeat music, and move around with pep in your step. Pretend life is a music video.
- Combine the two previous ones, and dance *while* cleaning.
- Never squint to see something—just walk over and see it!
- Rather than yelling at the top of your lungs or texting your family member on the other side of the house, go find them personally.
- While standing in line, stand on one leg or step side to side or clench random muscles. Who cares if you look like a nervous flamingo.
- Sit on an exercise ball rather than a chair. This will force your body to constantly maintain balance and posture, stimulating more NEAT than normal sitting.
- Consider a standing desk. If that's too $$, just stand at your desk. Or make a standing desk out of an IKEA diaper-changing station.
- Walk around while listening to an audiobook.
- Consider squatting at the toilet rather than sitting. You might do this anyway in public restrooms! (Or is that just me? TMI?)
- Keep things in order. See the objects lying around your room as potential NEAT implementation. Never again shall thy jeans rest on the floor, or thy mail be scattered on the desk!
- Embrace seemingly mundane tasks as NEAT, fat-burning adventures! Do them with *passion*, as the increased energy will further increase NEAT. *Oh yes, let me take out this trash! Oh yes, let me do my server side work! Oh yes, let me properly dispose of my gum rather than litter! Oh yes, let me save the world!*

BODY WEIGHTS

While you can always partake in gym-style strength training, I prefer a sneaky shortcut: Wear body weights to maximize strength building from daily movement. Simply strap on one- to two-pound wrist weights and three- to four-pound ankle weights, with perhaps an occasional weighted vest, and *presto*! Just like the pumpkin became Cinderella's carriage, daily life becomes strength training! I even wear my weights with pride to the grocery store. (In LA, no one really gives it a second glance, but at home in the South, people are like . . . umm #weirdo.) With body weights, every movement you do, from cleaning to picking up a magazine to making dinner, automatically burns more fat *and* builds muscle. It also strengthens the muscles you *actually* use, making it quite applicable to life, rather than just stroking vanity.

HOW?

FOOD QUALITY GUIDE

As a struggling actress/writer who just wants to eat healthy, nontoxic food that's also good for the environment (is that *so* much to ask?), I'm right there with you if ya think buying organic, grass-fed, and/or pasture-raised food costs a pretty penny, or that fishing practices and their corresponding labels ("Wild caught!" "Responsibly farmed!" "Farm raised!") are insanely confusing when the extent of your related experience caps at childhood fishing trips and *Finding Nemo*. (Or maybe sport fishing is totally your thing? If so—that's pretty cool!)

In this section, we'll evaluate the nutritional differences of various agriculture practices, so you can judge where to invest your hard-earned (gluten-free) dough.

BEEF

Despite its current manifestation as an expensive novelty, essentially all beef until the 1940s was grass fed, and we were likely much better off for it! While both grass-fed and grain-fed beef feature comparable total amounts of saturated and polyunsaturated fats, grass-fed beef is leaner overall, with better *types* of fat to boot. On the saturated side of things, grass-fed beef features more stearic fatty acids, which do not detrimentally affect cholesterol levels, whereas grain-fed contains more potentially cholesterol-raising myristic and palmitic fatty acids. Grass-fed beef also contains significantly higher levels of the anti-inflammatory polyunsaturated omega-3 fats. In fact, the *more* grains the cattle eat, the *less* omega-3s they generate. (For more on the omega-6-to-omega-3 ratio, check out "Fat Problems" on page 28.) Lastly, grass-fed beef can yield two to three times more conjugated linoleic acid (CLA), which may discourage weight gain, diabetes, and cancer.

On the flip side, grain-fed beef *does* typically contain higher levels of healthy monounsaturated fats (MUFA) than grass-fed beef, likely because that's how its *excess* fat materializes. (As discussed, grain-fed beef tends to be fattier than grass-fed.). In any case, I'd much rather embrace the overall leaner, healthier saturated and polyunsaturated fat of grass-fed beef than turn to grain-fed for more MUFA. (Go to avocados for those!)

As for vitamins, grass-fed beef contains around seven times more carotene—the precursor for vitamin A—which gives the beef its characteristic yellow tone. Vitamin A is key for bone health, vision, the immune system, cell reproduction, and membranes throughout the body, from the eyes to the lungs to the nether regions! Grass-fed beef also contains around three times the amount of the antioxidant vitamin E, specifically its potent α-tocopherol form, which can combat free radicals and toxins in the body. These vitamin E levels discourage oxidation, meaning grass-fed varieties may last longer in your fridge. Oh hey, money saving!

Other antioxidants boosted by the pasture include glutathione, superoxide dismutase (SOD), and catalase (CAT), thanks to their presence in grass. Glutathione, akin to the Superman of antioxidants, regulates inflammation, attacks free radicals, and protects DNA and proteins throughout the cells of the body. SOD and CAT are more like Batman and Robin: SOD attacks with hydrogen peroxide, while CAT breaks down the hydrogen peroxide. Pretty nifty.

On par with the importance of what grass-fed beef contains is what it *doesn't* contain. Since living bodies often shuttle toxins into fat stores to protect vital systems, cattle dining on the pesticides, hormones, genetically modified organisms (GMOs), and other toxins in grain-fed cows' food easily accumulate in beef fat. Studies even find things such as dioxins, PCBs, and flame retardants in conventional beef—yikes!

BUTTER

The makeup of butter's four hundred-ish fatty acids (oh my!) is largely determined by the lactating animal's diet and gut microbiome. You want your milkers going to town on nutrient-rich food while not being exposed to gut-disrupting antibiotics and hormones. Butter from grass-fed cow milk features more omega-3 fats (including the bioavailable forms of EPA and DHA), vitamin A, vitamin K_2, and around 500 percent more CLA. When you begin consuming rich, golden grass-fed butter (which isn't much more expensive, all things considered), I'll bet you'll never go back to the lackluster conventional butters that pale, quite literally, in comparison.

CHICKEN AND EGGS

Like beef, conventional agriculture practices encourage a host of yucky things in chicken meat, from pesticides to GMOs to arsenic! Studies even suggest the prevalence of antibiotics in chicken feed fuels the growing problem of antibiotic resistance and disease in humans. (A 2015 Vietnamese study found antibiotic residues in around one-fifth of all chicken tested.)[1] Chickens that eat chicken feed are also often promoted as having been "fed a vegetarian diet" as if that's a good thing. But chickens aren't vegetarian! They naturally scuttle around for a host of critters to provide vital proteins and nutrients. Feeding them a vegetarian diet can impede nutrition and yield insufficient protein, particularly the amino acid methionine.

Like chicken meat, pesticide residues can also accumulate in eggs, at levels officially leading to health risks. Pastured eggs, on the other hand, have been shown to contain around twice as much vitamin E, 2.5 times more omega-3s, as well as more vitamin A, lutein, lycopene, and zeaxanthin. And since these chickens can frolic in sunlit fields rather than camp out 24/7 in indoor cages, pastured eggs may contain anywhere from 30 to 600 percent more vitamin D.

Unlike pre–World War II days of selecting healthy live chickens for dinner, today we often purchase prepackaged portions in vacuum-sealed containers. A lot of funky business can go on behind the scenes to produce these chickens that reach market weight with larger breasts in *half* the time. Not surprisingly, it takes less-than-pleasant situations to engineer such a feat. Which brings us to . . .

STRESS EFFECTS

While it may seem a bit hocus-pocusy to say a departed animal's stress can affect your pot roast or chicken dinner . . . there's actually some truth to it. When an animal is killed, its muscle glycogen transforms into lactic acid, which keeps the meat plump and juicy. Stressful situations (such as from cramped, dark growing conditions and other treatment methods) release adrenaline and reduce muscle glycogen, resulting in less lactic acid and flavorless, off-colored meat. Lactic acid also protects against spoilage, so conventionally stressed meat is more likely to contain bacteria, go rancid, and instigate food poisoning. Less lactic acid also leads to more acidic meat and free radicals—yikesabee!

So while you may want to raise an eyebrow when a server pushes an expensive cut of grass-fed Wagyu, or a farm brags about its happy chickens . . . know there's something to that! Eating fear for dinner may not taste the best, and it can weigh on your conscience to boot!

ORGANIC PRODUCE

I used to view "organic" as a charlatan label promising coolness while secretly fueling a fast-growing billion-dollar industry. Surely if you're just buying veggies in the first place, you're doing well enough, right? Maybe. Or maybe not.

Studies pretty consistently find that organic practices yield produce that is significantly richer in nutrition—particularly magnesium, phosphorus, iron, carotenoids, and vitamin C, as well as phenolic antioxidants and flavonoids. (Since plant polyphenols serve as defense mechanisms, it makes sense that organic produce with fewer "protective" pesticides would naturally generate more of these compounds.) Studies have also found more potent anticancer action in organic versions.

That said, a multitude of factors can affect a plant's nutritional status, including an area's weather in a given year, soil mineral availability, and airborne exposure to neighboring pesticides. And while U.S. government regulations mandate that organic practices must be implemented for three years before produce can be certified organic, it can take up to a decade for diluted soil to regain its richness. Thankfully, the longer a location is organic, the more nutritious its produce becomes, as nutrients build up in the soil, while pollutants and pesticides diminish.

Speaking of the latter, organic produce does drastically reduce exposure to pesticides, herbicides, and fungicides. While these compounds are "generally recognized as safe," studies increasingly find an underestimated toxicity. Up to sixty of these chemicals have been determined carcinogenic. No big deal. And they're linked to all types of cancer, from ovarian to brain to connective tissue, as well as cancer in children. Other negative pesticide effects include developmental, central nervous system, immune, and cardiac problems. Reproductive toxicity is a particular concern, including reduced fertility, deterred fetal growth, and even natural abortion. Pesticides can also be genotoxic, affecting genes and cellular DNA, as well as endocrine disruptors, which alter hormones throughout the body. And on the foundational digestive side of things, pesticides may affect the oral and gut microbiome.

Unfortunately, most pesticides are tested solely for *acute* toxicity. While pesticide poisoning lamentably continues to occur upon immediate exposure worldwide, chronic long-term, lower-grade exposure may be a more expansive problem. Exposure to different types of pesticides from different produce further heightens toxicity, so if you're eating various types of pesticide-covered veggies every day, we may have a problem!

Perhaps most notably, pesticides are judged by the toxicity of their "active" ingredient rather than their entire formulation, which typically contains multiple compounds. These can include confidential "adjuvants," which, despite being labeled "inert," strengthen the pesticide and add their own toxicity. Such a farce! When a 2014 study looked at the effects of the entire composition of nine pesticides on three types of human cells, it found they were up to *a thousand times* more cytotoxic than the active ingredient used to qualify them, and were even more toxic at lower concentrations than those used in agriculture.[2] Pesticide testing is also performed on animals, though human cells, such as those of the umbilical cord, can be substantially more sensitive.

It can be pretty difficult to escape these assailants. Though only an estimated 0.1 percent of pesticides may reach their intended bug target (not a typo!), the remaining 99.9 percent can be anywhere and everywhere—including across continents! Even organic produce can be contaminated with preexisting pesticide residues from the air and soil. (This means greenhouse-grown produce may be particularly able to avoid pesticides, as well as heavy metals from the soil.) That said, organic produce *does* feature an estimated one-third to three-quarters less residue than conventional forms.

And yep, these pesticides can accumulate in humans, with a particular fancy for fat, liver, brain, and breast tissue. Studies have even found pesticide residue in breast milk! A Seattle study also found that preschoolers who ate conventional foods had six times more pesticide residues in their urine than those who ate organically. (Props to those organic moms!) Thankfully, switching the preschoolers' diets to organic foods successfully reduced their pesticide pee.

THE TAKEAWAY?

If all this grass-fed/grain-fed/organic/pesticide business has you nervously clutching your wallet as you eye the steak and spinach, I got you covered! While I obviously suggest purchasing the best you can afford, here are some realistic tips.

MEAT: Since toxins accumulate in fat, favor organic and grass-fed for fattier cuts. When buying conventional, consider lean beef and chicken. (You can then add healthy fats such as avocado, coconut oil, or organic, grass-fed butter/ghee.) Avoid conventional ground beef, since you have no way of skipping around the fat.

DAIRY/BUTTER: Really try to stick to grass-fed and organic on this one, as milk products are ripe for toxin and hormone accumulation. Trust me, the extra dollar or two is totally worth it!

EGGS: Pastured eggs are way more nutritious, and increasingly more affordable. That said, if you *have* to skimp on this, I understand.

PRODUCE: For fruits and vegetables with edible surface areas (think leafy greens, broccoli, and strawberries), try as best as you can to go organic. Save conventional purchases for produce where you just consume the inside, such as avocados or pineapple. Root vegetables (such as sweet potatoes, turnips, and carrots) tend to absorb pesticides and heavy metals from the soil, so try to go organic on those as well. You can consult the Environmental Working Group's website for a current list of produce highest and lowest in pesticides.

As a final note, conventional produce and meat is still better than processed foods, sugar, and grains any day! "I can't afford organic, so I'll just buy pasta" is not the way to think here.

SEAFOOD

Growing up, I never fancied fish, unless it was disguised in carbolicious salmon patties or fried popcorn shrimp, yet I now eat it many (if not most) nights of the week! Thankfully, my obsession has benefits, as seafood provides many oft-lacking, *key* nutrients, such as iodine, selenium, a multitude of vitamins (including some vitamin D!), and, perhaps most important, the vital EPA and DHA forms of omega-3s. Our ability to fish was likely a major catalyst in the evolution of our species, and seafood is a primary constituent in the diets of many centenarian populations. Basically, seafood is da bomb.

That said, things get tricky. As per usual.

Thanks to us humans having polluted our oceans, heavy metals (such as mercury), radioactive isotopes, and other toxins easily accumulate in wild fish. Farm-raised versions are also typically awash in antibiotics, grain and GMO feed, and disgusting by-products. (Think sewage sludge. Ew.) Overfishing also taxes natural fish populations, spelling trouble for future generations.

So what's a fish-loving modern-day hunter-gatherer to do?

For starters, I wholeheartedly recommend you check out the Environmental Defense Fund's "Seafood Selector" for the current sustainability, mercury, and omega-3 status of different fish. In general, fish lower in the food chain tend to feature fewer toxins, which have less time to build up in their systems. (Salmon, anchovies, flounder, rainbow trout, and shellfish are often good choices, but step away from the ahi tuna, orange roughy, and swordfish!)

When it comes to labels of "wild caught" versus "farm raised," it's vital that you research the specific fish, producer, and home body of water (such as Atlantic versus Pacific cod). While we'd generally like to think "wild-caught" fish is best, those from polluted waters would not be ideal. On the flip side, though I suggest you stay away from most farm-raised fish, some producers implement sustainable, healthy practices without the use of antibiotics or problematic feed. (I regularly consume some farm-raised, responsibly sourced tilapia and barramundi.)

Frozen fish is often a better alternative to fresh fish; the latter are often sprayed with unnecessary additives to keep them looking pretty in the case. (Think: polyphosphate, sodium tripolyphosphate, nitrates, and many others!) Such additives are slightly less common in frozen fish, which can be flash-frozen for preservation. Frozen food also grants access to labels to check for such nefarious substances. (I personally like to stock up on some good frozen fish brands available at Costco.)

The takeaway? Seafood is one area where you're gonna have to do some fishing for info before purchasing, but know that your health, the environment, and future generations will thank you! (Or they would if they could.)

TRANSLATING FOOD LABELS

While you can totally know how you *want* your food to be raised, the plethora of supermarket labels may or may not mean what they imply. Here's the low-down on those stickers!

USDA ORGANIC

Bearing the label most regulated by the United States Department of Agriculture, "USDA organic" products are kept separate from conventional ones. Organic growing processes seek to preserve natural resources, encourage biodiversity, and mimic natural conditions of these crops in the wild.

Organic crops are grown in "safe" soil, with no synthetic fertilizers, synthetic pesticides, sewage sludge, GMOs, or irradiation within the prior three years. (That said, a long list of questionably approved substances *can* be used.) For organic livestock, ruminants must dine in the pasture the entire grazing season, for a minimum of three months, with 30 percent of supplemental feed from pasture. Poultry must be provided constant access to the outdoors. Both consume organic feed with no antibiotics or growth hormones.

Keep in mind that, given the rigorous application process, many farmers may practice organic methods without the official seal. I recommend conducting your own research on individual producers, particularly at local farmers markets. In fact, I'd probably prefer fresh produce and meat from a responsible local farmer than large-scale "organic" products from a mainstream grocery store.

SUSTAINABLE

"Sustainable" is an agricultural philosophy supporting the well-being of the environment and community without jeopardizing future generations. It is similar to "organic" in that both aim to minimize toxic practices, though "sustainable" is not regulated. Not all sustainable agriculture is organic. (For instance, "sustainable" use of nonorganic antibiotics or fertilizers.) On the flip side, not all organic agriculture is sustainable. (For instance, an organic farm could still be large and industrialized, therefore taxing resources.) In any case, I encourage you to individually research the companies and farms producing your food, and invest your money where you see fit. Labels are just labels, but a farm's actions speak louder than its words.

BIODYNAMIC

Arguably the crème de la crème of environmentally friendly practices, biodynamic agriculture extends organic and sustainable practices into even more philosophical terrain. The Demeter Association enforces the standards, and includes USDA organic certification rules in their stipulations. Biodynamic practices encourage biodiversity and are holistically in tune with nature, utilizing cyclical environmental patterns (such as the lunar cycle) and natural animal fertilization, among many other things. (Note: Biodynamic winemaking *does* allow added sulfites up to one hundred parts per million.)

GRASS-FED

This label is key for the nutritional content of beef, as it indicates that the cattle dined on their natural, nutrient-rich diet. However, the USDA withdrew their official definition of the term in January 2016.[3] While still regulated, farmers can now assume more individual standards, which infuses a bit of ambiguity. The label also does not address the use of antibiotics, pesticides, or GMOs, and supplemental grains could potentially still be used. Look for the less common term "grass finished" if you want to assure a 100 percent grass-fed diet.

FREE-RANGE

This USDA term simply means the poultry were not caged, and had access to the outdoors during their laying cycle. Whether they actually ventured outside is up for debate, while the "outside" area itself could be small and netted.

CAGE-FREE

This evasive USDA term signifies the poultry were provided constant access to food and water, with no literal cages. That said, the poultry likely didn't have outdoor access, and might have resided in cramped interior spaces. "Cage free" also says nothing of their diet, which was likely grain- or soy-based.

VEGETARIAN-FED

This misleading term rests on vegetarianism's positive reputation. Vegetarian feed could still be GMO, and is likely grain-, corn-, or soy-based. As discussed, chickens *aren't* naturally vegetarian, making "vegetarian-fed" simultaneously unnatural and less nutritious.

NATURAL

This USDA term means the meat is "minimally processed" with no artificial ingredients or colors. Vague.

PASTURE-RAISED

This one sounds great in theory, but isn't regulated at all, so do your research.

NO ADDED HORMONES

These animals were raised without added hormones. (Surprise, surprise.) It's really only applicable to beef or dairy products, since federal regulations have never allowed steroids or hormones in poultry, pork, or goat. Yep, chicken with "no added hormones" is just a trick to get your money. Sneaky devils.

SHOPPING GUIDE

Just because you won't be living off ramen noodles and cereal doesn't mean your new lifestyle has to be difficult or expensive. In favoring fresh foods, you'll be shopping on a more intuitive basis, rather than stocking up on tempting, overpriced goodies. And while packaged grains and processed foods may *seem* cheaper, you'll get a *ton* more nutrition from whole foods, while warding off future doctor visits. (There's a money saver!) Plus, buying organic, pastured food from the store is usually cheaper (and healthier!) than conventional food from a restaurant any day! #perspective. With all that in mind, utilize these tips for epic shopping and money saving, Paleo-style!

WHERE TO SHOP

REDRAW YOUR MAP

Consider grocery store geography! When going Paleo, you'll mostly stick to your store's outer perimeter, seeking fresh meat and produce. Only venture into the aisles for the occasional cold-pressed oils, special-occasion nut flours, or a nice bottle of red wine. The freezers are also up for grabs for meat and produce!

SHOP WHOLESALE

This is a big one, pun intended. Wholesale clubs are excellent for stocking up on fruits, veggies, meat, and even things such as coconut oil in bulk. (I'm *quite* a Costco lover, myself!) Become besties with your freezer! Many Paleo peeps even invest in an extra freezer to store large, grass-fed meat shipments ordered online, and find the investment quickly pays for itself!

FARMERS' MARKETS

Farmers' market adventures provide access to super fresh food, often at great prices, and are likely grown with love. Plus, you can inquire about growing practices straight from the source, rather than Googling/emailing the company after the fact. Use these tips to make the most of your adventures!

- Go early to beat crowds and get access to everything before it sells out, and for things that spoil, such as meat and fish.
- Go late to beat crowds and for potentially lower prices and discounts! (But keep in mind that many things may be sold out.)
- Go in great weather for a rosy good time, or in bad weather for potentially better prices!
- Don't immediately buy the first thing you see. Depending on the size of the market, consider surveying everything first.
- Don't be scared to barter!
- Even if an item isn't labeled organic, ask the farmer *why*. It may essentially be organic, just without the certification.
- Research the characteristics of individual produce—such as texture, weight, and color—to know which will taste best. You can also ask the farmers for advice!
- Check out the "uglier," misshapen produce for cheaper prices—just make sure it's not damaged or moldy.
- Consider buying in bulk to save money.
- Favor whole rather than precut produce to save money *and* extend shelf life. The greens on root vegetables are edible as well!

- Remember the available food will be determined by what's in season, which you can research ahead of time. (And even if there's some produce *not* in season, your best bet for taste and nutrition is still sticking to what's in season.)
- Many markets are cash only: Bring small bills and change.
- Engage with the farmers to learn about the growing practices, as well as cooking and preparation recommendations!
- Bring your own sturdy, reusable (potentially insulated!) bags.
- Consider bringing a stroller or cart as well.
- If you plan on getting dairy, meat, fish, or fermented foods, consider bringing a cooler.
- Don't be scared to try the unique, weird stuff you can't find at your normal grocery store. That's half the fun!
- Bring a friend! Or even consider making it a date!
- And of course, have fun!!

BUTCHER SHOPS

Seek out local butcher shops for quality meat at potentially better prices. These are also great for off-kilter cuts, organ meats, and bones for bone broth!

CO-OPS

Growing up, I raised an eyebrow at my seemingly crazy relatives' conspiratorial-sounding co-ops. Nowadays, I'm totally on board! Co-ops, which are becoming increasingly popular, allow you to join forces with like-minded people to purchase healthy, sustainable whole foods at decent prices.

ONLINE

Consider shopping online for oils, spices, supplements, and even groceries. Not gonna lie, Amazon Prime's two-day free shipping is seriously my obsession.

Or try out the membership-based Thrive Market, which features many Paleo-friendly goods at wholesale prices.

DELIVERY SERVICES

Many online delivery meal-preparation services can provide organic, diet-tailored ingredients and recipes, shipped straight to your door. Plus, the competition keeps the costs down!

HOW TO SHOP

LABELS

Try buying foods that (arguably) shouldn't need labels. That said, *do* check those labels when present, and look for sneaky substances. You may be shocked by things added to foods you'd *think* would be just one ingredient. Once you start seeing labels (and not for the calories!), it's hard to look back. Don't automatically believe the promises. If a package proclaims "all natural," confirm on the back. It's probably not. Just saying.

DON'T PAY FOR CONVENIENCE

Ya know what's convenient? Having more money. Don't be fueled by the apparent ease of "ready-made" foods. It doesn't take *that* much longer to chop a head of lettuce. (Plus you get an arm workout thrown in! #Functionalexercise)

PLAN AND RESEARCH

After your Paleo honeymoon period in which you view the grocery store with newfound wonder (*So many new food experiences!*), you might want to adopt a more regimented mindset. Know what you like, what you need, and stick to it. Research various producers to know which are most friendly for your health and budget needs. Keep in mind that some brands are essentially organic but don't sport the official seal. (I've found many greenhouse-grown produce lines to be great, despite not being officially organic.)

WHAT TO SHOP

FROZEN FOODS

Frozen food can save time and money, discourage spoilage, and enhance nutrition. While fresh produce is often picked prematurely to allow ripening time in transport, frozen produce is typically frozen at its peak nutritional state, and can actually contain higher levels of antioxidants and nutrients, particularly the volatile vitamin C. Frozen fish is also less likely to contain preservatives, unlike its "fresh" counterparts, which are often sprayed with nefarious sulfites, sorbates, and nitrites to maintain their alluring shine.

NEW THINGS

You don't have to stick to sirloins and chicken breasts! As your taste buds begin to change, you may discover an appreciation for different (often more nutritious yet cheaper) types and cuts of meat than before. Ponder the culinary adventures of shank, oxtail, London broil, organ meats, bison, etc. The list goes on and on! (Check out the "Recipes" on page 269 for some cooking methods!)

WHOLE CHICKENS

Why pay a premium for a single-serve, vacuum-sealed breast when you can get cheaper, enhanced nutrition from a whole pastured chicken that lasts for days! Think: the meat entrée, then soup from the broth, then broth from the bones!

OILS

While I don't advocate slathering everything in refined fats, healthy cold-pressed oils and animal fats can enliven a meal, and also provide a lot of bang for their buck, calorie-wise. Think about how much energy is stored in a single jar of coconut or olive oil!

CARBS

If you're currently more of a carb lover than keto lover, you can get a ton of food for cheap from Paleo-approved sources such as sweet potatoes, as well as potential Paleo candidates such as white rice and potatoes, depending on your personal tolerances. (Definitely try to go organic on these.) Check out the "Personal Paleo Guide" on page 48 for more on all that!

SPICES

Organic spices are one of the cheapest, easiest paths to tasty variety, while providing their own potent health benefits. Spices for the win!

WATER

You can make vast improvements in your well-being by forgoing fluorinated, toxic tap water and/or pricey, plasticky bottled water. Try filling your own glass gallons with filtered water, available at many health food stores (I get mine at Whole Foods). You'll get a *ton* more water for a fraction of the price, while squeezing in some functional exercise carrying those jugs! Once you make the switch, it's *insanely* easy and awesome, in a "Why didn't I do this earlier?" type way. Plus, you're going to the store anyway, so why not?

SUPPLEMENTS

Avoid supplement black holes, as health comes primarily through food and lifestyle, rather than a pill. (I sigh at all the money I've wasted on the latter.) Research a supplement before purchase, evaluate its effects when you get it, and only keep it if it truly enhances your life.

COOKING GUIDE

Do you get high on home-cooked aromas while Instagramming self-created food masterpieces? Perhaps you're more a romancer of restaurant dates and to-go food? Or maybe you're somewhere in between—open to a bit of cooking if convenient and reasonably tasty? In any case, the time has come to explore the magical and liberating world of food preparation, which can seriously be as simple or as complex as you like! Get ready for healthier and yummier meals that save money, recover your sanity, and *still* could make your favorite restaurant green with envy! In this section, we'll explore tips and tricks for home cooking, as well as the specific benefits and downsides of various cooking methods, so you can cultivate a Paleo culinary world worthy of your inner Julia Child (she's in there somewhere!).

COOKING TIPS

LEARN

If you're not already savvy, invest the time to learn how to chop, grate, mince, simmer, sauté, and #allthethings for yourself. With a bit of practice, these invaluable (and easy!) skills welcome a whole new world of food that tastes awesome, boosts health, and fits your schedule!

FEEL FREE TO GO SIMPLE

Keep in mind not every (or even *any*) meal need be a Michelin candidate. While experimentation can be a blast (and the yummy "Recipes" section on page 269 features a range of complexity), you can eat as simply as you like, as often as you like. (I eat simply most of the time.)

REDEFINE MEALS

Don't be confined by convention. Who says breakfast has to be pancakes? You can totally do meat and veggies for breakfast, or eggs for dinner!

MAKE YOUR OWN

Though making your own condiments, sauces, or food novelties may seem a smidge daunting, it's actually easy, fun, and cost-effective! Plus, you can adjust ingredients and macros to your liking, while knowing *exactly* what's going on in that Caesar dressing or coconut ice cream.

GROW YOUR OWN

You don't have to go hard-core Old MacDonald, but consider growing some of your favorite spices or even veggies here and there! It costs barely anything but patience, eradicates pesticides and toxins, and generates a feeling of connection to your food.

SMART RECIPES

Make recipes you know you like, with ingredients you know you'll use. Sure, that complicated thirty-ingredient soup will probably taste fantastic, but will you ultimately use those thirty ingredients later? Except for the chemistry of baking, you can also *usually* play around with things. Experiment and substitute! If a recipe calls for a spice you'll never use again, consider omitting it, or substituting one you already know you love!

FREEZERS

For the ultimate convenience, fancy your freezer! You can easily cook in bulk, and freeze individual portions for homemade Paleo frozen dinners!

COOKING METHODS

The many cooking methods available today welcome a world of different tastes, textures, and times. Even seemingly foreign methods (Hi, pressure cooker!) can rival the convenience of the microwave, with substantially more flavor at that! Consider adding the following techniques to your culinary arsenal, and keep in mind that initial investment costs quickly pay for themselves!

OVEN

Okay, most people are probably familiar with this one, which almost always comes built in with your house! For this traditional method, favor lower temperatures (up to 300°F) to discourage advanced glycation end products (AGEs), oxidation, and nutrient breakdown (more on all that in a bit!). Convection ovens, by the way, recirculate air to evenly distribute heat, allowing speedier cooking at lower temperatures.

STEAMER

Steamers gently cook meat and veggies with water. While some people perceive steamed food as bland, I find it quite yummy! Plus, many steamers feature delayed timers, "keep warm" settings, and drip pans, rendering them highly convenient.

SLOW COOKER

Slow cookers are the oxymoron of cooking methods: easy, quick meals that take a long time. Basically, you throw in your ingredients in the morning and come home to a delicious dinner that's instantly ready! Slow cookers are great for soups, stews, whole chickens, shanks, pot roasts, and bone broths!

PRESSURE COOKER

Sort of like a slow cooker on steroids, a pressure cooker *drastically* reduces cooking times by cooking with (you guessed it!) pressure. They're sort of magical; they're capable, for example, of turning tough, collagen-rich shanks—which would take all day in a slow cooker—into delicious tenderness in under an hour! In fact, if you invest in just *one* kitchen appliance, I wholeheartedly recommend the Instant Pot, which can function as a slow cooker, steamer, *and* pressure cooker, with ridiculously easy cleanup to boot!

MICROWAVE

For the darling of convenience and controversy, look no further than the microwave! While the jury might forever be out, microwaves *may* not be the demon they're often perceived to be. By cooking food for brief periods of time,[4] microwaves can reasonably preserve nutrients (particularly vitamin C and anti-oxidants) while encouraging less AGE and amine formation (more on those in the next section!).[5] As for health concerns, microwaves work by simply vibrating (rather than ionizing) food particles via electromagnetic waves, which are shorter than visible light. Most of these waves are contained entirely within the unit, and rodent studies show they're likely not particularly cancer promoting. That said, I probably wouldn't stand by the microwave and stare at your food, and I also reserve the right to change my stance if future research reveals more deleterious effects. Downsides to microwave cooking include uneven cooking temperatures, less-than-ideal textures, and temptations to embrace TV dinners.

BLENDER

Though you may associate them with shakes and smoothies, blenders are also great for sauces, condiments, veggie mashes, and soups (including hot ones in powerful enough models). And blending frozen fruits can create instant, Paleo-friendly sorbets!

ICE CREAM MAKER

If you're an ice cream lover, you've got to get one of these! Making your own ice cream frees you from the many fillers, gums, and sweeteners in mainstream products. You can easily make dairy-free frozen goodies, or more traditional ice creams from grass-fed, organic, and even probiotic-rich dairy sources. Check out the "Recipes" on page 269 for a basic, dairy-free coconut milk ice cream recipe!

FERMENTING

Fermentation is *sort of* a cooking method, in that food is broken down and transformed, not by heat, but by bacteria. The process creates foods (such as sauerkrauts) rich in beneficial probiotics, which support the gut microbiome, immune system, and digestive health. I wholeheartedly encourage you to explore the (fun!) world of home fermentation, to create live, raw concoctions free of excess salt and pasteurization. A basic sauerkraut recipe is provided in the "Recipes" section on page 281. Please visit MelanieAvalon.com/fermentationguide for more tips on fermenting at home, or check out books such as *Wild Fermentation* by Sandor Ellix Katz. (Note: Fermented foods can be rich in histamine, and also may be problematic based on one's individual gut microbiome.)

HEALTHIEST COOKING METHODS?

By rendering energy and nutrients more available, the ability to cook cata-pulted the evolution of the human species, separating the men from the monkeys (and their smaller brains fueled by raw plant-based diets). That said, just like there is no single perfect diet, it seems there is no single perfect cooking method either. While you may want to pledge allegiance to #teamgrill or #rawfood, studies consistently find nutrient availability levels vary based on the specific food and cooking method. Cooking also holds the potential to generate inflammatory by-products, but also to break down problematic compounds in foods.

MEAT

While cooking meat kills potential pathogens and enhances nutrient availability, it can produce unpleasant by-products, such as heterocyclic amines (HCAs), polycyclic aromatic hydrocarbon (PAHs), advanced glycation end products (AGEs), and oxidized fats. These can promote stress, inflammation, and disease in the body. With meat, you might *not* want to perfectly reenact the caveman tableau, since cooking "rustically" with dry heat, high temperatures (above about 300ºF), fire grilling, charring, and for longer times tends to encourage these compounds. On the other hand, cooking in a more modern style, with lower temperatures, for shorter times, or with moist heat, discourages their formation.

You can significantly decrease AGEs by marinating meats in acidic mediums, such as lemon juice, vinegar, or wine (Yay!), and/or adding antioxidant spices such as garlic or ginger. (Garlic's antioxidants are particularly resilient to cooking.) The polyphenols found in red wine have also been shown to combat AGEs, so consider pairing a glass of wine with that steak!

The takeaway? Totally keep cooking your meat, but consider marinating your cuts, and learning to love rare to medium-rare steaks and sashimi, instead of, say, BBQ and fried fish. (Many people find they acquire a taste for rarer steaks and seafood when going Paleo.) Avoid frying, broiling, smoking, grilling at high temperatures (definitely not above 400ºF), and anything that creates a natural residue, such as searing or blackening. Instead, favor baking below 300ºF, braising, poaching, and steaming.

FATS

Dietary fats can oxidize when cooked, rendering them unstable and toxic within the body. While saturated fats, such as those found in meats and coconut oil, tend to be relatively stable, polyunsaturated fats, found in fatty fish and seed and vegetable oils, are quite prone to oxidation. Avoid cooking fatty fish at high temperatures, and try to stick to butter, ghee, coconut oil, and tallow when it comes to oils. When using olive oil, stick to lower temps. (The "Recipes" in this book take this all into account.)

VEGGIES

Here's where things *really* get complicated! Studies show that various cooking methods can both increase *and* decrease the nutrients in produce (such as vitamins, antioxidants, and polyphenols), depending on the type of veggie and cooking method used. While many foods feature heightened enzymes and nutrients in raw form, others are rendered more digestible and bioavailable when cooked, which breaks down the cell walls locking them up.

For example, cooking tends to increase antioxidants in celery, but decrease them in Swiss chard. It can increase carotenoids in carrots, but decrease polyphenols. Boiling doesn't seem to affect zucchini's carotenoids, but steaming does. One study proposed that cooking with water best preserved antioxidants, while another literally ends with "Water is not the cook's best friend when it comes to preparing vegetables."[6] Oh. My. Goodness.

Though we shouldn't draw any concrete conclusions when it comes to cooking and nutrient preservation, here are some general findings:

- Cooking at super high temperatures tends to break down nutrients. Try to bake below about 300°F.
- Cooking for longer periods of time tends to break down nutrients.
- Steaming may generally preserve the most nutrients, providing gentle cooking without leaching them into water. (For example, steam-

ing is particularly effective for broccoli, completely preserving its cancer-protecting glucosinolates.)

- Cooking doesn't tend to destroy minerals, but water can usher them out. While boiling or slow cooking may seem gentle, use these when you plan to consume the broth or make a soup.
- Because pressure-cooking utilizes pressure rather than heat, it can preserve nutrition while still breaking down problematic compounds.
- Fat-soluble vitamins (A, D, E, K) tend to be more resilient than water-soluble B and C vitamins, though veggies aren't a big source of the Bs anyway. (Turn to meat for that!) While the highly volatile C might be slightly preserved when microwaving or pressure-cooking, I recommend turning to raw fruits for your daily dose!
- While quick frying can minimize the amount of time to heat exposure, it can decrease antioxidants and encourage fat oxidation. I recommend avoiding too much of this one.
- Roasting and baking may preserve some nutrients, but going *too* high in temp can increase AGEs.

All that said, cooking at higher temperatures and for longer amounts of time can help break down problematic compounds, such as goitrogens found in cruciferous veggies, or phytates found in green beans. For people with digestive distress, cooking can render veggies much more digestible and less fermentable. So if you're an IBS and/or SIBO sufferer, you might want to go to town with cooking, until your bacterial dysbiosis is resolved (which is totally possible—check out MelanieAvalon.com for tons more on that!).

THE TAKEAWAY?

I suggest switching things up to ensure a variety of nutrients, while mostly avoiding particularly damaging methods such as high heat, frying, and grilling. Otherwise, prepare your food the way you're craving, and don't sweat it. That said, if you've got digestive distress, you might want to cook those veggies more, until your gut is more of a happy camper!

RESTAURANT GUIDE

Dining at restaurants Paleo-style is quite doable once you get the hang of it—you just gotta think outside the box! With a bit of tweaking, most restaurants have viable options, and many have gluten-free menus. Of course, these do make you realize just how many things *aren't* gluten-free. ("You mean this chicken isn't gluten-free? Oh.") Keep in mind that with Paleo, you don't have to gauge calories or scrutinize portion sizes! Can I get an amen?

QUICK PALEO RESTAURANT PROTOCOL

1. Inform the waiter you are gluten-free.
2. Pick a Paleo-esque entrée you like, such as chicken, steak, or fish.
3. Ask for the meat to be grilled, broiled, or steamed, etc., with no refined cooking oils. (You can ask for butter or olive oil, if ya like.)
4. Ask for no sauce, or sauce on the side.
5. Substitute sides with veggies, either steamed or sautéed in butter or olive oil.

   Done.

DETAILED PALEO RESTAURANT PROTOCOL

Oftentimes, the primary Paleo restaurant obstacle isn't *finding* something to eat, but rather gaining confidence in meal requests. You sit there *knowing* what you want to order in theory, but you are silenced by a hesitancy to ask questions and a fear of being annoying. So when the time comes to order, you mumble a disheartened "I'll take the chicken," and then silently pray the sauce isn't sugar or gluten infested. (It likely is.) If this is your predicament, have no fear! As a moonlighting waitress myself, I assure you, *it's okay to be picky.* Just please be nice. With practice, you'll learn how to minimize hassle while maximizing return on investment. Now on to the restaurant tips!

HOW TO PREP

LOOK AT THE MENU ONLINE

Most restaurants have online menus, so you can always mentally prepare your choice (and salivate over it!) ahead of time. Also check out online reviews to gauge a given restaurant's friendliness to dietary accommodations.

CHECK FOR A GLUTEN-FREE MENU

Always inquire about gluten-free menus. That said, remember these are your starting point, not destination, as you'll likely be tweaking things further.

LET THE WAITSTAFF KNOW WHAT'S UP

Don't just modify the entrée to make it *seemingly* Paleo and gluten-free: Make sure the server and kitchen *know* you *need* to be gluten-free. Otherwise, the server may modify the meal to your liking, but it could still be cooked in gluten-containing dishware. If the kitchen knows there's a gluten allergy, they're more likely to use pots and pans free of gluten residue.

ASK QUESTIONS

You might be shocked at just how many things go into seemingly simple entrées and accompaniments, including refined oils, flavorings, soy sauce, and vague seasoning blends with questionable additives. (IHOP puts pancake batter in their omelets—just saying.) Channel grade school's "The only stupid question is the one you didn't ask." Ask if the meats are prepared in anything (marinades, breading, sauces, oils, rubs, etc.) Ask about gluten and added sugar. Ask what type of cooking oil they use. (It's often canola, which we'd like to avoid.) Ask what the "mixed vegetables" entails. While this may sound like a lot of questions, it's not *that* bad. Besides, you'll be tailoring the questions to your potential entrées, not running down the entire menu.

BLAME ALLERGIES

Blaming allergies eradicates feelings of pickiness, while encouraging the waitstaff to honor your wishes. (No one wants to get sued!) How extreme you go is up to you. Want to make it life-threatening? Go for it. I mean, problematic foods *do* arguably threaten the quality of your life, so there's that.

WHAT TO ORDER

FIND THE FOUNDATION

Search the menu for the most foundational Paleo entrée you're craving, even if it's not in seemingly "Paleo" form. I'm talking basics, such as chicken, steak, fish, veggie medleys, salad, and so on. Don't worry, you're not committing to its current manifestation—we'll fix things from there!

TWEAK PREPARATION METHODS

Inquire about the preparation of your selected entrée, and adjust accordingly. Avoid methods such as fried and battered, and request that your meal be steamed, broiled, or grilled, without refined oils, additives, marinades, or braising. I typically ask for completely plain, but you of course can do simple spices, olive oil, or butter, if including dairy in your protocol.

SUBSTITUTE

Ask to substitute any sides, such as fries or mashed potatoes, with vegetables. Peruse the entire menu to see what sides accompany *other* dishes (including specials), and request what looks best. Even if you don't see a specific side item, they still might have it! Ask away! You can also ask for sandwiches and burgers served over lettuce. If they're adamant about no substitutions, ask for no sides, and hope they ramp up the entrée.

SIMPLIFY

You can usually get simpler versions of "complicated" vegetables. If they've got creamed spinach, they can probably do sautéed or steamed. The special has a mushroom roulade? Ask for mushrooms!

FIX SAUCES AND MARINADES

Sauces and marinades are *perfect* concoctions for hidden sugar, gluten, fillers, and processed stuff. Inquire about sauces' ingredients, omit them entirely, or ask for them on the side, if you want to give a nod to the chef, in an "I appreciate this sauce you have concocted" type way. Don't stress about the inconvenience—there's often an easy "sauce on the side" button for the waitstaff.

FIX SALAD DRESSINGS

Most salad dressings contain some sort nefarious ingredient, particularly if they're not made in-house. Oil and vinegar is a good go-to choice.

AVOID SOUPS

Most soups contain thickening agents, accompanied by other unfriendly ingredients. I recommend going the salad route instead.

REEVALUATE DESSERT

Some restaurants have fruit dessert plates, and many do cheese plates, if you're including dairy in your protocol. I typically just munch on my family's leftover meat while they eat dessert. I'm not kidding. But then again, I'm a crazy carnivore. Of course, sipping on wine totally qualifies as dessert as well!

FINAL THOUGHTS

DON'T FEEL BAD

For the love of an elk, do not feel bad about being picky. Consider this: If you ask a question, the server will either know or not know the answer. If they know, then what's the worry? If they don't know, they'll know *next* time somebody asks! You're saving them future trouble, and potentially from a *rude* guest, whereas you're a nice one! Being specific up front also means you'll more likely be satisfied with the end result. (Trust me, sending entrées back is where the *real* server headache comes in!) Most important, why pay good money for food that will make you feel yucky afterwards?

CHOOSE YOUR BATTLES

All this said, sometimes it's not worth it to go insane with everything. If you're really only hungry for the main "Paleo" portion of your dish anyway, just go ahead and order it. (But always ask about gluten, marinades, and oils, and emphasize you're gluten-free!)

DON'T STRESS

Please don't stress about what you're eating. Fear only hampers digestion and clouds fun times. Do the prep work, and accept it. You're doing great most of the time (I know you are!), so enjoy that restaurant moment!

SHOW GRATITUDE

Please be sincerely grateful, and show it accordingly in your gratuity. Servers literally live on tips.

RESTAURANT GENRES

Believe it or not, you can make many restaurants work in the Paleo lifestyle. Here's a guide to the genres!

EASIER RESTAURANTS

Self-Proclaimed "Healthy" Restaurants
Any restaurant that prides itself on its organic, sustainable, or farm-to-table options is usually a winner, featuring more Paleo-friendly choices and a staff "understanding" of dietary accommodations.

Steakhouses
Show me a steakhouse that doesn't have meat and veggies. Enough said.

Seafood Restaurants
The aquatic alternative to steakhouses. Totally doable!

Casual American Restaurants

Like steakhouses, most American cafés and diners feature a wide variety of salad, meat, and veggie options. They are, however, more likely to use pre-prepared, preservative, and additive-rich ingredients. Ask questions!

Italian, French, Mediterranean

In my experience, these places usually have steak, veal, fish, poultry, and/or seafood options, with veggies as well, though you may need to implement a few extra steps to avoid marinades and sauces. And skip the bread course, obvi.

MORE DIFFICULT RESTAURANTS

BBQ

Many BBQ joints feature meats with unavoidable rubs and seasonings. I suggest calling ahead to see if you can get your meat without them.

Korean BBQ

You'd *think* Korean BBQ would be easy, since you're cooking meat yourself (control!), but cross contamination seems to be a thing. Avoid marinated meats, and try to cook on your own "section" of the grill, no matter how weird it feels. The type of Korean BBQ where you cook in water is a safer bet.

Mexican

Staple Mexican dishes feature tortillas, sauces, Spanish rice, and beans, none of which are quite Paleo-friendly. Consider salads, fajitas without the tortilla, carne asada, guacamole, ceviche, and carnitas. (Though I wish you the best with avoiding gluten exposure.) Some Mexican chains do feature gluten-free menus.

Asian

Asian restaurants can be a mixed bag, with many dishes featuring rice, noodles, MSG, and precombined meat and veggies with unavoidable sauces. Soups can look promising, but good luck tracking down the ingredient list. Soy sauce is overwhelmingly prevalent, so consider bringing your own coconut aminos if you want to sneak in a super tasty substitute! Cross contamination can also be a problem at cook-in-front-of-you places.

Traditional (rather than Americanized) Asian restaurants may feature more friendly options, though some chains provide gluten-free menus. Potential options include sashimi, chicken/pork and broccoli without the sauces, steamed fish, and white rice, if you're including it in your protocol.

German

I realize most people don't typically dine German-style, but since I'm German, I thought I'd include it for grins. German is pretty difficult, featuring sausages with questionable additives and breaded meats. So this section is massively unhelpful, I guess. Sorry 'bout it.

Tapas

Since tapas restaurants prepare tiny portions with sauces, seasonings, and specific ingredients, substituting can be a bit awkward. You also may feel more self-conscious if sharing with other people. And if you're practicing IF, one-meal-a-day-style, it can be a bit pricey to fill up with enough food. I basically view tapas restaurants as a tasting, rather than eating, experience.

Vegan, Vegetarian

While at first you may think #healthy!, vegan and vegetarian places can actually be quite tricky. The lack of meat dishes leaves a lot of room for grains, soy, legumes, rice, potatoes, and processed faux meats. While you can likely find *something* to eat (hi, salads!), you may walk away less than satisfied.

OTHER RESTAURANT CONSIDERATIONS

$$$

While not a blanket statement, more expensive restaurants may be more accommodating of special requests, since they're essentially sucking up to you. They're also more likely to make their dishes in-house with fewer additives, and may even feature wild-caught fish or grass-fed steaks. That said, I see no reason to pay an arm and a leg for USDA Prime steak, which says *nothing* about growing practices. (Especially when I could purchase a grass-fed steak from the store at one-fifth of the price!) Fixed-price menus and pretentious entrées at fancy-schmancy places can also be unkind to substitutions.

CHAINS

Many sit-down chains regulate their menus to minimize the hassle of dealing with picky eaters, making them surprisingly Paleo-friendly and often understanding of substitutions. Some even feature easy mix-and-match-type menus with the whole meat and veggie thing, and many chains provide gluten-free menus. That said, be wary of additives and emphasize your gluten-free-ness.

FAST FOOD

While I shudder stepping foot in these restaurants, Paleo can occasionally be done fast food–style, with the added bonus that you can typically look up "nutrition" and ingredient lists online. When dining on fast food, favor salads, and avoid condiments. Places where you construct your own sandwiches or "bowls" are an instant win! Some fast-food places even have more Paleo-friendly *secret menus*, which often ramp up the protein. (Google is your friend here!)

DISNEY DINING

Because I'm obsessed with Disney, it gets its own section! You can always order off the kids' menu, which typically features simple concoctions. Customizing meals can also save you money: Asking for no sides at counter-service places makes the meal cheaper! Also, never buy bottled water in the parks, as they'll give you free cups of water at all counter-service places! Actually, this really has nothing to do with Paleo. I just love Disney. So. Much.

WINE PAIRING GUIDE

Like a series of first dates with someone you already know, or a new ending to a favorite movie, the wonderfully nuanced world of wine interfuses the comforts of home with the novelty of new frontiers. As we delight our eyes with swirling red and white hues, and enliven our nose and taste buds with essences of fruit, chocolate, and spices, we sharpen our senses, rediscovering familiar flavors in new combinations. When paired with food, wine gains even more potential, able to enhance the sensory wonders lying therein. On a less esoteric note, wine can also aid digestion, help mitigate toxic byproducts generated from cooking, and just make ya feel good! Basically, wine + food = #winning.

While today's overwhelming wine options navigated by lofty wine critics and well-schooled sommeliers can be intimidating, it need not be! Sure, knowing unique details and #allthethings can invariably enhance one's vino appreciation and aid in securing that *perfect* pairing experience, but in the end, it's all about what *you* experience, label aside. Yep, *you* are always right! So whether you're a wine novice who simply sticks to red or white, or a more experienced wine lover seeking rare varietals and specific appellations, I wish you the same: that you may find those wines that delight your senses and color your evening with magic.

WINE PROFILES

There are *thousands* of wine varietals out there. That's a lot of wine! That said, if you know the basics of a few key varietals, you'll be good to go in nearly any raise-a-glass setting.

THE REDS

CABERNET SAUVIGNON: If you only know one wine, chances are you know Cabernet. Cabs tend to be big and bold, with full body and high tannins. (Tannins are naturally occurring, organic compounds found in wine that give it a bit of bite—see "Longevity and Antioxidants and Polyphenols, Oh My!" on page 150 for more on that!) Common flavors found in Cabernet include black cherry, blackcurrant, and blackberry, with potential vegetal notes such as pepper and mint. Oak aging can yield tones of vanilla, coffee, and smoke. Famous old-world Cabernets call the French Bordeaux region home, while new-world Cabernets dominate California.

MERLOT: While Merlots got a bad rap from the movie *Sideways*, they can be wonderful wines! Softer than Cabernets (and often blended with such), they tend to be medium to full-bodied, with medium tannins. They feature flavors of blackberry and plum, with accents of chocolate, fruitcake, vanilla, and coffee. Merlots are a primary constituent of Bordeaux blends in France.

PINOT NOIR: One of my personal favorites, Pinot Noirs are known to be sensually light and delicate, yet complex. Often low in tannins, they feature red fruit flavors such as cherry and strawberry. Old-world Pinots (such as from Burgundy) tend to take on more earthy and gamey flavors, such as mushrooms and meaty aromas, whereas new-world Pinots (from California and Oregon) may be slightly fuller in body, with more sweet and jammy notes.

SYRAH: For Syrahs, think bold and spicy, like barbecue! These reds are typically full bodied, with medium or high tannins, and common flavors of dark fruits mixed with peppery spice, smoke, cooked meats, vanilla, and licorice. Syrahs famously hail from Australia (where they're called "Shiraz"), while premium versions are provided by the Northern Rhone in France.

THE WHITES

CHARDONNAY: Chardonnays are incredibly versatile. They can be light to full bodied, with a range of potential flavors: from citrus and green fruits such as lime, apple, and pear, to stones fruits such as peach with bits of melon, to tropical notes such as pineapple and banana. Chardonnays are also known for taking on creamy, buttery notes (which come from a process called malolactic fermentation), as well as pronounced oaky and smokey flavors, as Chardonnays are one of the few whites often aged in oak. Chardonnays are particularly famous in Burgundy and throughout California.

SAUVIGNON BLANC: Sauvignon Blancs are known for being dry, clean, and crisp, with striking citrusy green fruits such as apple and lime, as well as potential tones of gooseberry and passionfruit. They're often high in acidity, and can take on particularly herbaceous and grassy notes. New Zealand is the go-to region for premium Sauvignon Blancs.

RIESLING: Rieslings are difficult to pin down, taking on a variety of flavors depending on their climate and growing season. They can range from citrusy green fruits of apple and grape, to citrusy stone fruits of peach, to tropical fruits of pineapple and mango. Rieslings can be dry and crisp, semi-sweet, or super sweet (dessert-wine style!), and are categorized by their level of sweetness in their home country of Germany. (From driest to sweetest, these are *Kabinett, Auslese, Spätlese, Beerenauslese,* and *Trockenbeerenauslese.*) Rieslings do tend to be highly aromatic, with floral notes.

PAIRING FOOD WITH WINE

Like two starry-eyed lovers, wine and food should selflessly complement each other, each accentuating the other, with neither stealing the spotlight. The wine reveals hidden nuances in the food, while the food renders the wine all the more worthy of savoring (rather than guzzle-worthy!). Basically, you want to experience both the wine *and* the food, not just one or the other.

BASIC WINE PAIRING GUIDE

- In general, you can go for a "two peas in a pod" or an "opposites attract" approach when pairing wine and food, though the former tends to be a safer bet.
- The body and intensity of the food and wine should be balanced: you don't want one to overpower the other. That said, err on the side of making sure your wine is up to the challenge, as food is more likely to overpower wine, rather than the other way around.
- Sweetness should be similar, though the wine should be at *least* as sweet at the food, otherwise it may seem a bit bitter. This is especially important with desserts.
- Typically, acidity should be matched. While acidic food (such as citrusy or vinegary dishes) can make wine seem more approachable and fruity, if the wine isn't acidic enough, it may feel flat and dull. That said, high acid wines can go nicely with low acid, rich, fatty foods, as the wine can feel like it "cuts through" the fat. If a wine seems too bitter or acidic compared to a food, consider adding some salt or citrus to the dish.
- Spicy foods can make wine taste more alcoholic and bitter, and typically need some sweetness in the wine to balance them. Heat, alcohol, and tannins in wine tend to amplify heat in a dish, so unless you want to render your dinner sauna-worthy, avoid pairing overly intense wines with spicy dishes.
- Foods high in the "umami" flavor (the savory taste, found in things such as mushrooms, asparagus, and many cheeses) can be difficult to pair, as they make wine taste harsher.
- Keep in mind that age changes the flavor profile of wines—"softening" them, as fruity flavors give way to more nuanced, earthy notes.

- Heavier red meats and wild game typically pair well with reds, while chicken and fish dishes favor whites. That said, a wine's body can be more important than color, as delicate reds can suit some lighter dishes, while full-bodied whites might overpower them. On the food side of things, sauces and accompaniments are equally important: You'll often want to match wine to the dish's main flavor (such as a mushroom-y marsala sauce) rather than its main protein (such as the chicken underneath).

- Use extreme caution when pairing red wine with seafood, as the tannins in red wine can react with the iodine in fish, making it taste metallic.

- Food and wine from the same region often go together. Think grilled Spanish meats with Rioja, or Italian pasta with Chianti.

- If you're cooking a dish with wine, you can totally drink that wine with the meal as well!

- If you have an evening that's more about the wine than the food, you can go simple with the food preparations, and let the wine be the star. On the flip side, if the evening is all about showing off your cousin's new culinary skills, feel free to bring a simple, unoaked wine that won't steal the spotlight.

- All that said, when in doubt, eat the food and drink the wine you know you like! If you like them individually, chances are you'll still like them together. (Whereas if you don't like them on their own, that's unlikely to change from a pairing alone.) Want to order a super intense Zinfandel with a salad, or light Pinot Grigio with a grilled steak? Do it.

THE PROPER SETTING

While you can totally drink wine out of a solo cup, college-style, choosing the appropriate glassware and serving conditions can truly enhance a wine's potential. People love to do pretentious mock-swirling, sniffing, and tasting . . . but there's actually a reason for all of that! Use these tips and trick to get the most bang for your buck, wine wise!

- Choose crisp, clean, thin glasses for the ultimate tasting experience. Wider barrels are good for reds, as they allow the aromas to open up, while narrower glasses suit whites, concentrating the lighter, fruity flavors. Flutes are ideal for sparkling wines, as they prevent too much CO_2 from escaping.
- Light-bodied reds are best served lightly chilled (around 55°F), while all other reds do well on the cooler side of room temperature (around 59 to 64°F). Whites are served more chilled, from 45 to 50°F, depending on the body. (Serve lighter wines at lower temperatures.) A great tip noted in *What to Drink with What You Eat* is to refrigerate red wine for 15 minutes before serving, but take white wine out of the fridge 15 minutes before serving.

TASTING STEPS:

1. Swirl the wine in the glass to evaluate its color and body.
2. Slowly smell the wine. A large percentage of taste—somewhere between 75 and 95 percent—is actually due to smell. This will enhance your wine experience, while allowing you to check for any "off" aromas, such as mustiness or cork taint.
3. Take a sip of the wine, swirling it around your mouth to reach all the flavor receptors on your taste buds, and journey up into your nasal passage. In a world where we're quick to guzzle down food and wine like it's going out of style, this slow step of appreciation is key!

RECIPES

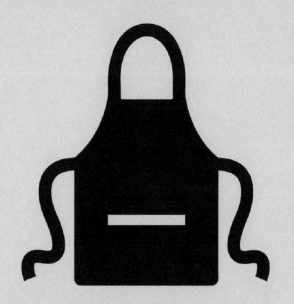

RECIPE FYI

I'm thrilled to bring you the following Paleo-friendly recipes, created by the insanely talented special diet chef and certified nutritionist Ariane Resnick, author of *The Bone Broth Miracle* and *The Thinking Girl's Guide to Drinking*. Ariane has cooked for many celebrities and appeared in tons of media outlets, from ABC News to *Cosmopolitan*! (Check out arianecooks.com for all the details!) Get ready to enter a Paleo-friendly cooking world that will delight your taste buds and make conventional food cravings not even a thing!

All recipes are grain- and gluten-free! Each recipe also indicates if it is low-carb, keto, dairy-free, a variation of vegetarian, vegan, low FODMAP, and/or AIP (Autoimmune Paleo).

Recipe descriptions and wine pairings are provided by Melanie.

CATEGORY NOTES

LOW-CARB/KETO: Carbs are a tricky business, as everyone has different perspectives on what constitutes "low-carb" or "keto." For our purposes, "low-carb" recipes contain fewer than 10 carbs per serving. "Keto" recipes contain fewer than 5 carbs per serving, as well as 5 percent or fewer carbs as a total macronutrient.

DAIRY-FREE: Recipe contains no milk products or eggs.

VEGETARIAN: Recipe contains no meat or dairy products.

LACTO-VEGETARIAN: Recipe contains no meat or eggs, but may contain milk products.

OVO-VEGETARIAN: Recipe contains no meat or milk products, but may contain eggs.

LACTO-OVO VEGETARIAN: Recipe contains no meat, but may contain milk products or eggs.

PESCATARIAN: Recipe contains no meat, but may contain fish, milk, or egg products.

VEGAN: Recipe contains no animal products, including honey.

LOW-FODMAP: Recipe is low in FODMAPs. See page 67 and visit Melanie Avalon.com/guides for more information on this!

AIP: Recipe is Autoimmune Paleo-friendly. See page 67 for more on this! Note: AIP recipes may include the following gray-area ingredients: avocado oil, coconut butter, honey, MCT oil, or nutritional yeast.

INGREDIENT NOTES*

For all ingredients marked with a *, visit MelanieAvalon.com/recommendations for Melanie's suggested Paleo-friendly versions!

COOKING TEMPERATURES

In general, it's best to avoid high heat and extended cooking times for meats and oils, to minimize toxic by-products and oxidation, as discussed in the

"Cooking Guide" on page 246. These recipes keep that in mind. That said, an occasional entrée on the hotter side won't kill you, and I'd rather you chow down on some well-cooked meat than a processed, addictive treat any day!

FOOD QUALITY

Try to favor organic, grass-fed, and pastured versions of the ingredients when realistically possible for you. I *definitely* recommend choosing organic spices, organic produce, organic nuts, and grass-fed versions of fattier meats and bone. Please see the "Food Quality Guide" on page 229 for details on the various growing practices, and for guidance on where to best invest your money.

COOKING OILS

Many of these recipes utilize avocado oil due to its high smoke point, versatile nature, and neutral flavor. This is how Ariane intends for the recipes to be cooked. That said, Melanie personally recommends substituting coconut oil, if you like the taste, in recipes up to 350°F, or refined coconut oil for a more neutral flavor and/or in higher-temperature recipes. In addition to having a high smoke point, coconut oil is a saturated fat less prone to oxidation, with many health benefits to boot!

SALT

Most conventional salt contains dextrose and anticaking agents. Favor pink, Himalayan, or sea salt to maximize nutrition and avoid additives.

PEPPER

In case you're wondering, black pepper is *not* a nightshade.

SUPERFOODS

Bone Broth

LOW-CARB/KETO, DAIRY-FREE, LOW-FODMAP, AIP

SUGGESTED WINE PAIRING: **MADEIRA OR SHERRY**

(Note: Do not pair with wine if consuming as part of a specific gut-healing protocol.)

A basic bone broth is a solid foundation for gut healing, strong hair and nails, and combating inflammation. Use it as a base for soups, added to sauces, or as a warm, soothing drink on a cool night or morning! It's a particularly FANTASTIC way to break your fast at the beginning of your eating window, for ultimate gut healing. You can enhance this basic recipe with any aromatics or herbs you like, such as onions, garlic, rosemary, ginger, or celery root. Avoid delicate herbs such as basil, as they will break down too much in cooking. Where to get the bones? You can save them in the freezer from your own steaks and chickens, ask your butcher for some, or even find them in the frozen aisle at health-conscious mainstream grocery stores such as Whole Foods. This is an instance where you definitely want to use organic, grass-fed bones if at all possible.

Store leftover bone broth in glass jars in the freezer. You can also freeze bone broth in an ice cube tray, then transfer the cubes to a larger container, for easy, small servings! MAKES APPROXIMATELY 1 QUART

1 pound beef or other animal bones (bison, lamb, chicken, turkey, etc.), preferably grass-fed

1 quart spring or filtered water

1 teaspoon salt

1 tablespoon apple cider vinegar*; substitute lemon juice if concerned about glutamines

* Visit MelanieAvalon.com for Paleo-friendly versions of all * ingredients.

continued

1. Brown bones to increase flavor by roasting them in a pan or caramelizing them on the stovetop in a pot or large pan. Skip this step if using bones that have been cooked.
2. Add the remaining ingredients and cook for 12 to 24 hours in a slow cooker, 1 to 2 hours in a pressure cooker, or on the stove for up to 24 hours if that can be done safely in your home.
3. Strain bones, and add additional salt to taste if desired.

FOR MEAT BROTH: Still building up your bone stockpile? You can totally make meat broth in the meantime. (Those with particularly sensitive guts may also want to start with meat broth before transitioning to bone broth.) Simply use meat instead of bones in the above recipe, and maintain the same quantity of water, salt, and vinegar/lemon juice. Strain the resulting broth into glass containers, and feel free to eat the meat as is, or reserve it for other dishes, such as soups or homemade chicken salad featuring Paleo-friendly mayo (see page 289 to create your own). And of course, store any bones in the freezer for bone broth!

Kombucha Probiotic Gummies

LOW-CARB* (DEPENDING ON SUGAR CONTENT OF KOMBUCHA), DAIRY-FREE, AIP* (OMIT STEVIA)

SUGGESTED "WINE" PAIRING: **THE KOMBUCHA USED IN THE GUMMIES**

. . . .

While perhaps a smidge tougher than your commercial versions, these gummies are delicious and super nutritious, full of gelatin for your gut and probiotics for your gut microbiome—thanks to the fermented tea drink known as kombucha. With all the versions of kombucha now available, the flavor possibilities are endless! Also feel free to use flavored coconut kefir instead of kombucha if you like.

MAKES AROUND 18 TO 24 SERVINGS, DEPENDING ON MOLD USED

. . . .

> 2 cups kombucha,* any flavor
> ¼ cup grass-fed gelatin*
> Liquid stevia*

1. In a saucepan, add 1 cup kombucha, then pour gelatin over it. Allow to bloom for 5 minutes.
2. Place the saucepan over low heat and stir until the gelatin dissolves, taking care not to heat kombucha too much or the probiotics will be killed. (Don't let it get hotter than warm to the touch, and definitely not simmering!)
3. Once the gelatin is dissolved, remove from heat and add the remaining 1 cup kombucha, plus stevia to taste.
4. Pour into molds or into an 8-by-8-inch baking dish, and refrigerate until set, about 4 hours.
5. Remove gummies from molds or cut into shapes from the pan.

Grass-Fed Gelatin Marshmallows

DAIRY-FREE

SUGGESTED WINE PAIRING: **SWEET SPARKLING ROSÉ OR ANY LATE-HARVEST WINE**

They're not the quickest or tidiest dessert, but these homemade grass-fed marshmallows are a scrumptious and healthful treat that can't be found in stores, and also provide a feeling of accomplishment when all's said and done! Gelatin is awesome for gut repair, pain-free joints, and strong hair and nails, and it can also help balance the amino acid profile of muscle meats. (So consider having these as a dessert after your chicken or steak entrée!) It's possible to make these marshmallows with stevia, but the texture won't be ideal, and they may deflate within a few hours. In any case, this recipe makes a full 9-by-13-inch pan, so the effort will be totally worthwhile!

MAKES 24 TO 30 MARSHMALLOWS

⅓ cup grass-fed gelatin*

½ cup ice water

¼ cup boiling or simmering hot water

¾ cup room-temperature water

¾ cup honey*

¾ cup maple syrup*

1 teaspoon vanilla extract*

½ teaspoon salt

Arrowroot starch,* as needed

1. In the bowl of an electric mixer, add gelatin and pour ice water over it. Allow to bloom for 5 minutes, then pour in boiling water and stir well, until no lumps remain.

2. In a medium saucepan over medium heat, heat room-temperature water, honey, and maple syrup until simmering. Turn heat low enough that mix-

ture continues to simmer gently, without stirring, until mixture reaches 235°F on a candy thermometer, about 20 minutes. (If not using a candy thermometer, then simmer until a soft-ball candy stage is reached, in which a bit of the mixture dropped into cold water forms a soft ball.) Swirl pan as needed to incorporate any drops on the sides.

3. Turn the electric mixer on low and begin pouring syrup, in a slow and steady stream, over gelatin mix. Add vanilla and salt.

4. Turn mixer up to high and whip until a marshmallow fluff consistency is reached, about 10 minutes.

5. Pour fluff into a 9-inch-by-13-inch pan that has been rubbed with arrowroot starch, and refrigerate until firm, about 30 minutes.

6. Cut marshmallows in a grid of six across and four or five wide, and toss each in arrowroot starch before storing.

Chicken Liver Pâté

LOW-CARB

SUGGESTED WINE PAIRING: **SAUTERNES OR BEAUJOLAIS**

Milder than beef liver, chicken livers are a sound intro to the insanely nutritious but potentially intimidating world of organ meats. Caramelizing the onions adds a balancing quality of sweetness, while eggs mellow the liver. Though the quantity of butter may seem high, this recipe has less than most recipes for chicken liver pâté, and averages one tablespoon per good-sized serving. Choose grass-fed, organic versions of these ingredients and you're looking at a veritable fat-soluble vitamin-rich superfood!

MAKES 6 SERVINGS

1 sweet onion, chopped

6 tablespoons butter*

1 pound chicken livers

2 eggs, hard boiled

¾ teaspoon salt

¼ teaspoon black pepper

1. In a large frying pan, sauté onion with 1 tablespoon butter until caramelized, about 10 minutes.
2. Add livers and sauté until cooked through, 3 to 4 minutes. Let cool slightly.
3. In a food processor, combine the sautéed livers with the rest of the ingredients until desired pâté texture is reached.

Raw Live Sauerkraut

BASIC KRAUT: **LOW-CARB/KETO, DAIRY-FREE, VEGAN, LOW-FODMAP* (OMIT LEEKS), AIP**

SUGGESTED WINE PAIRING: **DRY GERMAN RIESLING OR ALSATIAN GEWÜRZTRAMINER**

Fermented foods have been around since approximately 6000 BC, appearing in almost all societies, and for good reason! Originally used as a method of food preservation, fermented foods are epic for gut health and digestion, especially in our present antibiotic-driven times, as antibiotics often do a number on our gut bacteria. Unfortunately, most grocery store krauts are pasteurized, which kills the beneficial bacteria and kinda defeats the purpose. So why not make your own? Home fermentation is not just cooking—it's a creative adventure, and a potential new hobby to boot! Many basic lacto-fermented krauts use a neutral base of cabbage, which you can totally play around with, Harry Potter potions class–style. Feel free to experiment with other veggies and herbs—the possibilities are endless! ("Sour" mashed sweet potatoes are my favorite!) Check out MelanieAvalon.com/fermentationguide for recommended tools and more on home fermentation.

MAKES TWO 32-OUNCE JARS

BASIC KRAUT
¼ head cabbage, sliced thinly
1 carrot, grated
½ leek, sliced thinly
3 tablespoons horseradish, grated
½ tablespoon salt
2 cabbage outer leaves, whole

1. In a mixing bowl, add sliced cabbage, carrot, leek, and horseradish, and sprinkle with salt. Massage salt into veggies until they begin to release water, then let them sit for 10 to 15 minutes until liquid covers the vegetables.

continued

2. Divide contents into two 32-ounce mason jars; cover with cabbage leaves, then weights. (You can order weights specific for sauerkraut, or construct DIY versions. See MelanieAvalon.com/fermentationguide.)

3. Cover with either a loosely fitting lid, or a piece of cloth tied with string or a rubber band. Note that you do not want a tight seal, as contents will release gases. (You can also order special lids for this. See MelanieAvalon.com/fermentationguide.)

4. Put jars in a cabinet or dark corner of your kitchen to ferment. Begin checking them after three days, when fermentation should have occurred. Taste every one to two days until desired level of tang is achieved.

Alternate Flavors

Feel free to adjust the base ratio of the cabbage and carrot foundation to your liking, or use only one if you like. You can also swap out the horseradish and leek for any of the ingredients below for an entirely different-tasting end product, mixing and matching as you desire. Or try other ingredients as well!

....

½ Granny Smith apple, grated

1 teaspoon caraway seeds

1 tablespoon fresh dill, chopped

1 teaspoon fennel seeds

2 garlic cloves, minced

2 tablespoons fresh ginger, grated

1 jalapeño, minced

DRESSINGS, SAUCES, AND CONDIMENTS

Caesar Dressing

LOW-CARB, DAIRY-FREE, VEGAN* (OMIT ANCHOVIES)

SUGGESTED WINE PAIRING: **LIGHTLY OAKED CHARDONNAY OR A DRY ROSÉ**

Friends, Romans, countrymen, lend me your ears! Caesar dressing need not be a bastion of trans fats, dairy, and nefarious additives! This delicious rendition replaces Parmesan and MSG-laden Worcestershire sauce with nutritional yeast (totally cheesy tasting, I promise!) and coconut aminos (totally delicious, I promise!), while receiving a luxuriously rich, buttery flavor from olive oil. In other words, you can now totally praise Caesar, rather than bury him. MAKES APPROXIMATELY 1 CUP

¼ cup extra-virgin olive oil*

3 tablespoons lemon juice

2 tablespoons minced garlic (about 2 to 3 cloves)

1 tablespoon nutritional yeast*

1 tablespoon white wine vinegar*

1½ teaspoons coconut aminos*

1 teaspoon Dijon mustard*

2 anchovies, optional

Pinch of salt (omit if using anchovies)

Pinch of black pepper

Blend all ingredients on low in a blender until smooth.

Immune-Boosting Italian Dressing

LOW-CARB/KETO, DAIRY-FREE, VEGAN, LOW-FODMAP* (OMIT GARLIC)

SUGGESTED WINE PAIRING: **VERDICCHIO OR SAUVIGNON BLANC**

. . . .

Not feeling #down for a cold? This salad dressing is *the* powerhouse for immunity! Between the allicin-rich raw garlic, carvacrol-rich oregano, and malic-acid-and-probiotic-rich apple cider vinegar, this dressing is sure to help ya beat any nefarious invader! Choose your favorite Paleo-friendly mustard, and feel free to play with the ratio of cider to wine vinegar. You can also swap out half of the olive oil for coconut or MCT oil, which will yield a slightly less Italian but slightly more antimicrobial version, thanks to the lauric and/or caprylic acid! MAKES APPROXIMATELY 1 CUP

. . . .

¼ cup extra virgin olive oil*

2 tablespoons white wine vinegar*

1 tablespoon apple cider vinegar*

1 garlic clove, minced

1 teaspoon stone-ground, Dijon, or whole-grain mustard*

½ teaspoon oregano

½ teaspoon parsley

½ teaspoon basil

¼ teaspoon salt, or more to taste

Pinch of black pepper

Whisk all ingredients or shake in a mason jar until emulsified, and let sit for 15 minutes before using.

Cheesy Sauce

DAIRY-FREE, VEGAN

SUGGESTED WINE PAIRING: **UNOAKED CHARDONNAY OR DOLCETTO**

. . . .

Not gonna lie—one of my first thoughts when compiling a recipe list for Ariane was "I need a cheesy sauce." Because cheese. Some people get high on sugar, others on fat, and then there's us cheese monsters. Since cheese is debatable in the Paleo world, and notably encourages the release of addictive opioid-like peptides {sigh}, a cheese-free alternative is much desired. Use this recipe for your cheesy sauce needs, from zoodles to veggie-chip nachos to a dip for crudités! Whenever your inner cheese demon rears its head, this sauce has got you covered! By the way, don't omit the nutritional yeast, which is key for the cheesy flavor, and also provides B_{12} for all my vegetarians out there! MAKES APPROXIMATELY 2 CUPS

. . . .

½ cup cashews, soaked for around 2 to 3 hours, rinsed, and drained (about ¾ cup once soaked)

½ cup sliced red bell pepper (about ¼ pepper)

3 to 4 tablespoons lemon juice

1 tablespoon nutritional yeast*

1 tablespoon coconut aminos*

1 teaspoon ground turmeric

1 teaspoon smoked paprika

⅛ teaspoon black pepper

Pinch of salt

Water

Combine all ingredients in a high-speed blender, then add enough water to just cover ingredients. Blend until smooth and creamy.

Teriyaki Sauce

DAIRY-FREE, VEGETARIAN

SUGGESTED WINE PAIRING: **BEAUJOULAIS OR ROSÉ**

Growing up, I was a teriyaki fiend. I was also always disappointed by my inability to satisfactorily recreate a version of the sauce that was on par with the ones at my favorite restaurants. Who could have guessed that if I had taken a Paleo approach to the sauce, I probably would have been happier? The secret here is the coconut aminos, which provide all the tastiness of this Asian goodie with none of the MSG or soy. Oh hey! You can use this sauce as both a marinade and a finishing or dipping sauce.   MAKES APPROXIMATELY ¾ CUP

¼ cup coconut aminos*

3 tablespoons fresh orange juice

2 tablespoons honey*

1 garlic clove, minced

1 tablespoon fresh ginger, grated

1 tablespoon fresh turmeric, grated, optional

1 tablespoon toasted sesame oil*

1 teaspoon to 1 tablespoon chili paste,* optional

1 teaspoon arrowroot starch* dissolved in 2 teaspoons water, optional

1. Combine all ingredients in a small saucepan and bring to a boil, then reduce to a simmer.
2. Simmer for 5 minutes until slightly thickened.
3. If using arrowroot starch slurry, add that to the pot and stir until thickened, less than 30 seconds. If not using, simmer an additional 2 to 3 minutes until sauce has thickened slightly further on its own.

Alfredo Sauce

DAIRY-FREE, VEGAN* (USE VEGETABLE STOCK)

SUGGESTED WINE PAIRING: **BEAUJOULAIS OR ROSÉ**

Paleo-ness aside, my all-time favorite dish in life is chicken pasta Alfredo. For reals. When I first went low-carb, I even went through a phase where I simply slathered chicken in Alfredo sauce, sans pasta. So. Much. Alfredo. Thankfully, Alfredo sauce can still be done Paleo-style! This dairy-free version maintains a satisfying richness, without relying heavily on nuts or seeds, by embracing the lighter alternative of cauliflower—chock-full of vitamins C, K, and B$_6$. Pretty cool! Don't omit the nutritional yeast, which is important for the flavor. **MAKES APPROXIMATELY 2 CUPS**

1 cup cauliflower florets

¼ cup Bone Broth* (see page 275 to create your own) or vegetable stock* for a vegan version

¼ cup raw cashews, soaked for at least 2 hours, then rinsed and drained

3 tablespoons Nut Milk* (page 345)

1 tablespoon olive oil*

1 teaspoon nutritional yeast*

1 teaspoon onion powder

½ teaspoon salt

1. Steam cauliflower until tender, 5 to 10 minutes. Let cool.
2. Add all ingredients to a blender and blend on high until smooth.

Ten Mayonnaises!

BASIC VERSION: **LOW-CARB/KETO, OVO-VEGETARIAN, LOW-FODMAP**

SUGGESTED WINE PAIRING: **CHAMPAGNE OR CHABLIS**

. . . .

From canola oil to stabilizers to preservatives, commercial mayonnaise can be pretty sinister stuff. Thank goodness you can totally make a delicious version yourself, along with *tons* of variants to suit any mayo hankering! It's like shopping at the Mayo Mall of America! Make sure to add the oil very slowly to the blender, as pouring it in too quickly will make the sauce break.

MAKES 1 CUP

. . . .

BASIC MAYO

1 egg yolk (room temperature is best)

1 tablespoon lemon juice, or more to taste

1 teaspoon Dijon or German mustard*

¼ teaspoon salt, or more to taste

⅛ teaspoon white pepper, optional

1 cup avocado oil or olive oil, or a mix*

1. Blend all ingredients except oil together on low in a blender until smooth.
2. *Very* slowly drizzle in oil, keeping blender on low and pausing frequently to let oil incorporate.

Variations

Add these ingredients in with all the others at the start of blending.

. . . .

AIOLI MAYO: **2 garlic cloves, chopped**

CHIPOTLE MAYO: **¾ teaspoon chipotle powder**

continued

FIESTA MAYO: 1 tablespoon cilantro, ½ seeded jalapeño, 1 teaspoon lime juice

GINGER MAYO: 1 teaspoon fresh ginger, grated

HERB MAYO: 1 tablespoon fresh dill, tarragon, oregano, and/or parsley

HORSERADISH MAYO: 1½ teaspoons fresh horseradish, grated

PESTO MAYO: 1 tablespoon Pesto (page 314)

ROASTED GARLIC MAYO: 4 garlic cloves, roasted

WASABI MAYO: 1 teaspoon wasabi powder rehydrated per package instructions, 1 teaspoon lime juice

Guacamole

LOW-CARB/KETO, DAIRY-FREE, VEGAN, LOW-FODMAP, AIP* (OMIT CUMIN AND CHIPOTLE)

SUGGESTED WINE PAIRING: **CHILEAN SAUVIGNON BLANC OR TORRONTÉS**

Avocados are delicious, nutritional powerhouses, low in carbs but rich in monounsaturated fats and fat-soluble vitamins. Not only is guac the quintessential avocado dish, it's also super versatile! Use it as a dip for veggies or veggie chips, as a topping for meat or burgers, as an enhancer for chimichurri or pesto, or even eat it plain! The key is using good avocados: Check for ripeness by evaluating color and texture. Darker avocados tend to be riper, and the perfect avocado should yield just slightly and softly to gentle pressure. Ripe avocados are ready to eat right away; firm, unripe avocados will ripen at room temperature over a few days. (Put them in a paper bag with a banana to speed up the process!) Avoid mushy avocados, which are likely past their prime. MAKES 4 SERVINGS

3 medium avocados

2 tablespoons chopped onion, optional

1 tablespoon chopped cilantro, optional

3 to 4 tablespoons lemon juice

½ teaspoon cumin powder

½ teaspoon salt

¼ teaspoon chipotle powder, optional

Mix all ingredients together in a mixing bowl, choosing optional ingredients based on how you like your guac. Guacamole can be left with large chunks of avocado, or mashed into nearly a paste, depending on your preference.

ENTRÉES

Steak with Red Wine Reduction

STEAK: **LOW-CARB/KETO, DAIRY-FREE, LOW-FODMAP, AIP**
RED WINE REDUCTION: **LOW-CARB**

SUGGESTED WINE PAIRING: **THE WINE USED IN THE REDUCTION
(BOLD CALIFORNIA CABERNETS AND SYRAHS ARE AWESOME FOR THIS!)**

This perfect date-night entrée brings a fancy steakhouse feel to a home-cooked meal! Choose a filet if you love luxuriously lean and tender, a rib-eye for flavorful marbling, or a strip if you fancy a firmer cut. For extra flavor, choose steaks on the bone. (My all-time favorite cut of steak is a bone-in filet. Yum!) This recipe's red wine reduction features super nutritious bone broth, and the wine can help mitigate any toxic by-products formed from grilling meat, especially if you prefer your steaks more well-done than rare. While Ariane used a Zinfandel in concocting this recipe, feel free to use whatever quality red wine you prefer—particularly bold ones for intense flavor! MAKES 2 SERVINGS

STEAK

2 (5-ounce) filet mignon, rib-eye, or New York strip steaks
1 tablespoon butter*
Salt
Pepper

RED WINE REDUCTION

½ cup Bone Broth* (see page 275 to create your own)
½ cup red wine
1 teaspoon garlic powder
1 teaspoon onion powder
½ teaspoon thyme
¼ to ½ teaspoon salt (depending on saltiness of broth)
⅛ teaspoon cracked black pepper
½ teaspoon arrowroot starch* dissolved in 1 teaspoon water, optional

continued

1. Sprinkle both sides of steak with salt and pepper to taste. Allow steak to rest and come to room temperature while you make the red wine reduction.

2. For reduction, heat all ingredients except arrowroot slurry in a medium saucepan.

3. Bring mixture to a boil, then reduce to a simmer; cook for 15 to 20 minutes, until reduced and thickened by at least one-third.

4. Add arrowroot slurry if using and stir briefly; mixture will thicken. Remove from heat.

5. In a frying pan, heat butter over medium-high heat; once melted and bubbling, add steaks.

6. Cook steaks until well caramelized on both sides, which will yield a medium-rare result. If you want them more cooked, place in a preheated 375°F oven for 10 to 15 minutes, or a 400°F oven for 5 to 10 minutes.

7. Before serving, bring reduction back to a simmer over heat, then spoon sauce over cooked steaks.

Braised Beef Shanks with Marrow Butter

SHANK: **LOW-CARB, DAIRY-FREE**

MARROW BUTTER: **LOW-CARB/KETO, LOW-FODMAP**

SUGGESTED WINE PAIRING: **BAROLO OR SYRAH**

. . . .

Beef shank is definition #winning. Due to its intimidation factor, you can typically get organic, grass-fed shanks way cheaper than other cuts—yay! But there's nothing to fear anyway. In the spirit of the famed osso buco (which utilizes veal, rather than beef), this recipe transforms a tough cut of meat into health-supporting lusciousness. A shank's initial toughness is thanks to its high amount of connective tissue rich in collagen, which supports bone, joint, and gut heath while balancing the potentially inflammatory amino acid profile common in muscle meat, such as chicken breasts and filets. The proper slow-cooker or pressure-cooker techniques, however, break down this collagen into gelatin, which coats the meat and creates a mouthwatering meal you can eat without a knife! Oh hey!

Beef shanks also come with a stellar bonus: the marrow bone. Not only is marrow rich in monounsaturated fat, protein, and fat-soluble vitamins, it's sinfully delicious! You can totally eat the marrow plain, or you can use it in the provided Marrow Butter recipe. You can pair this butter with the shank, or save it as a condiment for other things—on the Root Veggie Mash (page 332), steamed veggies, scrambled eggs, or perhaps to spice up a simple steak on another night. On top of all that, you can save the bone in the freezer, to build up your collection for Bone Broth (page 275)! Basically, shank is just the gift that keeps on giving. MAKES 2 SERVINGS

. . . .

BRAISED SHANKS

2 beef shanks

1 tablespoon avocado oil*

1 onion, chopped

3 garlic cloves, minced

continued

2 celery stalks, chopped

1 cup red wine

1 cup Bone Broth* or beef broth* (see page 275 to create your own)

1 tablespoon coconut aminos*

3 to 4 sprigs fresh thyme, optional

1 sprig rosemary, optional

½ teaspoon salt

¼ teaspoon pepper

1. In a pan, brown shanks until golden, about 5 minutes; remove from pan. (You can also do this directly in your slow cooker or pressure cooker, if supported by your appliance.)
2. Add oil, then onions once oil is hot; sauté for 5 minutes, until just beginning to turn golden. Add garlic and sauté for an additional 2 minutes.
3. Return shanks and add all remaining ingredients. Stir well.
4. Transfer (if applicable) and cook in a pressure cooker for 1 hour or in a slow cooker on high for 4 hours, then remove shanks from pot. Scoop out marrow from bones to create marrow butter, if desired.

MARROW BUTTER

3 tablespoons bone marrow, cooked

2 tablespoons butter*, softened

1 tablespoon fresh parsley, chopped

Pinch of salt, optional

In a food processor, blend all ingredients until incorporated. Serve as is, or refrigerate in a mold until firm.

Bison Meatloaf

MEATLOAF: **LOW-CARB/KETO, LOW-FODMAP* (OMIT SCALLIONS AND GARLIC)**
MARINARA (OPTIONAL): **DAIRY-FREE, VEGAN**

SUGGESTED WINE PAIRING: **MERLOT, CABERNET, OR BORDEAUX BLEND OF THE TWO!**

This likely isn't your mother's meatloaf! (If it is, can I please be friends with your mother?) While you can substitute regular ground beef, ground bison is becoming increasingly available at mainstream grocery stores and is leaner than ground beef, with a richer, sweeter flavor. The best part? Unlike for cattle, U.S. federal regulations prohibit the use of growth hormones and antibiotics in bison, which roam freely with a pastured diet for a majority of their lives (though they may be grain-finished). This meatloaf is also a fantastic way to optionally sneak grass-fed liver into your diet—a Paleo superfood rich in fat-soluble vitamins, minerals, protein, and essential fatty acids! Feel free to top with the marinara from the Chicken Parmesan recipe on page 303!

MAKES 4 SERVINGS

1 pound ground bison (substitute 1 pound ground beef if desired; choose a leaner ratio if you want to mimic bison)

½ cup grass-fed beef liver, chopped, optional

½ cup carrots, grated

¼ cup scallions, sliced

1 large egg

2 tablespoons fresh parsley, chopped

2 tablespoons almond flour* (see page 347 to create your own)

1 garlic clove, minced

1 tablespoon fresh rosemary, chopped

1 teaspoon salt

¼ teaspoon cracked black pepper

1 cup Marinara Sauce (page 303), optional

continued

1. Preheat oven to 375°F.
2. In a large mixing bowl, mix all ingredients except marinara together; your hands are the best tool for this job!
3. Form in a loaf pan; this quantity will work for a half-size loaf pan or a thin loaf in a full-size pan.
4. If using marinara, pour over the top.
5. Bake about 45 minutes, until cooked through and browned.

Chimichurri Steak

LOW-CARB/KETO, DAIRY-FREE, LOW-FODMAP* (OMIT GARLIC), AIP*
(AVOID NIGHTSHADE AND SEED SPICES)

SUGGESTED WINE PAIRING: **ARGENTINIAN MALBEC OR GRENACHE**

. . . .

For days when filet isn't in the budget, this tasty marinade can tenderize even the cheaper cuts, thanks to citric-acid-rich lemon juice. Its garlic component not only ramps up the flavor, it also helps minimize toxic by-products from cooking with heat. You can choose whatever fresh herbs you like, both for taste and for their various health benefits! Feel free to replace the MCT oil with coconut oil, if desired, which will yield a slightly thicker marinade. As a final note, the marinade is fantastic as a finishing or dipping sauce!

MAKES 1 LARGE OR 2 SMALL SERVINGS

. . . .

1 (6-ounce) skirt steak

1 cup fresh herbs, such as basil, dill, cilantro, and mint

3 to 4 tablespoons lemon juice

1 garlic clove, minced

1 tablespoon avocado oil*

½ teaspoon salt

Pinch of black pepper

2 teaspoons MCT oil*

1. In a blender on low, blend all marinade ingredients except MCT oil until mixture has the texture of a thick sauce; pieces of herbs are fine.
2. Add half of the marinade to steak and refrigerate for one hour, or up to overnight.
3. Cook steak on a grill, in a grill pan, or in a skillet to desired temperature.
4. Whisk MCT oil into the remaining half of the marinade and serve with cooked steak.

Chicken Marsala

LOW-CARB/KETO, DAIRY-FREE

SUGGESTED WINE PAIRING: **PINOT NOIR OR CHIANTI CLASSICO**

. . . .

THIS CLASSIC ITALIAN DISH FEATURES FORTIFIED WINE FROM SICILY'S MAR-
SALA REGION. USE WHATEVER MUSHROOMS YOU LIKE! (CHECK OUT THE
MARINATED MUSHROOM RECIPE ON PAGE 331 FOR HEALTH BENEFITS!) THE
SAUCE'S GELATIN SUPPORTS GUT HEALTH AND BALANCES THE AMINO ACID PRO-
FILE OF THE CHICKEN.

. . . .

    2 chicken breast cutlets, pounded to ½-inch thickness
    ½ teaspoon salt
    ⅛ teaspoon cracked black pepper
    1 tablespoon avocado oil*
    1 tablespoon grass-fed gelatin*
    ½ cup Marsala wine
    3 cups assorted mushrooms, cut into manageable pieces
    ½ cup Bone Broth* (see page 275 to create your own)

1. Sprinkle salt and pepper over both sides of the chicken.
2. In a large frying pan, heat avocado oil over medium-high heat and sauté chicken until golden on both sides, about 2 minutes per side.
3. Set chicken aside, covered, to stay warm.
4. Sprinkle gelatin over ¼ cup wine and set aside to bloom.
5. Add mushrooms to pan, combining with as much of the pan scrapings as possible, and cook for 5 minutes.
6. Add remaining wine, gelatin-wine mix, and broth to pan; once boiling, reduce heat to a simmer.
7. Simmer mushrooms in sauce until thickened, about 5 more minutes.
8. Return chicken to pan and toss with sauce.

Jerk Chicken with Digestive Pineapple Salsa

CHICKEN AND MARINADE: **LOW-CARB/KETO, DAIRY-FREE, LOW-FODMAP* (OMIT GARLIC)**

SALSA: **DAIRY-FREE, VEGAN, LOW-FODMAP**

SUGGESTED WINE PAIRING: **LATE-HARVEST RIESLING OR GEWÜRZTRAMINER**

Jerk chicken gets its heated intensity from habanero peppers, which have loads of vitamin C and boost the metabolism. The accompanying raw salsa is rich in digestion-aiding ingredients: pineapple, which contains the enzyme bromelain, as well as ginger. Feel free to use the salsa in other dishes as well!

MAKES 2 SERVINGS

½ habanero pepper, seeded and chopped

2 garlic cloves, chopped

2 tablespoons ginger root (about 1-inch piece), grated

¼ cup chopped scallion (about ½ scallion)

1 teaspoon refined coconut oil*

1 teaspoon coconut aminos*

½ teaspoon thyme

½ teaspoon cinnamon

½ teaspoon allspice

¼ teaspoon salt

⅛ teaspoon nutmeg

2 tablespoons lime juice

2 tablespoons orange juice

2 chicken breasts or 4 chicken thighs, skin on, with bones

1. Puree all ingredients except chicken, and coat chicken in marinade. Let sit, refrigerated, for 1 to 4 hours.

continued

2. Preheat oven to 350°F.

3. Place chicken pieces on a lined baking sheet and bake until fully cooked, about 45 minutes.

4. If desired, once cooked, put under broiler for 2 to 3 minutes to darken and crisp.

SALSA

1 small red bell pepper, chopped

½ cup fresh pineapple, chopped

½ cup fresh papaya, chopped

2 tablespoons mint, chopped

2 tablespoons cilantro, chopped

3 to 4 tablespoons lemon juice

2 tablespoons lime juice

Pinch of salt

Combine all ingredients in a mixing bowl and refrigerate for at least 15 minutes before serving.

Chicken Parmesan

DAIRY-FREE

SUGGESTED WINE PAIRING: **BARBERA OR SANGIOVESE**

. . . .

Chicken parmesan without the cheese and breading, yet still über-delicious? Yes please! And if nightshades don't bother you, the marinara in this recipe has many other awesome uses as well: It can be used as a topping for Bison Meatloaf (page 297), as an ingredient in Lasagna (page 316), to instantly spice up other meat and fish dishes, or perfectly paired with zoodles or spaghetti squash! MAKES 2 LARGE OR 4 SMALL SERVINGS

. . . .

MARINARA

MAKES APPROXIMATELY 3 CUPS

1½ tablespoons avocado oil*

1 onion, chopped

4 garlic cloves, minced

1 tablespoon dried oregano

1 tablespoon dried basil

¾ teaspoon salt

4 ounces tomato paste*

1 (16-ounce) jar crushed tomatoes

1. Heat oil in a medium saucepan over medium-high heat; add onion and cook until just golden, about 10 minutes.
2. Add garlic, oregano, basil, salt, and tomato paste to pot; stir well.
3. Add crushed tomatoes, stir well, and reduce heat to a simmer.
4. Remove marinara from heat and let cool slightly.

continued

CHICKEN

2 chicken breasts, pounded to ¾-inch thickness

2 zucchini, sliced lengthwise into four slices each

⅓ cup almond flour* (see page 347 to create your own)

1 tablespoon dried oregano

1 tablespoon dried basil

¼ teaspoon salt

Pinch of black pepper

1½ teaspoons avocado oil*

2 tablespoons nutritional yeast*

1. Preheat oven to 400°F.
2. While the marinara cooks, prep chicken and zucchini. Mix almond flour with oregano, basil, salt, and pepper; dredge the chicken and zucchini in this almond flour mix, then place them on a cookie sheet with avocado oil.
3. Bake chicken and zucchini slices about 15 minutes, until golden, then flip and bake an additional 5 to 10 minutes.
4. Assemble in a casserole dish by layering as follows: a quarter of the marinara sauce, zucchini, a quarter of the nutritional yeast; a quarter of the marinara, a quarter of the nutritional yeast, chicken; half of the marinara, and half of the nutritional yeast.
5. Bake 15 minutes at 375°F.

Orange Duck

DAIRY-FREE

SUGGESTED WINE PAIRING: **GERMAN AUSLESE RIESLING OR TEMPRANILLO**

Fancying poultry but want to branch out beyond the stereotypical chicken? Though duck is daunting for many because it can dry out easily, this quick-prep method yields succulent results! Duck is notably high in saturated and monounsaturated fat, making it a nice bridge between chicken and red meat, and it's lower in omega-6 than other poultry. It's also very high in thyroid-supporting selenium and detox-supporting glutathione! Garam masala is a spice mix available at major grocery stores, and it includes blood-sugar-stabilizing cinnamon, antifungal cloves, and digestion-enhancing nutmeg. MAKES 2 SERVINGS

DUCK
2 duck breasts, skin on
¼ teaspoon salt

ORANGE GLAZE
½ cup orange juice
1 tablespoon honey*
½ teaspoon garam masala

1. Sprinkle duck breasts with salt. Place a medium frying pan or skillet over medium-high heat and add duck breasts, skin side down.
2. Sauté 10 minutes, then drain most of the fat from the pan. Flip and cook an additional 4 to 5 minutes.
3. While duck cooks, make glaze. In a small saucepan, heat orange juice, honey, and garam masala together over medium heat until boiling, then reduce to a simmer. Simmer for 5 minutes, then remove from heat.
4. Let duck rest for 10 minutes, then return to pan and add glaze. Stir well and serve.

Turkey with Apple-Cranberry Chutney

TURKEY: **LOW-CARB/KETO, LOW-FODMAP, AIP* (SUBSTITUTE REFINED COCONUT OIL FOR GHEE)**

CHUTNEY: **DAIRY-FREE, VEGETARIAN**

SUGGESTED WINE PAIRING: **FRUITY ZINFANDEL OR BEAUJOLAIS**

. . . .

While you can totally enjoy this sweet and savory dish any time of year, it's fantastic to have in your arsenal for the holidays! Plus, cranberries are high in thyroid-supporting iodine, can positively modulate the gut microbiome, and are also a go-to source for D-mannose, which is great for attacking UTIs. (Who needs that during the holidays?) The pectin in apples helps slow sugar absorption, which is a nice side benefit. Feel free to use the chutney with other entrées, or pair it with charcuterie and/or cheese if you're including dairy in your personal Paleo protocol. See page 339 for the perfect Paleo Pumpkin Pie happy ending!

MAKES 2 SERVINGS

. . . .

TURKEY

1 tablespoon ghee*

½ teaspoon salt

¼ teaspoon cracked black pepper

1 small turkey breast

CHUTNEY

1 Granny Smith apple, peeled and grated

1 cup fresh or frozen cranberries

½ cup orange juice

⅓ cup honey*

¼ cup raisins

2 tablespoons apple cider vinegar*

2 tablespoons grated ginger (about 1-inch piece)

1 teaspoon mustard seeds

1. Preheat oven to 425°F.
2. Rub ghee, salt, and pepper all over turkey breast and place in a baking dish.
3. Put breast in oven and after 5 minutes reduce heat to 350°F.
4. Bake until done, about one hour for a small breast. If not cooked throughout, check every 10 to 15 minutes. (Turkey should reach an internal temperature of 165°F.)
5. Make chutney while turkey cooks. Combine all ingredients in a large saucepan and bring to a boil; reduce to a simmer and cook until cranberries are popped and apples are soft, about 15 minutes.

Slow-Baked Lemon-Dill Salmon with Sautéed Spinach

SALMON: **LOW-CARB/KETO, DAIRY-FREE, PESCATARIAN, LOW-FODMAP, AIP**

SPINACH: **LOW-CARB/KETO, LACTO-VEGETARIAN**

SUGGESTED WINE PAIRING: **SAUVIGNON BLANC OR CALIFORNIA CHARDONNAY**

. . . .

This simple-yet-flavorful, light-yet-satiating dish is swimming with digestion-aiding lemon, anti-inflammatory dill, and the vital EPA and DHA forms of omega-3 fatty acids. The spinach provides whole-food fiber, vitamin C, and antioxidants, and is cooked with just enough fat for optimal nutrient absorption! MAKES 1 SERVING

. . . .

SALMON

1 (6-ounce) fillet salmon

1 teaspoon avocado oil*

2 tablespoons chopped fresh dill

3 (¼-inch-thick) lemon slices

Pinch of salt

Pinch of black pepper

1. Preheat oven to 275°F.
2. Place salmon on a baking sheet drizzled lightly with avocado oil, and sprinkle dill, salt, and pepper over salmon; drizzle with remaining oil.
3. Bake salmon until opaque, about 16 to 25 minutes, depending on thickness of fillet. Serve with lemon slices.

SPINACH

1 tablespoon ghee*

3 ounces baby spinach

1 clove garlic, minced

1. Heat a medium pan over medium-high heat; once hot, add ghee and allow to melt.
2. Add spinach and garlic and stir frequently until spinach is wilted fully, 2 to 3 minutes.

Coconut Black Cod

LOW-CARB/KETO, DAIRY-FREE, PESCATARIAN, AIP* (SUBSTITUTE AVOCADO OR
COCONUT OIL FOR SESAME OIL)

SUGGESTED WINE PAIRING: **BUTTERY CHARDONNAY OR SLIGHTLY SWEET PINOT GRIGIO**

Black cod—which is actually part of the sablefish rather than cod family—is one of the silkiest fish available. Its mild taste pairs perfectly with coconut, which provides its own luxurious crunch, additional sweetness, and metabolism-boosting MCTs! MAKES 1 SERVING

1 (6-ounce) fillet black cod

1 tablespoon coconut aminos*

2 tablespoons small dried coconut flakes*

Pinch of white pepper

Small drizzle toasted sesame oil*

1. Preheat oven to 375°F.
2. Place black cod on a baking sheet.
3. Pour coconut aminos over fish and let marinate for 16 to 18 minutes.
4. Pat away any excess liquid, then cover with coconut flakes, patting them into the fish firmly.
5. Top with pepper.
6. Bake 12 to 14 minutes, depending on thickness of fillet, until opaque.
7. Drizzle lightly with toasted sesame oil.

Tropical Shrimp and Scallop Ceviche

DAIRY-FREE, PESCATARIAN

SUGGESTED WINE PAIRING: **SANCERRE SAUVIGNON BLANC OR ALBARINO**

Ceviche is a Latin American dish that uses citrus juice to "cook" seafood, bypassing any issues of cooking with heat. Yay! Shellfish are a particularly excellent source of many oft-lacking nutrients, including B_{12}, iodine, selenium, and zinc. This rendition features the refreshing sweetness of mango and just enough heat to feel authentic. With no raw onion, raw whitefish, or cilantro, it's sure to please even a picky eater! MAKES 2 SERVINGS

6 large scallops
6 large shrimp
½ red bell pepper, diced
½ small mango, diced
1 jalapeño, minced
1 scallion, thinly sliced, optional
½ teaspoon garlic salt
⅓ cup orange juice
⅓ cup lime juice
Plantain chips* or avocado

1. Mix all ingredients except the plantain chips together in a mixing bowl, then cover and refrigerate for one hour.
2. Stir and discard soaking liquids. Serve in a bowl with plantain chips, or hollow out avocado halves and fill with ceviche.

Deviled Egg Tuna Salad
(or Tuna Salad Deviled Eggs)

LOW-CARB/KETO, PESCATARIAN, LOW-FODMAP

SUGGESTED WINE PAIRING: **ROSÉ OR UNOAKED CHARDONNAY WITH THE TUNA;
SPARKLING ROSÉ OR CHAMPAGNE WITH THE DEVILED EGGS**

Tuna salad is near and dear to my heart, as it was a quick go-to meal in my family. This recipe offers a nice spin on it, using soft-boiled egg yolks to replace much of tuna salad's traditionally used mayo. Not only do the yolks add texture and flavor, but they're also akin to a whole-foods multivitamin, rich in B_{12}, A, D, E, and K, zinc, selenium, choline, the anti-inflammatory omega-3 DHA, the highly antioxidant cysteine, and lecithin! So many things! Plus, bringing deviled eggs to parties always looks fancy. MAKES 3 SERVINGS

3 large soft-boiled eggs, halved

1 (6-ounce) jar tuna* in oil or water

1 tablespoon mayonnaise* (see page 289 to create your own)

1 teaspoon yellow mustard*

½ teaspoon salt

¼ teaspoon dill weed

Pinch of black pepper

1. Separate egg yolks from whites.
2. Combine all ingredients except egg whites in a mixing bowl and stir until well combined.
3. For deviled egg tuna salad, chop egg whites and add to tuna mix. For tuna salad deviled eggs, pile a large dollop of tuna salad into each egg white half.

Burger with Sweet-Potato-Slice Bun

DAIRY-FREE, AIP

SUGGESTED WINE PAIRING: PINOTAGE WITH LIGHTER CONDIMENTS, MALBEC WITH HEAVIER CONDIMENTS

. . . .

Craving a burger with its bun intact? Thankfully, sweet potatoes are totally Paleo, rich in vitamin A and C, potassium, manganese, and phenolic acids! Choose grass-fed beef to ramp up nutrition! You can top your burger with some homemade Mayo (page 289), Sauerkraut (page 281), Guac (page 291), Marinated Mushrooms (page 331), and round things out with homemade Paleo-friendly Jicama Fries (page 333)! Who needs fast food? MAKES 1 BURGER

. . . .

    1 sweet potato
    1 teaspoon avocado oil*
    ¼ teaspoon salt
    ½ teaspoon onion powder
    ¼ teaspoon garlic salt
    ⅛ teaspoon black pepper
    ⅓ pound 85/15 ground beef (or other protein/fat ratio if preferred)

1. Preheat oven to 400°F.
2. Slice two ¾-inch-thick slices from the sweet potato, either lengthwise or in disks depending on the size of your tuber—whatever shape holds the burger best. Place the slices on a cookie sheet lightly drizzled with half of the avocado oil, then drizzle remaining oil over slices and sprinkle with salt.
3. Roast sweet potatoes about 20 minutes, until browned and cooked.
4. Mix onion powder, garlic salt, and pepper into ground beef and form into a large patty.
5. Grill burger on a grill or in a grill pan to desired level of cooking—about 6 to 7 minutes for medium-rare, or 8 to 9 minutes for medium-well.

Pesto Spaghetti Squash

SQUASH: **LOW-CARB, DAIRY-FREE, VEGAN, LOW-FODMAP, AIP**

PESTO: **LOW-CARB/KETO, DAIRY-FREE, VEGAN, LOW-FODMAP* (OMIT GARLIC), AIP* (OMIT NUTRITIONAL YEAST)**

SUGGESTED WINE PAIRING: **ITALIAN UNOAKED CHARDONNAY OR PINOT GRIGIO**

Finding it hard to break up with spaghetti? This Paleo alternative will have you moving on like it was never a thing! Not only is this recipe delicious, but its zesty pesto is bursting with detoxifying lemon juice, antimicrobial garlic, and avocados, which provide vitamin E and richness, sans cheese! Store any leftover pesto sauce (which is great on other entrées as well!) with an extra squeeze of lemon juice on top, to prevent browning. MAKES 4 SERVINGS

1 small spaghetti squash, cut in half, seeds removed

PESTO
2 cups basil leaves
2 garlic cloves
3 to 4 tablespoons lemon juice
1 tablespoon nutritional yeast*
½ medium avocado
3 tablespoons extra virgin olive oil*
½ teaspoon salt
¼ teaspoon black pepper

1. Preheat oven to 375°F. In a baking dish, place squash skin side up in ½ inch of water, then bake 30 minutes.
2. Flip squash over with tongs and bake for about 15 more minutes, until tender, when threads separate easily with a fork. Once cooled, remove squash threads.
3. To make pesto, combine all remaining ingredients in a blender or food processor and blend or process until creamy, with bits of basil remaining.
4. Toss squash with pesto and serve.

Breaded Veggie Bake

LOW-CARB* (DEPENDING ON VEGGIES), DAIRY-FREE* (OMIT GHEE), VEGAN* (OMIT GHEE)

SUGGESTED WINE PAIRING: **CHARDONNAY OR PINOT NOIR, IF FEATURING MUSHROOMS**

. . . .

Wanting to go hardcore #teamveggie, and feel supersatiated in the process? This hearty vegan dish is awash in possibility, open to featuring any of your favorite veggies! Feel free to go as simple or as crazy as you like!

MAKES 2 SERVINGS

. . . .

> 2 cups mixed vegetables (broccoli, zucchini, carrots, etc.), cut into bite-size pieces
> ¼ cup Nut Milk* (page 345)
> Drizzle of melted ghee*
> 3 tablespoons Paleo Bread Crumbs (page 349)

1. Preheat oven to 375°F.
2. Dip veggies in milk, then in bread crumbs, then place on a lined cookie sheet.
3. Drizzle with a tiny amount of melted ghee and bake in the oven for about 15 minutes, until browned.

Lasagna

DAIRY-FREE, VEGAN (OMIT MEAT)

SUGGESTED WINE PAIRING: **SANGIOVESE OR PINOT NOIR**

Lasagna without cheese or noodles? Totally possible! The delicious flavors and textures in this dish can satiate your inner Italian any day, with far more nutrients than typical versions to boot! MAKES 4 SERVINGS

4 zucchini, sliced lengthwise into thin slices

1 teaspoon salt

2 cups Marinara Sauce (page 303)

½ pound cooked ground turkey, chicken, lamb, bison, or beef, optional

½ cup basil, chopped

1 cup Alfredo Sauce (page 288)

¼ cup Paleo Bread Crumbs (page 349)

1. In a colander, toss zucchini with ¾ teaspoon salt and let liquid drain from it for 20 minutes.
2. Preheat oven to 350°F.
3. Combine marinara with cooked ground meat, if using.
4. In a small casserole dish, layer as follows: a quarter of the zucchini slices, 2 tablespoons basil, a small sprinkle of salt, ½ cup marinara sauce, and ¼ cup Alfredo sauce. Do this four times, ending with marinara and Alfredo on top. Sprinkle with bread crumbs, then place in oven and bake for about 45 minutes, until Alfredo is golden.

Coconut Flour Pancakes

OVO-VEGETARIAN

SUGGESTED WINE PAIRING: **SPARKLING WINE OR VIOGNIER**

. . . .

This simple pancake recipe offers the joy of a short stack without the flour, or any of the starches or gums found in many gluten-free baking mixes. It's also rich in fiber, protein, metabolism-boosting MCTs from coconut oil, and the many nutrients of eggs. Consider topping with some honey (try Manuka honey from New Zealand if you want to get *real* medicinal!), maple syrup, or fresh berries. Skipping breakfast with intermittent fasting? You can totally have these for lunch or dinner! MAKES 16 TO 18 SILVER-DOLLAR PANCAKES

. . . .

½ cup plus 1 tablespoon coconut flour*

¼ cup coconut sugar*

¾ teaspoon baking soda

¼ teaspoon salt

6 large eggs

⅓ cup melted coconut oil*

⅓ cup Nut Milk* (page 345)

1. Combine dry ingredients (flour through salt) in a mixing bowl until free of lumps.
2. Add wet ingredients and whisk until uniform in texture. Mixture should be the thickness of standard pancake batter; if too thin, add an additional tablespoon of coconut flour; if too thick, add a tablespoon of nut milk.
3. Heat a pan or griddle on medium heat and drop 2 to 3 tablespoons of batter for each pancake, spreading out slightly with the back of a spoon. Cook several minutes until golden underneath and no longer forming bubbles, then flip and cook an additional several minutes until golden on the underside.

Prosciutto Mushroom Frittata

LOW-CARB/KETO, OVO-VEGETARIAN* (OMIT PROSCIUTTO)

SUGGESTED WINE PAIRING: **CHAMPAGNE OR PINOT BLANC**

. . . .

This delicious frittata is insanely rich in fat-soluble vitamins, omega-3 fatty acids, and choline, cysteine, and lecithin from eggs. The prosciutto enhances flavor and gives the dish a heartier feel, while the assorted mushrooms add both a classic quiche element and immune-boosting properties. (Check out the Marinated Mushroom recipe on page 331 for more on mushrooms' benefits!) Feel free to add in other veggies or spices to really make this frittata your own! You can also make this dish ahead of time, refrigerate raw, and cook when ready, or reheat the cooked version for quick breakfasts on the go! MAKES 2 SERVINGS

. . . .

> 6 large eggs
> ½ teaspoon salt
> Pinch of black pepper
> 1 teaspoon avocado oil*
> 1 ounce prosciutto,* sliced or chopped
> 2 ounces maitake, shiitake, porcini, and/or oyster mushrooms

1. Preheat oven to 350°F.
2. Whisk the eggs with salt and pepper until smooth.
3. Heat a medium pan over medium-high heat, and add avocado oil.
4. Add prosciutto and sauté until crispy, about 5 minutes.
5. Remove prosciutto, set aside, and add mushrooms; sauté until tender, 3 to 4 minutes. Remove from heat and allow to cool.
6. In a pie plate or loaf pan, place mushrooms and prosciutto; top with whisked eggs and bake until fluffy and golden, about 25 minutes.

SOUPS

Boeuf Bourguignon

DAIRY-FREE, LOW-FODMAP* (OMIT ONIONS)

SUGGESTED WINE PAIRING: **THE SAME BURGUNDY USED IN THE SOUP**

Also known as beef Burgundy, *boeuf Bourguignon* is a fancy term for beef stew made with Burgundy wine, which comes from the eponymous region in France, known for its Pinot Noirs! Classic boeuf Bourguignon has a roux, tomato products, and a whole lot of wine; this gluten- and nightshade-free rendition keeps only the wine (the best part!), using healthful pureed vegetables in lieu of a roux. MAKES 4 SERVINGS

1 tablespoon bacon fat (lard)*
¾ teaspoon salt
1 pound beef stew meat, cubed
2 parsnips, sliced in thick coins
2 carrots, sliced in thick coins
1 onion, chopped
1 turnip, cubed
2 cups Burgundy wine
1 cup Bone Broth* (see page 275 to create your own)
1 bay leaf
2 sprigs fresh thyme
Pinch of cracked black pepper

1. Heat a saucepan to medium high and add bacon fat.
2. Sprinkle half of the salt over beef pieces and sauté until browned, about 5 minutes. (You can also do this directly in your slow cooker or pressure cooker, if supported by your appliance.)
3. Add parsnips, carrots, onion, and turnip, and sauté until slightly softened, about 5 minutes.

4. Transfer (if applicable) to pressure cooker or slow cooker. Add remaining ingredients and put lid on; in a pressure cooker, pressurize and then cook for one hour. In a slow cooker, turn to high and cook for 4 hours. Depressurize or turn off slow cooker and allow to cool slightly.

5. Remove 2 cups of cooked vegetables along with a small amount of broth, and puree in blender until smooth. Alternately, simply remove and then mash vegetables with a potato masher.

6. Return pureed or mashed vegetables to cooker and stir to combine, creating a thick sauce for beef and remaining vegetables. Discard bay leaf and thyme sprigs.

Coconut Lemongrass Soup

LOW-CARB, DAIRY-FREE, VEGAN, AIP

SUGGESTED WINE PAIRING: **OFF-DRY GERMAN RIESLING OR NEW ZEALAND SAUVIGNON BLANC**

In this delicious Thai soup, lemongrass transforms a simple vegetable stock into a lush, exotic adventure, while coconut butter provides plenty of coconut flavor without the need for coconut milk. Feel free to snazzy things up with some chicken, beef, or fish as well! MAKES 2 SERVINGS

2 cups vegetable stock*
1 (3- to 4-inch) stalk lemongrass
1½ tablespoons coconut butter*
1 teaspoon coconut aminos*
1 tablespoon scallions, sliced
1 tablespoon fresh cilantro, chopped

1. Heat vegetable stock in a medium saucepan until simmering; add lemongrass and let simmer gently for 15 minutes.
2. Add coconut butter and coconut aminos, and whisk to combine. Remove lemongrass stalk and discard.
3. Add scallions and cilantro, and remove from heat.

Variations

Desiring a heartier soup? Add any of the following optional proteins along with step 3.

1 dozen cooked shrimp
¾ cup cooked chicken breast or thigh
½ cup sliced steak
¼ cup cashews

Butternut Squash Bisque

DAIRY-FREE, VEGAN, AIP

SUGGESTED WINE PAIRING: **CHARDONNAY OR VIOGNIER**

Looking for a soothing, warm soup for a cool autumn or cold winter night? Look no further than this tasty bisque, featuring a fruit masquerading as a vegetable: butternut squash! Squash is rich in vitamin A, vitamin C, magnesium, potassium (more than a banana!), and much more, while being easy on digestion to boot. Though you can make this soup with steamed or baked squash, roasting yields a ton more flavor. Plus, you don't have to cube the squash, saving solid prep time! MAKES 4 SERVINGS

- 1 tablespoon coconut oil*
- ¾ teaspoon salt
- 1 small butternut squash, cut in half lengthwise with seeds removed
- 2 cups vegetable stock*
- ½ teaspoon ground sage
- ¼ teaspoon black pepper

1. Preheat oven to 375°F.
2. Drizzle oil and salt over butternut squash, then place skin side up in a baking dish.
3. Roast until soft, about 45 minutes. Let cool.
4. Scoop flesh out of squash skin halves and blend in a blender with remaining ingredients until smooth.

Stone Fruit Gazpacho

DAIRY-FREE, VEGETARIAN, AIP

SUGGESTED WINE PAIRING: **MOSCATO D'ASTI OR LATE-HARVEST GERMAN RIESLING**

Looking for a refreshing soup to combat the heat of summer? This gazpacho has totally got you covered! Though using in-season fresh fruit is awesome and quite Paleo in spirit, this recipe will also accommodate frozen fruit (which is typically picked in season anyway, and also preserves nutrients!). Choose a combo of whatever stone fruits you enjoy most, and peel them if you'd like a silkier texture. MAKES 4 SERVINGS

4 pieces stone fruit such as peaches, plums, large apricots, and/or nectarines, pitted

½ cucumber, seeded and peeled

½ cup fresh orange juice

1 to 2 tablespoons honey* (depending on sweetness or tartness of fruit)

1 tablespoon extra virgin olive oil*

1 tablespoon lemon or lime juice

1 tablespoon chopped shallot

Pinch of salt

2 tablespoons fresh herbs such as mint, basil, or rosemary, for garnish

Blend all ingredients except herbs in a blender until desired consistency—you can whip completely for a creamy soup, or leave some bits for texture. Garnish with chopped herbs.

Congee

DAIRY-FREE, VEGAN* (USE WATER), LOW-FODMAP

SUGGESTED WINE PAIRING: **CHARDONNAY OR RIESLING (CHOOSE BODY AND/OR SWEETNESS TO MATCH YOUR CONGEE VARIATION)**

(Note: Do not pair with wine if consuming as part of a specific gut-healing protocol.)

Congee is a traditional Asian porridge made from slow cooked rice and water. Wait a minute . . . a GRAIN on the recipe list? What is happening?! For starters, please see page 61 for a discussion on white rice, which is gluten-free and basically devoid of antinutrients (if organic). In its congee form, white rice is also typically very easy on digestion and free of fiber. It features carbs in the form of glucose (rather than fructose or sucrose), which is assimilated high up in the digestive tract, discouraging gut fermentation. While you might not be wowed by congee on its own, consider it a medicinal base to which Chinese herbs, meat, and/or vegetables can be added—which can make it super yummy! Congee can be great when you're under the weather or looking to sooth digestion, or you can try it out to potentially address SIBO or IBS issues, depending on your personal constitution. Of course, you may find you just fancy this stuff as an easy, simple, cheap go-to meal any way! MAKES 2 SERVINGS

½ cup organic Jasmine rice*

3 cups water or Bone Broth*, or more if desiring a thinner porridge (see page 275 to create your own)

Salt to taste, optional

ON THE STOVETOP

1. In a small pot, combine rice and water or broth; bring to a boil, then reduce to a simmer.

continued

2. Stir occasionally and simmer for about 1½ hours, until rice is broken down into a silky porridge, then salt to taste if desired. More stirring will create more soft results; less stirring will keep rice grains more intact.

IN A PRESSURE COOKER

1. In a pressure cooker, combine rice and water or broth.
2. Cook 30 to 45 minutes, on high pressure or "multigrain" setting, if available.
3. Sauté in pressure cooker to further thicken, if desired.

Additions

Feel free to experiment and make congee your own! Add any additional ingredients while the congee is cooking.

Chinese herbs: astragalus, ginseng, ginger, reishi, etc.

Spices: ginger, garlic, lemongrass, mustard, cilantro, etc.

Coconut aminos*

"Chicken soup" veggies: carrots, celery, onions, mushrooms, etc.

Greens: spinach, Chinese broccoli, collards, etc.

Kimchi* or Sauerkraut* (see page 281 to create your own)

Shredded chicken breast

Shredded beef shank

Bacon and poached egg

Fish

Cinnamon, chopped apple, and coconut sugar

SIDES

Garlic Broccoli Sauté

LOW-CARB/KETO, DAIRY-FREE, VEGAN, AIP

SUGGESTED WINE PAIRING: **NEW-WORLD CHARDONNAY OR SAUVIGNON BLANC**

Why overcomplicate things? If you're craving nutrition, this simple side dish is *the* place to be. There's a reason broccoli consistently maintains its healthy reputation: It's brimming with vitamins (particularly vitamin C and folate), antioxidants, antimicrobials, and cancer-preventing sulforaphane. This sauté also has the added benefit of immune-supporting garlic, and coconut oil's metabolism-boosting MCTs. You seriously can't go wrong!

MAKES 2 SERVINGS

1 tablespoon refined coconut oil*
2 cups broccoli florets
3 garlic cloves, sliced thinly
½ teaspoon salt
⅛ teaspoon black pepper
Squeeze of lemon

1. Heat oil in a large sauté pan over medium-high heat.
2. Add broccoli florets and sauté, stirring occasionally, for 5 minutes.
3. Add garlic, salt, and pepper, and sauté an additional 2 to 3 minutes until broccoli is tender-crisp and garlic pieces are golden.
4. Turn off heat and add lemon to pan, then stir well to incorporate into the broccoli.

Slow-Cooked Black Kale

LOW-CARB/KETO, LACTO-VEGETARIAN

SUGGESTED WINE PAIRING: **ALSATIAN PINOT BLANC OR RIESLING**

. . . .

Think ya don't love kale? Think again! Slow cooking the green just may change your mind, thanks to the resulting incredibly tender texture. This version also minimizes oil by replacing it with heavier ghee. Of course, be prepared to hang out near the stove for a bit! Shorter cooking time, less fat, or skipping the blanching are all allowed, but won't yield as tender of a result . . . which is so worth it! MAKES 3 SERVINGS

. . . .

2 bunches black kale, thinly sliced
2 tablespoons ghee*
½ large sweet onion, thinly sliced
2 garlic cloves, thinly sliced
½ teaspoon smoked salt
¼ teaspoon black pepper

1. Blanch kale in boiling water for 2 minutes, then drain and squeeze out all moisture. Set aside.
2. In a medium pot, heat 1½ tablespoons ghee over medium-high heat.
3. Add onion and sauté until softened, about 5 minutes.
4. Add garlic and sauté an additional 5 minutes.
5. Add remaining ghee, kale, and seasonings, and reduce heat to medium low.
6. Stirring frequently, cook until kale is blackened, very withered, and soft, about 45 minutes.

Spinach Salad with Bacon Dressing

LOW-CARB/KETO, LOW-FODMAP

SUGGESTED WINE PAIRING: **PINOT NOIR OR MERLOT**

. . . .

Nothing livens up vitamin-K-packed leafy greens like bacon! This quick and easy dressing is rich enough to be an entrée-worthy salad on its own, but feel free to add chicken, steak, or other additions to really beef things up—no pun intended! You can also swap out spinach for chard, kale, or whatever leafy green you fancy! **MAKES 2 SERVINGS**

. . . .

8 slices nitrate-free bacon*

¼ cup red wine vinegar*

1 tablespoon Dijon mustard*

½ teaspoon salt

¼ teaspoon cracked black pepper

4 cups spinach leaves

½ cup diced tomatoes

2 large hard-boiled eggs

1. Preheat oven to 375°F.
2. Line a baking sheet with parchment and place bacon slices on it, then cook 10 to 15 minutes until desired level of doneness. Reserve fat.
3. Whisk ⅓ cup bacon fat with vinegar, mustard, salt, and pepper.
4. Place spinach in a large mixing bowl and top with half of dressing, giving it a couple minutes to wilt slightly.
5. Divide spinach into two bowls and top with tomatoes, bacon slices, and 1 egg each. Drizzle with remaining dressing.

Marinated Mushrooms

LOW-CARB/KETO, DAIRY-FREE, VEGAN

SUGGESTED WINE PAIRING: **OREGON PINOT NOIR OR BARBERA**

Mushrooms are actually one of the only plants to contain vitamin D, B12, and conjugated linoleic acid. Well, they're technically not plants! These medicinal fungi wield a ton of health benefits, from immune support to blood sugar and cholesterol regulation to Candida mitigation to #allthethings. Use whichever mushrooms you like, such as traditional button, crimini, or shiitake, or more adventurous adrenal-supporting reishi or iron-rich oyster. (Fun fact: The carnivorous oyster mushrooms chemically attack worms!) Marinated mushrooms actually work great if you don't cook them first, as they'll soften, but won't turn mushy as leftovers! MAKES 4 SERVINGS

1 pound mushrooms, cut into bite-size pieces

1 garlic clove, crushed

1 sprig rosemary, chopped (remove stem first)

3 tablespoons apple cider vinegar*

3 tablespoons extra virgin olive oil*

2 tablespoons balsamic vinegar*

1 tablespoon dill weed

1 tablespoon MCT oil*

½ teaspoon salt

Pinch of cayenne pepper

Mix all ingredients together in a large mixing bowl and let marinate for at least 30 minutes before serving, or up to a couple hours for more intense flavor!

Root Veggie Mash

LACTO-VEGETARIAN* (USE VEGETABLE BROTH), AIP

SUGGESTED WINE PAIRING: **BUTTERY CHARDONNAY OR YELLOW MUSCAT**

. . . .

The possibilities for Paleo-friendly mock mashed potatoes are limited only by your root vegetable imagination! This is the perfect opportunity to branch out and try some of those *strange-looking* tubers you've been wondering what to do with. For a sweeter mash, try sweet potatoes and yams. For something more traditional, consider name root or boniato (if ya can find them), turnips, or celery root. Want to go crazy with the colors? Add some heirloom carrots or purple sweet potatoes! If you know you enjoy the peel of a certain veggie, feel free to leave it on for more of a smash than a mash.

MAKES 2 SERVINGS

. . . .

¾ cup sweet root vegetables such as white sweet potato and/or parsnip, peeled and cubed

¾ cup savory root vegetables such as turnips, rutabagas, and/or celery root, peeled and cubed

½ cup Bone Broth* (see page 275 to create your own) or vegetable broth,* or more to taste

2 tablespoons butter*

½ teaspoon salt

⅛ teaspoon black pepper

Herb seasoning such as 1 tablespoon fresh rosemary, 1 teaspoon dill weed, or 2 tablespoons fresh parsley, optional

1. Steam root vegetables together until tender, either in a steamer or in a pot with a small amount of water. Let cool slightly.
2. Mash or blend vegetables with all remaining ingredients.

Jicama Fries

LOW-CARB, DAIRY-FREE, VEGAN, LOW FODMAP, AIP* (OMIT PAPRIKA)

SUGGESTED WINE PAIRING: **CHAMPAGNE OR PINOT GRIS**

Jicama is a crunchy, nutty, sweet tuber teeming with vitamin C, fiber, and assorted minerals, as well as prebiotics for your gut flora. Since these "fries" aren't even fried, they bypass the toxic by-products of traditional frying, while still becoming soft enough to mimic potatoes and make any fast-food clown or king jealous! MAKES 2 SERVINGS

> 2 cups jicama, peeled and sliced into matchsticks or other preferred french-fry size
> ¼ teaspoon paprika
> ¼ teaspoon salt, or more to taste
> ¼ teaspoon dried parsley
> 1 tablespoon avocado oil*

1. Preheat oven to 400°F.
2. Bring a pot of water to a boil and boil jicama until slightly softened, about 8 minutes.
3. Drain jicama and let cool slightly.
4. Toss jicama with seasonings and oil.
5. Place in a single layer on a cookie sheet and roast for 20 minutes, turning halfway through.

Cauliflower Rice

LOW-CARB, DAIRY-FREE, LACTO-VEGETARIAN

SUGGESTED WINE PAIRING: **CHENIN BLANC OR RICE WINE**

....

While riced vegetables once lurked on the eyebrow-raising fringe (flash-back to my low-carb days, eons ago!), they're becoming quite in vogue and are actually available (often frozen) in major grocery stores. This traditional cauliflower version features far fewer carbs than rice, but still yields a similar taste and texture. While a food processor works best, you can use a blender or box grater in a pinch (and get a nice functional arm workout in to boot!). MAKES 2 LARGE OR 4 SMALL SERVINGS

....

> 2 cups cauliflower florets
> 2 teaspoons butter*
> ½ teaspoon salt

1. In a food processor, pulse florets until they are broken up into approximately the size of rice kernels. If you don't have a food processor, chop by hand, grate on the outside of a box grater, or blend in a blender on low in multiple batches.
2. Steam cauliflower rice in a steamer until tender-crisp, 3 to 4 minutes. Alternately, add cauliflower to a medium saucepan with just enough water to cover the bottom and steam that way, then drain excess water.
3. In a mixing bowl, add cauliflower rice, butter, and salt, and stir well. Serve as you would white rice.

DESSERTS

Red Velvet Cake with Chocolate Frosting

CAKE: **OVO-VEGETARIAN**

FROSTING: **DAIRY-FREE, VEGETARIAN**

SUGGESTED WINE PAIRING: **RUBY PORT OR MOSCATO D'ASTI**

. . . .

Many a myth surround the origins of this Southern fav. Despite sciencey tales of chemical reactions causing its crimson hue, the cake typically utilizes artificial red dye. This recipe swaps that out for red beets, while maintaining the staple vinegar and cocoa powder. (Choose cacao for max health benefits!) While not as unnaturally bright, it'll still taste fantastic, and be better for ya to boot! The unique chocolate frosting perfectly pairs with the cake's cocoa accents, and is fantastic to have on hand for other Paleo desserts!

MAKES 12 SERVINGS

. . . .

CAKE

1 large beet

¼ cup almond milk* (see page 345 to create your own)

1½ cups almond flour* (see page 347 to create your own)

⅓ cup coconut sugar*

¼ cup coconut flour*

1 tablespoon raw cocoa* or raw cacao powder*

1 teaspoon baking soda

½ teaspoon salt

2 eggs

½ cup avocado oil* (substitute coconut oil* for a heavier cake, if desired)

¼ cup honey*

1 teaspoon vanilla extract*

1 teaspoon chocolate extract*

2 tablespoons apple cider vinegar*

1. Preheat oven to 350°F.
2. Make 2 cups of a beet puree by steaming or boiling the large beet, then blending with the almond milk.
3. Combine all dry ingredients in a mixing bowl, removing any lumps.
4. Add all the remaining ingredients, except cider vinegar, and mix well.
5. Once thoroughly mixed, add cider vinegar and fold in until swirled through.
6. Place batter in an 8-inch square or 8-inch round cake pan and bake until firm in the center, approximately 35 minutes.

FROSTING

3 medium avocados

½ cup coconut oil*

½ cup honey*

⅓ to ½ cup cocoa* or raw cacao powder,* depending on desired chocolate intensity

1 teaspoon vanilla extract*

1 teaspoon chocolate extract*

Pinch of salt

1. Combine all ingredients in a stand mixer or hand mixer and blend on high speed until smooth and creamy in texture.
2. Once cake has cooled, apply frosting.

Snickerdoodle Cookies

LACTO-OVO VEGETARIAN

SUGGESTED WINE PAIRING: **MUSCAT OR SAUTERNES**

When that adorable Girl Scout comes a-knocking, stay strong and turn to this recipe, which is equally reminiscent of childhood. The coconut sugar provides a delicious caramel flavor, while almond and coconut flours perfectly combine for delicious taste and texture. MAKES 12 COOKIES

1 tablespoon cinnamon

1 cup coconut sugar*

1½ cups almond flour* (see page 347 to create your own)

½ cup coconut flour*

1 teaspoon baking soda

¾ teaspoon salt

2 large eggs

⅓ cup butter,* softened

1. Preheat oven to 350°F.
2. Mix cinnamon and ¼ cup coconut sugar together in a small bowl and set aside.
3. Mix all remaining dry ingredients in a mixing bowl until free of lumps.
4. Add wet ingredients to the dry ingredients and whisk until smooth in texture.
5. Form into small balls and flatten slightly, then place on a cookie sheet.
6. Sprinkle 1 teaspoon cinnamon-sugar mix on top of each cookie. (Alternately, toss entire cookie ball in cinnamon sugar prior to flattening for a more strongly cinnamon-flavored cookie.)
7. Bake about 15 minutes, until golden.

Pumpkin Pie

LACTO-OVO VEGETARIAN

SUGGESTED WINE PAIRING: **TAWNY PORT OR TOKAJI**

What better way to round out that Turkey with Apple-Cranberry Chutney (page 306) or impress at a holiday party than with a deliciously healthy pumpkin pie? This quintessential, nostalgic fall dessert provides the vitamins and antioxidants of pumpkin, along with blood sugar–regulating cinnamon and anti-inflammatory cloves! MAKES 8 SERVINGS

1 Paleo Piecrust (page 350)

2 cups pumpkin puree*

1 cup full-fat coconut milk*

3 extra-large eggs

½ cup coconut sugar*

1½ tablespoons pumpkin pie spice

1½ teaspoons stevia powder*

¼ teaspoon salt

1. Prepare the Paleo Piecrust according to the recipe on page 350.
2. Mix all remaining ingredients together in a large mixing bowl until uniform in texture, then pour into cooled piecrust.
3. Bake until set, about 50 minutes.

No-Bake Chocolate Brownies

VEGAN

SUGGESTED WINE PAIRING: **SHERRY P.X. OR BANYULS**

. . . .

If you pledge allegiance to #teamchewy rather than #teamcakey (and perhaps are looking to save on your electrical bill?), then these raw brownies are totally for you! Rather than turning to chocolate's typically commercialized processed forms, these goodies are made with antioxidant-rich cocoa or cacao power. They also feature walnuts, which contain far more omega-3s than most nuts, and have been shown to support cardiovascular health. If you really want to go to chocolate town, you can add the Chocolate Frosting from the Red Velvet Cake on page 336. MAKES 12 BROWNIES

. . . .

1½ cups pitted dates (soften in water for ten minutes if hardened)

1 cup raw walnuts

⅓ cup cacao* or cocoa* powder (this quantity will result in a dark chocolate flavor—use less for a sweeter taste if desired)

1 tablespoon maple syrup,* or more to taste

½ teaspoon vanilla extract*

Pinch of salt

1. In a food processor, combine all ingredients until a uniform, crumbly texture is achieved.
2. Press mixture into a pan and refrigerate for at least one hour before serving.

Banana Bread

OVO-VEGETARIAN

SUGGESTED WINE PAIRING: **MADEIRA OR MUSCAT DE BEAUMES-DE-VENISE**

This throw-it-all-together banana bread recipe is denser, moister, and easier than many! If ya fancy big pieces of banana, you can even skip the step of mashing them first. Err on the side of caution in regards to baking time (more rather than less) for a pristine end result. MAKES 10 SERVINGS

3 very ripe bananas, mashed

4 large eggs

⅔ cup coconut flour*

⅓ cup coconut oil*

2 tablespoons maple syrup,* optional

1 dropperful liquid stevia*

1 teaspoon baking soda

¼ teaspoon salt

1. Preheat oven to 350°F.
2. In a mixing bowl, combine all ingredients until thoroughly mixed; lumps from bananas are acceptable.
3. Pour mixture into standard loaf pan and bake 45 to 50 minutes, until a knife or toothpick inserted comes out clean. Let cool before slicing.

Dreamy Dairy-Free Vanilla Ice Cream

DAIRY-FREE, VEGETARIAN

SUGGESTED WINE PAIRING: **CREAM SHERRY OR MUSCAT**

. . . .

Thanks to coconut milk's richness, it's easy to make a dairy-free ice cream as indulgent as its commercial, cow-derived alternative. (Choose a coconut milk without added gums!)

. . . .

>   2 cans full-fat coconut milk*
>   ½ cup coconut sugar*
>   ¼ cup honey*
>   1 teaspoon vanilla extract*
>   Scrapings of one vanilla pod, optional
>   ½ teaspoon salt

1. Prefreeze ice cream maker bowl.
2. Blend all ingredients in a blender until completely smooth.
3. Add mixture to ice cream maker and process according to maker's instructions. Eat as is for soft serve, or freeze until firm. Honey will help prevent overfreezing, but ice cream will still freeze pretty solid if frozen overnight, so take out a few minutes ahead of time before serving.

For Fruity Flavors

After blending ice cream base mixture, add one cup of cooked fruit. Fruit should be sweetened to taste. Stir in cooked fruit mix for a swirled ice cream, or blend briefly in the blender for a more uniform texture and color.

For Chocolate Chips

After blending ice cream base mixture, add ½ cup Paleo-friendly, unsweetened chocolate chips, or more to taste.

Sangria Gelatin

SUGGESTED WINE PAIRING: **ICE WINE OR SANGRIA**

Time to bring back the 1960s! Remember Jell-O salads? This red-wine-and-berry-rich adult dessert is full of antioxidants and gut-supporting gelatin! Use whatever red wine you fancy, and feel free to switch up the fruit if you aren't specifically going for a red theme—stone fruit or other berries would both be excellent. Be sure to avoid raw pineapple, as its enzymes can prevent gelling. MAKES 3 SERVINGS

½ cup raspberries (frozen fruit is okay)

¼ cup honey*

¼ cup water

1 tablespoon plus 1 teaspoon grass-fed gelatin*

1 cup red wine

½ cup chopped strawberries (choose fresh for best texture; if using frozen, thaw and drain)

1. In a small saucepan, bring raspberries, honey, and water to a boil together.
2. Reduce heat to a simmer and stir occasionally until berries are broken down, 5 minutes for fresh berries, 10 for frozen.
3. While berry syrup is cooking, bloom gelatin in wine.
4. Strain berry syrup and add gelatin-wine mix to it. Return to heat if gelatin does not dissolve into a glossy liquid, taking caution to not overheat or you'll lose the alcohol in the wine.
5. Add strawberries and pour into a bowl, pan, or molds.
6. Refrigerate for one hour, then stir gently to help berries fall down into the gelatin. Let chill until firm, about 3 hours more.

BASICS

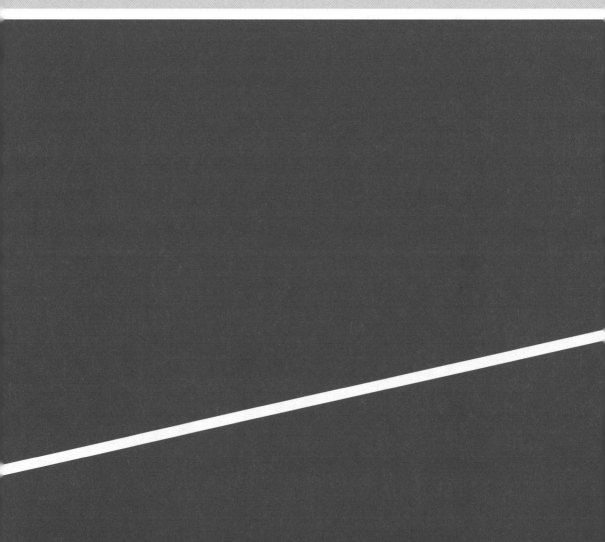

Nut Milk

LOW-CARB* (DEPENDING ON NUTS/SWEETENERS), DAIRY-FREE, VEGAN* (DEPENDING ON SWEETENERS), LOW-FODMAP* (DEPENDING ON NUTS/SWEETENERS)

Nut milks are delicious, nutritious alternatives to cow's milk, and can satisfy all your related baking and drinking needs! Unfortunately, almost all commercially available forms contain preservatives, thickeners, and sweeteners, so thank goodness it's super simple and inexpensive to make your own version at home! You can use whatever nuts you like, and can even try out seeds such as flax or pumpkin (which took my homemade nut milk virginity). Do avoid peanuts, which are actually a legume, highly allergenic, and sometimes moldy. Also make sure you get raw, organic versions, so you don't end up with a drink rich in pesticides and other potential nasties.

Soaking the nuts beforehand is key to deactivating enzyme inhibitors and phytic acid, which can bind to nutrients and inhibit digestion, and also yields a tastier, creamier milk. You can play with the ratio of nuts to water to reach your desired consistency. For baking recipes, make unsweetened versions; for beverages, you can experiment with Paleo-friendly sweeteners (such as honey and stevia) and flavorings (such as vanilla extract, cinnamon, or cocoa/cacao powder) to really make it your own! You can also save the leftover almond pulp to add to other goodies, or even turn it into almond meal. So many things!

MAKES ABOUT 4 CUPS, DEPENDING ON PREFERRED CONSISTENCY

1 cup unsalted, raw, organic nuts or Paleo-friendly seeds (almonds, cashews, hazelnuts, macadamia, pistachios, pumpkin seeds, walnuts, etc.)

3 to 4 cups water, depending on preferred consistency

1. Soak nuts in a bowl with filtered water for 8 to 24 hours. (Note: Macadamia and pine nuts are generally not soaked.)
2. Rinse the nuts, discarding the soaking liquid.

continued

3. Add nuts and fresh filtered water to blender.

4. Pulse and then blend on high for around 2 minutes, until milk reaches creamy, milky-white consistency.

5. Strain nut milk through a nut milk bag or a strainer with a cheesecloth laid on top. (This step is optional, but it's best for a smooth, drinkable version.)

6. Store nut milk in a covered container in the fridge for up to 3 or 4 days. Milk may separate, so shake before serving.

Additions

For sweetened or flavored nut milks, add Paleo-friendly ingredients to taste.

Honey* or stevia*
Vanilla extract* or vanilla bean
Cocoa/cacao powder*
Salt

For Almond Pulp

If desired, save leftover pulp from strained milk to add to shakes, baked goods, etc. You can store the pulp in the freezer for later use.

Nut Flour

Almond nut flour is a wonderfully versatile grain and gluten-free baking ingredient, but it can be quite expensive and hard to find organic. Thankfully, as with nut milks, you can totally make your own! Though homemade versions will be slightly more textured and brown-flecked in appearance compared to commercial versions, the taste is still totally delicious! (You can blanch your almonds beforehand for a more commercial flour consistency.) The soaking step is optional, but it helps remove antinutrients such as phytic acid and enzyme inhibitors, which can bind to nutrients and hamper digestion. Favor pulsing rather than blending, to avoid accidentally creating a nut butter rather than flour. MAKES ABOUT 1 CUP

1 cup unsalted, raw, organic nuts (almonds, cashews, hazelnuts, macadamia, pistachios, walnuts, etc.)

1. Soak nuts in a bowl with filtered water for 8 to 24 hours. (Note: Macadamia and pine nuts are generally not soaked.)
2. Rinse the nuts, discarding the soaking liquid. Dry nuts in dehydrator, or air dry.
3. Pulse dry nuts, ½ cup at a time, in a high-speed blender or food processor until desired flour consistency is reached.

Almond Meal

LOW-CARB*, DAIRY-FREE, VEGAN

Confused by a recipe calling for almond meal rather than almond flour? We got you covered! Almond meal tends to be slightly grittier than almond flour, and you can make it from your leftover Nut Milk's almond pulp (page 346). Impatient? You can also quickly whip some up from store-bought almonds, for all your Paleo-friendly baking needs! Like with the nut flour, the soaking step is optional, but great for de-activating antinutrients.

MAKES APPROXIMATELY 1 CUP

1 cup almond pulp from Nut Milk (page 346), or 1 cup unsalted raw organic almonds

FROM ALMOND PULP

1. Bake strained pulp on a baking sheet at 100°F for 2 to 5 hours until dry.
2. Pulse in a food processor or high-speed blender, until it reaches a medium-fine texture or desired consistency.

FROM ALMONDS

1. Soak almonds in a bowl with filtered water for 8 to 24 hours.
2. Dry in a dehydrator, or air dry thoroughly.
3. Pulse in a food processor or high-speed blender, until it reaches a medium-fine texture, or desired consistency.

Paleo Bread Crumbs

LOW-CARB*, DAIRY-FREE, VEGAN

These versatile gluten-free "bread" crumbs are perfect to have in your back pocket! They're key for the Breaded Veggie Bake (page 315), and can also be used to crust fish, make jalapeño poppers, top a dairy-free mock mac and cheese, and tons of other things! **MAKES APPROXIMATELY 3 TABLESPOONS**

¼ cup Almond Meal* (page 348)
½ tablespoon all-purpose salt-free seasoning*
½ teaspoon garlic powder
½ teaspoon salt

Mix all ingredients together.

Paleo Piecrust

LOW-CARB*, LACTO-VEGETARIAN

U se this tasty and versatile starch-free, gum-free, gluten-free crust for all your pie needs!

MAKES 1 PIECRUST

2 cups almond flour* (see page 347 to create your own)
⅓ cup butter*
1 tablespoon honey*
Pinch of salt

1. Preheat oven to 350°F.
2. Pulse all ingredients together in a food processor until mixture begins to form a ball.
3. Press mixture into a pie plate, then bake about 10 minutes, until just golden. Let cool.

A Concluding Confession

Time to get real for a second, if I may.

Perhaps the most daunting part of writing this book lay not in the eons of research and perpetual second-guessing of sentence constructions, but rather in tackling this seemingly simple conclusion. For when all's said and done, how does one select that final resounding thought for the dear reader? Should I choose fireworks, melodramatic tears, a CliffsNotes summary, or perhaps one last inspirational proclamation of "You got this"? (Note: You totally do!)

In the end (as I suppose this is the end), I have settled upon a more serious matter that lies behind this book's otherwise cheerful demeanor. It is a pivotal piece of the puzzle, which ultimately served to crystalize my resolve and clear my vision, testifying to the beauty of this lifestyle, not just for weight loss, but also for its influence on my experience of life at large. I hope this anecdote shall not only validate my testimony, but ultimately motivate you to cannonball into the deep end of a new dietary world, whatever your motivation may be.

So here we go!

I initially resolved to write *The What When Wine Diet* because I could not escape the implications of how the composition of food, and timing of eating it, so radically influences one's body. Paleo and intermittent fasting 100 percent changed my life, and with the veil lifted, I wanted to spread the word, regardless of whether I came across as a crazy zealot. Admittedly, my early enthusiasm was primarily aesthetic (*Wait . . . you mean weight loss and maintenance can be easy?*), secondarily based on how I began to *feel* (*Oh hi, in-the-zone energy!*), and finished with a glistening top coat of health improvements (*No more headaches! Clearer skin! Fewer colds!*).

And then in the middle of all the wonder and transformation, something slipped.

Ya see, for 90 percent of my life, I was a motivated, happy girl who essentially lived life like it was a musical. I clung to the beauty of each magical, fleeting #moment, equally savoring both the laughter and tears. (The latter often rested on less-than-dire foundations of unrequited puppy love and existential reflections on the meaning of life, materializing in written form à la my Sad Quote Book.) Perhaps I'm wearing rose-colored glasses in evaluating the past, but I do remember, despite momentary hiccups and moments of panic about the future, an immutable thread of optimism. Definition glass half full. I looked at my peers dealing with mood swings, apathy, melancholy, or fear, and wondered why they didn't just get off the struggle bus. Life was too grand to wallow!

Then a conglomerate of factors post-graduation flew together to form a tornado worthy of my inner Dorothy. (Had to sneak in one last Oz allusion!) I moved into an adorable apartment I selected, quite honestly, for its appearance. Little did I know that behind the shiny pink '50s façade crept insidious black mold in all its crevices—from the shower to the wall behind my bed. Or that the oven, which adorns the cover of the first version of this book, leaked carbon monoxide every single time I cooked my Paleo meals. And little did I know that, when I'd venture to downtown Los Angeles one fateful night with one of my dearest friends for Korean BBQ, my digestive tract would encounter *something* that would leave me moaning on the floor for nights on end, to the point that I willingly showed up to the set of *Parenthood* to play a bartender with my makeup barely done and my hair in a ponytail. (As I'm an appearance control freak hiding behind the security blanket of my hair, this is quite telling. Everything is relative!) Or little did I know that I'd get a diagnosis of SIBO (small intestinal bacterial overgrowth), for which I'd nervously take a small intestine–specific antibiotic to try and fix things, only to welcome seemingly worse dysbiosis, coupled with a newfound perpetual bloatedness. And little did I know that this perfect storm of maladies would launch a substantial hit on my thyroid.

So. Many. Things.

And despite my resilient and arguably effective efforts to maintain some semblance of fiery passion (one must always maintain appearances!), things weren't so easy anymore. Actually, they were downright difficult. I felt the grips of fatigue, my once-rosy temperament was suddenly fragile, and I became fixated on my bowel movements—or lack thereof. I now understood the struggle to feel sanguine as I searched madly for answers in the black holes of online message boards, taking small comfort in the large community of fellow sufferers. My glass half full got returned for a glass only full of 50 percent liquid, and no one had offered me the receipt.

But there was a silver lining.

While the tectonic plates of my health had shifted, so too did my diet priorities and perspective. I finally got the gut-health-influence side of things that I'd been preaching all along. I now *understood* what it was like to feel the immediate effects of foods, popping up physically via GI distress, or emotionally in my brain's neurotransmitters. Whereas in the past, the ramifications of my standard American diet had manifested as a generalized state of inflammation and moodiness that I simply interpreted as "normal," knowing no other alternative, these newfound troubles now contrasted sharply with the potential state of being I *knew* was possible, thanks to Paleo and intermittent fasting. I finally grasped the truth: The state of your gut affects everything. Everything.

And therein lies the purpose.

My fixation on the science of fat burning and my vanity about my appearance transitioned to a broader quest for knowledge—one involving the elemental and far-reaching effects of food, inflammation, genetics, and the gut microbiome. I can now confidently say that I truly appreciate the momentous importance of diet, not just to lose weight, but to shape the entirety of one's constitution (though these things often go hand in hand!).

My troubles also halted my search for some dietary panacea, replacing my overwhelming quest for an idealized, perfect solution, with a quest to find what actually worked for *me* specifically. For in tirelessly seeking answers, researching an overwhelming number of food sensitivities, and scrutinizing the *so many* protocols for gut healing, I eventually realized there likely is no single solution to be found. True, some foods are more inherently toxic than others—particularly those introduced relatively recently to our species (aka grains) or those appearing in bastardized forms (aka processed foods). But beyond these categories lies a vast spectrum of potentially *wonderful* diets, based on what works for each individual. And so I hope we may all sit around the proverbial and literal dinner table in peace, reveling in our personal choices while appreciating others' as well. And in doing so, may we ultimately focus on the nourishment of both food and fellowship, as we welcome the good into our life, whatever that personal good may be.

And if I can tell you one other thing, it's this: Through it all—fears and fixations aside—focusing on the "what" and the "when" has never forsaken me. Despite any momentary ailments, consuming whole foods compatible with my body catalyzes growth and healing, while a decent fast invariably results in a calm, content state of renewal. Seeing these effects, I am continually assured that the foundation of our health lies in the dietary and lifestyle choices we make each and every day. Yes, *choices.* For we are not destined for ill health or for continued struggle. Our bodies *want* to heal. They *want* to thrive—if we only may support them in these endeavors!

Of course, our mindset in all of this is key, capable of rapidly escalating progress or holding us back. In a world where the very sustenance of our being—our food—is often laced with toxins and temptations, is it any wonder we struggle with bodily distress, degenerative disease, and obesity? How could we not? Yet I encourage you not to jump to rash conclusions of doom or failure. You are *not* destined. You *can* change. The best years of your life can always be before you!

I pray you may see the world through new eyes. To eat the foods that make you feel wonderful, in the times that suit it. To raise a glass of wine in the company of your dearest friends. To rise with the sun and sleep with the darkness (or, if you're a night owl like me, to at least hack your light exposure to mimic nature!). To embrace movement like a child, filled with a simple, radiant desire to *move.*

But ultimately, I encourage you to love not just your friends, family, and the world, but yourself. We are much too hard on ourselves. Whatever your current weight, whatever your current state of mind—you are there because of the factors that brought you there. It cannot be any other way. Both you and your body have been and are doing the best you can toward a brighter future. Understanding the keys for positive change—embracing that which nourishes and letting go of that which hinders—will only add to that. In being your body's friend, not enemy, the two of you can team up toward resilient health.

I bid you nothing but warmth, love, and well-wishes in your journey. I hope you may see everything as a learning experience rather than a test. Every second can be a new beginning. Like me, I hope you may not seek to return to any past self, but rather embrace becoming your *new* self. Don't listen to what they say. Run with the wild abandon of your intuition, and cling to your health, knowing it is always waiting for you. Available to you. Your body's inner cells desire to live and thrive, which is overwhelmingly in your favor.

You got this.

Melanie Avalon

Gratitude

When I self-published the original *What When Wine Diet*, I fantasized about the day I could write my gushing acknowledgements in a "real" version of the book. (Sort of how I still fantasize about my tear-laden Oscar speech. #dreams). I truly cannot believe this moment is now transpiring. So. Much. Appreciation.

First of all, thank you to The Countryman Press at W. W. Norton for investing so much in this book, and bringing my crazy idea to reality. To my sparkling, fantastic editor Ann Treistman: From the second we first spoke, I knew you simply got it, which was increasingly confirmed by your intelligent design in the book's evolution. Thank you for guiding me in this adventure, putting up with all my requests, and championing the vision. I raise a glass to you! Also at Countryman, thank you to Aurora Bell for your warm help (especially with the reference madness!), and to Rebecca Caine for copy-editing. On the publicity side of things, thank you Devorah Backman and Maya Baran for promoting this project (even in the face of a maternity leave!), as well as to Justin Loeber and his team! Last but not least, to all the other people behind the scenes who designed, edited, held meetings behind closed doors about this book's future, and did who knows what else: I wish I could know you more, and I thank you!

To stay in the literary world for a bit, I am overwhelmingly humbled to be able to thank Celeste Fine, and her team at Sterling Lord Literistic, as well as the agency at large. When I first sat down to research literary agents, I immediately knew Celeste was my #1, it'll-never-happen-only-in-my-dreams-who-am-I-kidding agent. Celeste, you will forever hold a special place in my heart, and I shall sing you praises till the end of time! Thank you SO much for seeing potential in my vision—I had never cried from happiness until that first call with you. Sarah Passick: Thank you for responding to the query I spent a month writing (without which, none of this would be!), and then accompanying me for the beginning of the journey. You are awesome. Thank you to Megan Feulner for also assisting and joining the madness. (And I wish you the best in your new department!) Likewise to Jaidree Braddix, for jumping on board and subsequently dealing with #alltheemails and #allthethings. And thank you John Maas for talking me through contract craziness with comforting encouragement.

Collaborator time! Thank you Ariane Resnick for responding to my random tweet, and subsequently putting up with all my neuroticism about ingredients and cooking temperatures. I could not be happier with the recipes! To the wondrous Sarah Fragoso: Thank you for spending your valuable time reading my manuscript, and then writing such a fresh, funny, #onpoint foreword! I am ridiculously honored, and it makes me smile so!! Also thank you to Dr. Srini Pillay, Mahshid Shelechi, and Dr. Michael VanDerschelden for contributing your time and endorsements!

Now for my entertainment industry mentors! Andrew Mayne: Thank you for insisting that I write this book, providing constant guidance, and keeping the magic alive. Thank you Adam and Erin Borba for further enlightening my preparation. And Adam, please tell Jim Whitaker he's my ultimate entertainment industry role model: proof that success, talent, and genuine goodness can co-exist in Hollywood.

I also must thank my Paleo idol Robb Wolf. You were a key influencer in my journey, and I respect every word you speak to us guys and gals.

To my friends: I wish I could name every single one of you, yet I'd like to avoid creating a phone book that may still accidentally omit someone. So, to my dearest and insanely talented Carmen Emmi: Thank you for shooting the original cover of this book (fueled by the taste of vino and tunes of Lizzie McGuire) and providing feedback on everything. To my dietary adventure buddies: Ben Empey (IF!), Kara Kieffer (Paleo!), and Jason Kehe (Wine!).

Also to Kylie Clark and Kathryn Hendrickson (Tripod!), just because. More recently, to my co-host/IF-partner-in-crime Gin Stephens, for helping create our wonderful Intermittent Fasting Podcast.

Of course, I could never have done any of this without my foundation. Dear parents: I will never be able to truly express my undying gratitude for all you do. Thank you for raising me with morals and instilling in me passion and commitment, never failing to support my dreams and ambitions. Thanks Dad for cultivating my love of wine, dining, and Disney, and serving as my ultimate role model in life. Thanks Mom for always being there and talking me through all my problems and sending me random emojis. Thanks Danielle for our many life adventures and conversations, be they in the same room or across the country. And thanks Michael, for being the coolest little brother around. Which you seriously are.

Last but not least, this book can only exist in the mind of an audience. So, I must thank YOU, my dearest reader. Thank you for joining me in this journey through the crazy diet wonderland. May you always live vicariously through yourself. You got this!

Melanie Avalon

Notes

Hi friends! I sort of went overboard researching for this book! In order to keep this book from reaching #phonebook status, this list includes only studies directly discussed in the text. For a complete reference list of every study I read (sorted by category!), please see MelanieAvalon.com/references. Enjoy!

NOTES FOR FRONT MATTER, PAGES I–XLII

1. B. Alberts, et al. "Programmed Cell Death (Apoptosis)." *Molecular Biology of the Cell*, 4th edition (2002). https://www.ncbi.nlm.nih.gov/books/NBK26873.
2. Azevado, Fernanda Reis de, Bruno Caramelli, and Dimas Ikeoka. "Effects of intermittent fasting on metabolism in men." *Revista da Associação Médica Brasileira* 59, no. 2 (2013): 167–73, https://doi:10.1016/j.ramb.2012.09.003.
3. Davis, Caroline. "From Passive Overeating to 'Food Addiction': A Spectrum of Compulsion and Severity." *ISRN Obesity* (2013): 1–20, https://doi:10.1155/2013/435027.
4. Bronson, F. H. "Climate change and seasonal reproduction in mammals." *Philosophical Transactions of the Royal Society B: Biological Sciences* 364, no. 1534 (October 15, 2009): 3331–340, https://doi:10.1098/rstb.2009.0140.
5. Toops, Diane. "A History." *Food Processing*, October 5, 2010. http://www.foodprocessing.com/articles/2010/anniversary.
6. Kniffin, Kevin M., Mitsuru Shimizu, and Brian Wansink, "Death Row Nutrition. Curious Conclusions of Last Meals." *Appetite* 59, no. 3 (2012): 837–43, https://doi:10.1016/j.appet.2012.08.017.
7. Kanarek, Robin. "Psychological Effects of Snacks and Altered Meal Frequency." *British Journal of Nutrition* 77, no. S1 (1997): S105.
8. Graaf, Cees de. "Effects of Snacks on Energy Intake: An Evolutionary Perspective." *Appetite* 47, no. 1 (2006): 18–23, https://doi:10.1016/j.appet.2006.02.007.
9. Wansink, B. and C. S. Wansink. "The Largest Last Supper: Depictions of Food Por-

tions and Plate Size Increased Over the Millennium." *International Journal of Obesity* 34, no. 5 (2010): 943–44. https://doi:10.1038/ijo.2010.37.

10. Hirvonen, Matt D. and Richard E. Keesey. "Body Weight Set-Points: Determination and Adjustment." *American Society for Nutritional Services* 127, no. 9 (September 1, 1997): 1875S–883S.

11. Devecis, J., P. Greene, A. Skaf, W. Willett. "Pilot 12-Week Feeding Weight-Loss Comparison: Low-Fat vs. Low-Carbohydrate (Ketogenic) Diets." *Obesity Research* 11 (September 2003).

12. Feinman, Richard D. and Eugene J. Fine. "'A Calorie is a Calorie' Violates the Second Law of Thermodynamics." *Nutrition Journal* 3, no. 1 (2004): https://doi.10.1186/1475-2891-3-9.

13. Westerterp, Klaas R. "Diet Induced Thermogenesis." *Nutrition & Metabolism* 1, no. 5 (August 18, 2004): https://doi:10.1186/1743-7075-1-5.

14. "Butyrate as Therapy: Fatty Acid Produced by Gut Bacteria Boosts Immune System." News, Science 2.0. Accessed November 14, 2013. http://www.science20.com/news_articles/butyrate_therapy_fatty_acid_produced_gut_bacteria_boosts_immune_system-124388.

15. Antonio, Jose, et al. "The Effects of Consuming a High Protein Diet (4.4 g/kg/d) on Body Composition in Resistance-Trained Individuals." *Journal of the International Society of Sports Nutrition* (May 12, 2014): https://doi.org/10.1186/1550-2783-11-19.

16. Adelmant, Guillaume, et al. "Control of Hepatic Gluconeogenesis through the Transcriptional Coactivator PGC-1," *Nature* 413, no. 6852 (2001): 131–38, https://doi.10.1038/35093050.

17. Parker, Hilary. "A Sweet Problem: Princeton Researchers Find that High-Fructose Corn Syrup Prompts Considerably More Weight Gain." News, Princeton University. Accessed March 22, 2010. https://www.princeton.edu/news/2010/03/22/sweet-problem-princeton-researchers-find-high-fructose-corn-syrup-prompts.

Bocarsly, M. E. et al. "High-fructose Corn Syrup Causes Characteristics of Obesity in Rats: Increased Body Weight, Body Fat and Triglyceride Levels." *Pharmacology Biochemistry and Behavior* 97, no. 1 (2010): 101–06.

18. Dokken, Betsy B. and Tsu Shuen Tsao. "The Physiology of Body Weight Regulation: Are We Too Efficient for Our Own Good?" *Diabetes Spectrum* 20, no. 3 (June 2007): 166–70, https://doi:10.2337/diaspect.20.3.166.

19. Bouchard, Claude et al. "The Response to Long-Term Overfeeding in Identical Twins." *New England Journal of Medicine* 322, no. 21 (1990): 1477–482, https://doi:10.1056/nejm199005243222101.

20. Ravussin, E. et al. "Determinants of 24-Hour Energy Expenditure in Man. Methods and Results Using a Respiratory Chamber." *Journal of Clinical Investigation* 78, no. 6 (1986): 1568–578, https://doi.10.1172/jci112749.

21. Loeffelholz, Christian von. "The Role of Non-Exercise Activity Thermogenesis in Human Obesity." *Endotext* (June 5, 2014).

22. Chakraborti, Chandra Kanti. "New-Found Link Between Microbiota and Obe-

sity." *World of Journal of Gastrointestinal Pathophysiology* 6, no. 4 (2015): 110, https://doi:10.4291/wjgp.v6.i4.110.

NOTES FOR "WHAT?" SECTION, PAGES 1–76

1. Ross, A. Catharine. *Modern Nutrition in Health and Disease.* Philadelphia: Lippincott Williams & Wilkins, 2014.

2. Simopoulos, A. P. *Evolutionary Aspects of Nutrition and Health, Diet, Exercise, Genetics, and Chronic Disease.* Basel, Switzerland: Karger, 1999.

3. "Simple changes in diet can protect you against friendly fire." *Harvard Health Publications.* Accessed February 2007. https://www.health.harvard.edu/newsletter_article/simple-changes-in-diet-can-protect-you-against-friendly-fire.

   Anand, Preetha, et al. "Cancer Is a Preventable Disease that Requires Major Lifestyle Changes." *Pharmaceutical Research* 25, no. 9 (2008): 2097–116, https://doi:10.1007/s11095-008-9661-9.

4. Breslin, Paul A. S. and Mari A. Sandell. "Variability in a taste-receptor gene determines whether we taste toxins in food." *Current Biology* 16, no. 18 (2006). http://dx.doi.org/10.1016/j.cub.2006.08.049.

5. Cordain, Loren. "Cereal grains: humanity's double-edged sword." *World Review of Nutrition and Dietics* 84 (1999): 19-73.

6. Nikulina, M., et al. "Wheat Gluten Causes Dendritic Cell Maturation and Chemokine Secretion." *The Journal of Immunology* 173, no. 3 (2004): 1925-933. https://doi.org/10.4049/jimmunol.173.3.1925

7. Fasano, Alessio. "Zonulin, regulation of tight junctions, and autoimmune diseases." *Annals of the New York Academy of Sciences* 1258, no. 1 (2012): 25-33. doi:10.1111/j.1749-6632.2012.06538.x.

8. Dolfini, Ersilia. "Cytoskeleton reorganization and ultrastructural damage induced by gliadin in a three-dimensional in vitro model." *World Journal of Gastroenterology* 11, no. 48 (2005): 7597. doi:10.3748/wjg.v11.i48.7597.

9. Pruimboom, Leo, and Karin De Punder. "The opioid effects of gluten exorphins: asymptomatic celiac disease." *Journal of Health, Population and Nutrition* 33, no. 1 (2015). doi:10.1186/s41043-015-0032-y.

10. Uhde, Melanie, et al. "Intestinal cell damage and systemic immune activation in individuals reporting sensitivity to wheat in the absence of coeliac disease." *Gut* 65, no. 12 (2016): 1930–937. doi:10.1136/gutjnl-2016-311964.

11. Catassi, Carlo, et al. "Non-Celiac Gluten Sensitivity: The New Frontier of Gluten Related Disorders." *Nutrients* 5, no. 10 (2013): 3839-853. doi:10.3390/nu5103839.

12. Miller, Sara G. "Americans Claim Gluten Sensitivity More Than Others." *LiveScience*, May 08, 2017. Accessed August 08, 2017. https://www.livescience.com/59011-gluten-avoidance-different-countries.html.

13. "Diagnosis of Celiac Disease: Current State of the Evidence." *Effective Healthcare Program*, July 26, 2016. Accessed August 08, 2017. https://www.effectivehealthcare.ahrq.gov/search-for-guides-reviews-and-reports/?pageaction=displayproduct&productID

=2259&utm_source=AHRQ&utm_medium=AHRQDPI&utm_content=2&utm_term=Publication&utm_campaign=AHRQ_CELIAC_2016.

14. Duncan, Eric. "U.S. Gluten-free Foods Market—Statistics & Facts." *Statista*. Accessed August 08, 2017. https://www.statista.com/topics/2067/gluten-free-foods-market.

15. Dolan, Laurie C., Ray A. Matulka, and George A. Burdock. "Naturally Occurring Food Toxins." *Toxins* 2, no. 9 (2010): 2289–332. doi:10.3390/toxins2092289.

16. "Lack of Effect of a High-Fiber Cereal Supplement on the Recurrence of Colorectal Adenomas." *New England Journal of Medicine* 343, no. 13 (2000): 980. doi:10.1056/nejm200009283431321.

17. Rock, Cheryl L. "Primary Dietary Prevention: Is the Fiber Story Over?" *Cancer Prevention Recent Results in Cancer Research*: 171–177. doi:10.1007/978-3-540-37696-5_14.

18. Cummings, J. H., et al. "The effect of meat protein and dietary fiber on colonic function and metabolism. II. Bacterial metabolites in feces and urine." *American Journal of Clinical Nutrition* 32, no. 10 (October 1979): 2094–101

19. Tan, Kok-Yang. "Fiber and colorectal diseases: Separating fact from fiction." *World Journal of Gastroenterology* 13, no. 31 (2007): 4161. doi:10.3748/wjg.v13.i31.4161.

20. Guyton, Arthur C., and John E. Hall. Textbook of Medical Physiology. Philadelphia.: Elsevier Saunders, 2006.

21. Mohanty, Priya, et al. "Glucose Challenge Stimulates Reactive Oxygen Species (ROS) Generation by Leucocytes." *The Journal of Clinical Endocrinology & Metabolism* 85, no. 8 (2000): 2970-973. doi:10.1210/jcem.85.8.6854.

22. Sanchez, Albert, et al. "Role of Sugars in Human Neutrophilic Phagocytosis." *American Journal of Clinical Nutrition* 26, no. 1 (1973): pp. 1180–184.

23. Avena, Nicole M., Pedro Rada, and Bartley G. Hoebel. "Evidence for sugar addiction: Behavioral and neurochemical effects of intermittent, excessive sugar intake." *Neuroscience & Biobehavioral Reviews* 32, no. 1 (2008): 20–39. doi:10.1016/j.neubiorev.2007.04.019.

    Basciano, Heather, Lisa Federico, and Khosrow Adeli. "Fructose, insulin resistance, and metabolic dyslipidemia." *Nutrition & Metabolism* 2, no. 1 (2005): 5. doi:10.1186/1743-7075-2-5

24. Moerman, Clara J., H. Bas De Mesquita, and Sytske Runia. "Dietary Sugar Intake in the Aetiology of Biliary Tract Cancer." *International Journal of Epidemiology* 22, no. 2 (1993): 207–14. doi:10.1093/ije/22.2.207.

    Nöthlings, Ute, et al. "Dietary Glycemic Load, Added Sugars, and Carbohydrates as Risk Factors for Pancreatic Cancer: The Multiethnic Cohort Study." *American Journal of Clinical Nutrition* 86, no. 5 (2007): pp. 1495–501.

25. Asif, Mohammad. "The prevention and control the type-2 diabetes by changing lifestyle and dietary pattern." *Journal of Education and Health Promotion* 3, no. 1 (2014): 1. doi:10.4103/2277-9531.127541.

26. Basu, Sanjay, et al. "The Relationship of Sugar to Population-Level Diabetes Prevalence: An Econometric Analysis of Repeated Cross-Sectional Data." *PLoS ONE* 8, no. 2 (2013). doi:10.1371/journal.pone.0057873.

27. Frassetto, L. A., et al. "Metabolic and physiologic improvements from consuming a paleolithic, hunter-gatherer type diet." *European Journal of Clinical Nutrition* 69, no. 12 (2015): 1376. doi:10.1038/ejcn.2015.193.

28. Lindeberg, S., et al. "A Palaeolithic diet improves glucose tolerance more than a Mediterranean-like diet in individuals with ischaemic heart disease." *Diabetologia* 50, no. 9 (2007): 1795–807. doi:10.1007/s00125-007-0716-y.

29. Jönsson, Tommy, et al. "Beneficial effects of a Paleolithic diet on cardiovascular risk factors in type 2 diabetes: a randomized cross-over pilot study." *Cardiovascular Diabetology* 8, no. 1 (2009): 35. doi:10.1186/1475-2840-8-35.

30. Zeevi, David, et al. "Personalized Nutrition by Prediction of Glycemic Responses." *Cell* 163, no. 5 (2015): 1079–094. doi:10.1016/j.cell.2015.11.001.

31. Ibid.

32. Siri-Tarino, P. W., et al. "Meta-analysis of prospective cohort studies evaluating the association of saturated fat with cardiovascular disease." *American Journal of Clinical Nutrition* 91, no. 3 (2010): 535–46. doi:10.3945/ajcn.2009.27725.

33. Bailey, Regina. "Cell Membranes Function, Structure and Composition." *ThoughtCo.* August 4, 2017. Accessed August 08, 2017. https://www.thoughtco.com/cell-membrane-373364.

    Spector, Arthur A., and Mark A. Yorek. "Membrane lipid composition and cellular function." *Journal of Lipid Research* 26 (1985): 1015–035.

    Chang, C. Y., K. E. DS, and J. Y. Chen. "Essential fatty acids and human brain." *Acta Neurol Taiwan* 18, no. 4 (December 2009): 231–41.

34. Yehuda, Shlomo, et al. "Essential Fatty Acids Preparation (Sr-3) Improves Alzheimers Patients Quality of Life." *International Journal of Neuroscience* 87, no. 3-4 (1996): 141–49. doi:10.3109/00207459609070833

35. Stoll, A. L., et al. "Omega-3 fatty acids and bipolar disorder: a review." *Prostaglandins, Leukotrienes and Essential Fatty Acids* 60, no. 5–6 (1999): 329–37. doi:10.1016/s0952-3278(99)80008-8.

36. Hibbeln, J. R., and N. Salem, JR. "Dietary polyunsaturated fatty acids and depression: when cholesterol does not satisfy." *American Journal of Clinical Nutrition* 62, no. 1 (July 1995): 1–9.

37. Laugharne, J. D., J. E. Mellor, and M. Peet. "Fatty acids and schizophrenia." *Lipids*, March 1996, S163–5.

38. Bartoshuk, Linda. "Learning to Like Foods." *Association for Psychological Science.* Accessed August 08, 2017. http://www.psychologicalscience.org/observer/learning-to-like-foods#.WR5HNVKZOcY.

39. Esteve, Montserrat, et al. "Effect of a cafeteria diet on energy intake and balance in Wistar rats." *Physiology & Behavior* 56, no. 1 (1994): 65–71. doi:10.1016/0031-9384(94)90262-3.

40. Johnson, Paul M., and Paul J. Kenny. "Dopamine D2 receptors in addiction-like reward dysfunction and compulsive eating in obese rats." *Nature Neuroscience* 13, no. 5 (2010): 635–41. doi:10.1038/nn.2519.

41. Rettner, Rachael. "Obesity Rate in U.S. Women Climbs to 40%." *LiveScience.* June

07, 2016. Accessed August 08, 2017. https://www.livescience.com/54994-obesity-rate-women.html.

42. Valenstein, E. S., J. W. Kakolewski, and V. C. Cox. "Sex Differences in Taste Preference for Glucose and Saccharin Solutions." *Science* 156, no. 3777 (1967): 942–43. doi:10.1126/science.156.3777.942.

43. Lovejoy, J. C., et al. "Increased visceral fat and decreased energy expenditure during the menopausal transition." *International Journal of Obesity* 32, no. 6 (2008): 949–58. doi:10.1038/ijo.2008.25.

44. Fedewa, Amy, and Satish S. C. Rao. "Dietary Fructose Intolerance, Fructan Intolerance and FODMAPs." *Current Gastroenterology Reports* 16, no. 1 (2013). doi:10.1007/s11894-013-0370-0.

45. Sievenpiper, John L., et al. "Effect of Fructose on Body Weight in Controlled Feeding Trials." *Annals of Internal Medicine* 156, no. 4 (2012): 291. doi:10.7326/0003-4819-156-4-201202210-00007.

46. Stellman, Steven D., and Lawrence Garfinkel. "Artificial sweetener use and one-year weight change among women." *Preventive Medicine* 15, no. 2 (1986): 195–202. doi:10.1016/0091-7435(86)90089-7.

47. Colditz, G. A., W. C. Willet, M. J. Stampfer, S. J. London, M. R. Segal, and F. E. Spezizer. "Patterns of weight change and their relation to diet in a cohort of healthy women." *American Journal of Clinical Nutrition* 51, no. 6 (June 1990): 1100–5.

48. Fowler, Sharon P., Ken Williams, Roy G. Resendez, Kelly J. Hunt, Helen P. Hazuda, and Michael P. Stern. "Fueling the Obesity Epidemic? Artificially Sweetened Beverage Use and Long-term Weight Gain." *Obesity* 16, no. 8 (2008): 1894–900. doi:10.1038/oby.2008.284.

49. Swithers, Susan E., and Terry L. Davidson. "A role for sweet taste: Calorie predictive relations in energy regulation by rats." *Behavioral Neuroscience* 122, no. 1 (2008): 161–73. doi:10.1037/0735-7044.122.1.161.

50. Black, Richard M., Lawrence A. Leiter, and G.Harvey Anderson. "Consuming aspartame with and without taste: Differential effects on appetite and food intake of young adult males." *Physiology & Behavior* 53, no. 3 (1993): 459–66. doi:10.1016/0031-9384(93)90139-7.

51. Porikos, K. P., G. Booth, and T. B. Van Itallie. "Effect of covert nutritive dilution on the spontaneous food intake of obese individuals: a pilot study." *American Journal of Clinical Nutrition* 30, no. 10 (October 1977): 1638–44.

52. Mattes, Richard. "Effects of aspartame and sucrose on hunger and energy intake in humans." *Physiology & Behavior* 47, no. 6 (1990): 1037–044. doi:10.1016/0031-9384(90)90350-d.

53. Suez, Jotham, et al. "Artificial sweeteners induce glucose intolerance by altering the gut microbiota." *Nature*, 2014. doi:10.1038/nature13793.

54. Natoli, Sharon, et al. "Unscrambling the research: Eggs, serum cholesterol and coronary heart disease." *Nutrition & Dietetics* 64, no. 2 (2007): 105–11. doi:10.1111/j.1747-0080.2007.00093.x.

55. Abeyrathne, E. D. N. S., H. Y. Lee, and D. U. Ahn. "Egg white proteins and their potential use in food processing or as nutraceutical and pharmaceutical agents—A review." *Poultry Science* 92, no. 12 (2013): 3292–299. doi:10.3382/ps.2013-03391.

56. Sharma, Hari, Xiaoying Zhang, and Chandradhar Dwivedi. "The effect of ghee (clarified butter) on serum lipid levels and microsomal lipid peroxidation." *AYU (An International Quarterly Journal of Research in Ayurveda)* 31, no. 2 (2010): 134. doi:10.4103/0974-8520.72361.

57. Molan, P. C. "The potential of honey to promote oral wellness." *General Dentistry*, Nov. & Dec. 2001, 584–9. Accessed August 8, 2017.

58. Osato, Michael S. "Osmotic effect of honey on growth and viability of Helicobacter pylori." *Digestive Diseases and Sciences* 44, no. 3 (1999): 462–64. doi:10.1023/a:1026676517213.

59. Anovski, Susan. "Sugar and Fat: Cravings and Aversions." *The Journal of Nutrition* 133 (2003): 835S–37S.

60. Allen, Robin R., et al. "Daily Consumption of a Dark Chocolate Containing Flavanols and Added Sterol Esters Affects Cardiovascular Risk Factors in a Normotensive Population with Elevated Cholesterol." *The Journal of Nutrition* 138, no. 4 (April 2008): 725–31.

61. Balboa-Castillo, Teresa, et al. "Chocolate and Health-Related Quality of Life: A Prospective Study." *PLoS ONE* 10, no. 4 (2015). doi:10.1371/journal.pone.0123161.

62. Grassi, Davide, et al. "Short-term administration of dark chocolate is followed by a significant increase in insulin sensitivity and a decrease in blood pressure in healthy persons." *American Journal of Clinical Nutrition* 81, no. 3 (March 2005): 611–14.

63. Sunni, Ahmed Al, and Rabia Latif. "Effects of chocolate intake on Perceived Stress; a Controlled Clinical Study." *International Journal of Health Sciences* 8, no. 4 (October 2014): 393–401.

64. Vinson, Joe A., and Matthew J. Motisi. "Polyphenol antioxidants in commercial chocolate bars: Is the label accurate?" *Journal of Functional Foods* 12 (2015): 526–29. doi:10.1016/j.jff.2014.12.022.

65. "The Structures of Life: Chapter 1: Proteins are the Body's Worker Molecules." *National Institute of General Medical Sciences.* October 27, 2011. Accessed August 09, 2017. https://publications.nigms.nih.gov/structlife/chapter1.html.

66. Pal, Sebely, et al. "Milk Intolerance, Beta-Casein and Lactose." *Nutrients* 7, no. 9 (2015): 7285–297. doi:10.3390/nu7095339.

67. Crinnion, Walter J., ND. "Organic Foods Contain Higher Levels of Certain Nutrients, Lower Levels of Pesticides, and May Provide Health Benefits for the Consumer." *Alternative Medicine Review* 15, no. 1, 4–12.

68. Månsson, Helena Lindmark. "Fatty acids in bovine milk fat." *Food & Nutrition Research* 52, no. 1 (2008): 1821. doi:10.3402/fnr.v52i0.1821.

69. Fiocchi, Alessandro, et al. "Precautionary labelling of cross-reactive foods: The case of rapeseed." *Asthma Research and Practice* 2, no. 1 (2016). doi:10.1186/s40733-016-0028-4.

70. Tamura, Motoi, Chigusa Hoshi, and Sachiko Hori. "Xylitol Affects the Intestinal Microbiota and Metabolism of Daidzein in Adult Male Mice." *International Journal of Molecular Sciences* 14, no. 12 (2013): 23993–4007. doi:10.3390/ijms141223993.

71. Baudier, Kaitlin M., et al. "Erythritol, a Non-Nutritive Sugar Alcohol Sweetener and the Main Component of Truvia®, Is a Palatable Ingested Insecticide." *PLoS ONE* 9, no. 6 (2014). doi:10.1371/journal.pone.0098949.

72. Moyer, Melinda. "Food Wars: The Truth About Soy." *Self*, May 2015, 89–93.

73. Hilakivi-Clarke, L., J. E. Andrade, and W. Helferich. "Is Soy Consumption Good or Bad for the Breast?" *Journal of Nutrition* 140, no. 12 (2010). doi:10.3945/jn.110.124230.

74. "Adoption of Genetically Engineered Crops in the U.S." USDA.gov. July 12, 2017. Accessed August 10, 2017. https://www.ers.usda.gov/data-products/adoption-of-genetically-engineered-crops-in-the-us.aspx.

75. Gasnier, Céline, et al. "Glyphosate-based herbicides are toxic and endocrine disruptors in human cell lines." *Toxicology* 262, no. 3 (2009): 184–91. doi:10.1016/j.tox.2009.06.006.

76. "2015 Agriculture Chemical Use Survey: Soybeans." NASS.USDA.gov. May 2016. Accessed August 10, 2017. https://www.nass.usda.gov/Surveys/Guide_to_NASS_Surveys/Chemical_Use/2015_Cotton_Oats_Soybeans_Wheat_Highlights/ChemUseHighlights_Soybeans_2015.pdf.

77. Perry, George H., et al. "Diet and the evolution of human amylase gene copy number variation." *Nature Genetics* 39, no. 10 (2007): 1256–260. doi:10.1038/ng2123.

78. Key, T. J., et al. "Mortality in British vegetarians: results from the European Prospective Investigation into Cancer and Nutrition (EPIC-Oxford)." *American Journal of Clinical Nutrition* 89, no. 5 (2009). doi:10.3945/ajcn.2009.26736l.

79. Weyrich, Laura S., et al. "Neanderthal behaviour, diet, and disease inferred from ancient DNA in dental calculus." *Nature* 544, no. 7650 (2017): 357–61. doi:10.1038/nature21674.

80. Key, Timothy J., et al. "Mortality in vegetarians and non-vegetarians: a collaborative analysis of 8300 deaths among 76,000 men and women in five prospective studies." *Public Health Nutrition* 1, no. 01 (1998). doi:10.1079/phn19980006.

81. Pawlak, R., S. E. Lester, and T. Babatunde. "The prevalence of cobalamin deficiency among vegetarians assessed by serum vitamin B12: a review of literature." *European Journal of Clinical Nutrition* 68, no. 5 (2014): 541–48. doi:10.1038/ejcn.2014.46.

82. Pawlak, Roman, et al. "How prevalent is vitamin B12deficiency among vegetarians?" *Nutrition Reviews* 71, no. 2 (2013): 110–17. doi:10.1111/nure.12001.

83. "What Causes Pernicious Anemia?" *NIH National Heart Lung and Blood Institute.* April 01, 2011. Accessed August 10, 2017. https://www.nhlbi.nih.gov/health/health-topics/topics/prnanmia/causes.

84. Turner, Rufus, Carlene H. Mclean, and Karen M. Silvers. "Are the health benefits of fish oils limited by products of oxidation?" *Nutrition Research Reviews* 19, no. 01 (2006): 53. doi:10.1079/nrr2006117.

85. Yago, Marc R., et al. "Gastric Reacidification with Betaine HCl in Healthy Volun-

teers with Rabeprazole-Induced Hypochlorhydria." *Molecular Pharmaceutics* 10, no. 11 (2013): 4032–037. doi:10.1021/mp4003738.

86. Cunnane, Stephen C. "Origins and evolution of the Western diet: implications of iodine and seafood intakes for the human brain." *American Journal of Clinical Nutrition* 82, no. 2 (August 2005): 483.

NOTES FOR "WHEN?" SECTION, PAGES 77–142

1. Acheson, K. J., et al. "Glycogen storage capacity and de novo lipogenesis during massive carbohydrate overfeeding in man." *American Journal of Clinical Nutrition* 48, no. 2 (August 1988): 240–47.

2. Elia, M., et al. "The energy cost of triglyceride-fatty acid recycling in nonobese subjects after an overnight fast and four days of starvation." *Metabolism* 36, no. 3 (1987): 251–55. doi:10.1016/0026-0495(87)90184-3.

3. Izumida, Yoshihiko, et al. "Corrigendum: Glycogen shortage during fasting triggers liver–brain–adipose neurocircuitry to facilitate fat utilization." *Nature Communications* 4 (2013). doi:10.1038/ncomms3930.

4. Manninen, Anssi H. "Metabolic Effects of the Very-Low-Carbohydrate Diets: Misunderstood "Villains" of Human Metabolism." *Journal of the International Society of Sports Nutrition* 1, no. 2 (2004): 7. doi:10.1186/1550-2783-1-2-7.

5. Varady, Krista A., et al. "Alternate day fasting for weight loss in normal weight and overweight subjects: a randomized controlled trial." *Nutrition Journal* 12, no. 1 (2013). doi:10.1186/1475-2891-12-146.

6. Harvie, Michelle, et al. "The effect of intermittent energy and carbohydrate restriction v. daily energy restriction on weight loss and metabolic disease risk markers in overweight women." *British Journal of Nutrition* 110, no. 08 (2013): 1534–547. doi:10.1017/s0007114513000792.

7. Varady, K. A. "Intermittent versus daily calorie restriction: which diet regimen is more effective for weight loss?" *Obesity Reviews* 12, no. 7 (2011). doi:10.1111/j.1467-789x.2011.00873.x.

8. Richelsen, B. "Increased Alpha 2—but Similar Beta-Adrenergic Receptor Activities in Subcutaneous Gluteal Adipocytes from Females Compared with Males." *European Journal of Clinical Investigation*, vol. 16, no. 4 (1996): pp. 302–09.

9. Hatori, Megumi, et al. "Time-Restricted Feeding without Reducing Caloric Intake Prevents Metabolic Diseases in Mice Fed a High-Fat Diet." *Cell Metabolism* 15, no. 6 (2012): 848–60. doi:10.1016/j.cmet.2012.04.019.

10. Munsters, Marjet J. M., and Wim H. M. Saris. "Effects of Meal Frequency on Metabolic Profiles and Substrate Partitioning in Lean Healthy Males." *PLoS ONE* 7, no. 6 (2012). doi:10.1371/journal.pone.0038632.

11. Nair, Pradeepm.k, and Pranavg Khawale. "Role of therapeutic fasting in womens health: An overview." *Journal of Mid-life Health* 7, no. 2 (2016): 61. doi: 10.4103/0976-7800.185325.

12. Rizza, Wanda, Nicola Veronese, and Luigi Fontana. "What are the roles of calorie

restriction and diet quality in promoting healthy longevity?" *Ageing Research Reviews* 13 (2014): 38–45. doi:10.1016/j.arr.2013.11.002.

13. Anson, R. M., et al. "Intermittent fasting dissociates beneficial effects of dietary restriction on glucose metabolism and neuronal resistance to injury from calorie intake." *Proceedings of the National Academy of Sciences* 100, no. 10 (2003): 6216–220. doi:10.1073/pnas.1035720100

14. Azevedo, Fernanda Reis De, Dimas Ikeoka, and Bruno Caramelli. "Effects of intermittent fasting on metabolism in men." *Revista da Associação Médica Brasileira* 59, no. 2 (2013): 167–73. doi:10.1016/j.ramb.2012.09.003.

15. Longo, Valter D., and Mark P. Mattson. "Fasting: Molecular Mechanisms and Clinical Applications." *Cell Metabolism* 19, no. 2 (2014): 181–92. doi:10.1016/j.cmet.2013.12.008.

16. Lavin, Desiree N., et al. "Fasting Induces an Anti-Inflammatory Effect on the Neuroimmune System Which a High-Fat Diet Prevents." *Obesity* 19, no. 8 (2011): 1586–594. doi:10.1038/oby.2011.73.

17. Aksungar, Fehime B., Aynur E. Topkaya, and Mahmut Akyildiz. "Interleukin-6, C-Reactive Protein and Biochemical Parameters during Prolonged Intermittent Fasting." *Annals of Nutrition and Metabolism* 51, no. 1 (2007): 88–95. doi:10.1159/000100954.
    Faris, "Moez Al-Islam" E., et al A. Fararjeh, Yasser K. Bustanji, Mohammad K. Mohammad, and Mohammad L. Salem. "Intermittent fasting during Ramadan attenuates proinflammatory cytokines and immune cells in healthy subjects." *Nutrition Research* 32, no. 12 (2012): 947–55. doi:10.1016/j.nutres.2012.06.021.

18. Youm, Yun-Hee, et al. "The ketone metabolite β-hydroxybutyrate blocks NLRP3 inflammasome–mediated inflammatory disease." *Nature Medicine*, 2015. doi:10.1038/nm.3804.

19. Goodrick, Charles L., et al. "Effects of Intermittent Feeding Upon Growth and Life Span in Rats." *Gerontology* 28, no. 4 (2009): 233–41. doi:10.1159/000212538.

20. Raffaghello, L., et al. "Starvation-dependent differential stress resistance protects normal but not cancer cells against high-dose chemotherapy." *Proceedings of the National Academy of Sciences* 105, no. 24 (2008): 8215–220. doi:10.1073/pnas.0708100105.

21. Ibrahim, Wissam H. et al. "Effect of Ramadan Fasting on Markers of Oxidative Stress and Serum Biochemical Markers of Cellular Damage in Healthy Subjects." *Annals of Nutrition and Metabolism* 53, no. 3–4 (2008): 175–81. doi:10.1159/000172979.

22. Wegman, Martin P. et al. "Practicality of Intermittent Fasting in Humans and its Effect on Oxidative Stress and Genes Related to Aging and Metabolism." *Rejuvenation Research* 18, no. 2 (2015): 162–72. doi:10.1089/rej.2014.1624.

23. Sundqvist, T. et al. "Influence of fasting on intestinal permeability and disease activity in patients with rheumatoid arthritis." *Scandinavian Journal of Rheumatology* 11, no. 1 (1982): 33–38.

24. Umar, Shahid. "Intestinal Stem Cells." *Current Gastroenterology Reports* 12, no. 5 (2010): 340–48. doi:10.1007/s11894-010-0130-3.

25. Takahashi, Toku. "Mechanism of Interdigestive Migrating Motor Complex." *Journal of Neurogastroenterology and Motility* 18, no. 3 (2012): 246–57. doi:10.5056/jnm.2012.18.3.246.

26. Kanazawa, Motoyori, and Shin Fukudo. "Effects of fasting therapy on irritable bowel syndrome." *International Journal of Behavioral Medicine* 13, no. 3 (2006): 214–20. doi:10.1207/s15327558ijbm1303_4.

27. Remely, Marlene, et al. "Increased gut microbiota diversity and abundance of Faecalibacterium prausnitzii and Akkermansia after fasting: a pilot study." *Wiener klinische Wochenschrift* 127, no. 9–10 (2015): 394–98. doi:10.1007/s00508-015-0755-1.

28. Vega, V. L., R. De Cabo, and A. De Maio. "Age and Caloric Restriction Diets Are Confounding Factors that Modify the Response to Lipopolysaccharide by Peritoneal Macrophages in C57Bl/6 Mice." *Shock* 22, no. 3 (September 2004): 248–53.

29. Cheng, Chia-Wei et al. "Prolonged Fasting Reduces IGF-1/PKA to Promote Hematopoietic-Stem-Cell-Based Regeneration and Reverse Immunosuppression." *Cell Stem Cell* 14, no. 6 (2014): 810–23. doi:10.1016/j.stem.2014.04.014.

30. Harvie, Michelle et al. "The effect of intermittent energy and carbohydrate restriction v. daily energy restriction on weight loss and metabolic disease risk markers in overweight women." *British Journal of Nutrition* 110, no. 08 (2013): 1534–547. doi:10.1017/s0007114513000792.

31. Varady, K. A. et al. "Modified alternate-day fasting regimens reduce cell proliferation rates to a similar extent as daily calorie restriction in mice." *The FASEB Journal* 22, no. 6 (2008): 2090–096. doi:10.1096/fj.07-098178.

32. Raffaghello, L. et al. "Starvation-dependent differential stress resistance protects normal but not cancer cells against high-dose chemotherapy." *Proceedings of the National Academy of Sciences* 105, no. 24 (2008): 8215–220. doi:10.1073/pnas.0708100105.

33. Seyfried, Thomas N. and Purna Mukherjee. "Targeting Energy Metabolism in Brain Cancer: Review and Hypothesi." *Nutrition & Metabolism* 2, no. 1 (2005): 30. doi:10.1186/1743-7075-2-30.

34. Martin, Bronwen, Mark P. Mattson, and Stuart Maudsley. "Caloric restriction and intermittent fasting: Two potential diets for successful brain aging." *Ageing Research Reviews* 5, no. 3 (2006): 332–53. doi:10.1016/j.arr.2006.04.002.

35. Anson, R. M. et al. "Intermittent fasting dissociates beneficial effects of dietary restriction on glucose metabolism and neuronal resistance to injury from calorie intake." *Proceedings of the National Academy of Sciences* 100, no. 10 (2003): 6216–220. doi:10.1073/pnas.1035720100.

36. Brandhorst, Sebastian et al. "A Periodic Diet that Mimics Fasting Promotes Multi-System Regeneration, Enhanced Cognitive Performance, and Healthspan." *Cell Metabolism* 22, no. 1 (2015): 86–99. doi:10.1016/j.cmet.2015.05.012.

37. Miller, M. J. S., et al. "Exaggerated Intestinal Histamine Release by Casein and Casein Hydrolysate but Not Whey Hydrolysate." *Scandinavian Journal of Gastroenterology* 26.4 (1991): 379–84.

38. Tsenkova, Vera K., et al. "Anger, adiposity, and glucose control in nondiabetic adults:

findings from MIDUS II." *Journal of Behavioral Medicine* 37, no. 1 (2012): 37–46. doi:10.1007/s10865-012-9460-y.

39. Mousavi, Seyed Ali, et al. "Effect of fasting on mental health in the general population of Kermanshah, Iran." *Journal of Fasting and Health* 2, no. 2 (Spring 2014): 65–70.

40. Maryam, Javanbakht, et al. "The effect of Ramadan fasting on students' self-esteem and mental health." *The Quarterly Journal of Fundamentals of Mental Health*, 44th ser., 11, no. 4 (Winter 2010): 266–73. Accessed August 12, 2017.

41. Teng, Nur Islami et al. "Efficacy of fasting calorie restriction on quality of life among aging men." *Physiology & Behavior* 104, no. 5 (2011): 1059–064. doi:10.1016/j.physbeh.2011.07.007.

42. Loveman, E. et al. "The clinical effectiveness and cost-effectiveness of long-term weight management schemes for adults: a systematic review." *Health Technology Assessment* 15, no. 2 (2011): doi:10.3310/hta15020.

43. Johnson, J.B., S. John, and D.R. Laub. "Pretreatment with alternate day modified fast will permit higher dose and frequency of cancer chemotherapy and better cure rates." *Medical Hypotheses* 72, no. 4 (2009): 381–82. doi:10.1016/j.mehy.2008.07.064.

44. Varady, K. A., et al. "Short-term modified alternate-day fasting: a novel dietary strategy for weight loss and cardioprotection in obese adults." *American Journal of Clinical Nutrition* 90, no. 5 (2009): 1138–143. doi:10.3945/ajcn.2009.28380.

45. Varady, Krista A. et al. "Alternate day fasting for weight loss in normal weight and overweight subjects: a randomized controlled trial." *Nutrition Journal* 12, no. 1 (2013). doi:10.1186/1475-2891-12-146.

46. Baumeister, Roy F., et al. "Ego depletion: Is the active self a limited resource?" *Journal of Personality and Social Psychology* 74, no. 5 (1998): 1252–265. doi:10.1037//0022-3514.74.5.1252.

47. Vohs, Kathleen D., and Todd F. Heatherton. "Self-Regulatory Failure: A Resource-Depletion Approach." *Psychological Science* 11, no. 3 (2000): 249–54. doi:10.1111/1467-9280.00250.

48. Kahan, D., M. T. et al. "Conformity and dietary disinhibition: a test of the ego-strength model of self-regulation." *International Journal of Eating Disorders* 33, no. 2, 165–71. Accessed March 2003.

49. Danziger, S., J. Levav, and L. Avnaim-Pesso. "Extraneous factors in judicial decisions." *Proceedings of the National Academy of Sciences* 108, no. 17 (2011): 6889–892. doi:10.1073/pnas.1018033108.

50. Neal, David, Wendy Wood, and Jeffrey M. Quinn. "Habits—A Repeat Performance." *Current Directions in Psychological Science* 15, no. 4 (2006): 198–202. https://dornsife.usc.edu/assets/sites/208/docs/Neal.Wood.Quinn.2006.pdf.

51. Dickinson, Anthony, and Bernard Balleine. "Motivational Control of Instrumental Action." *Current Directions in Psychological Science* 4, no. 5 (1995): 162–67. doi:10.1111/1467-8721.ep11512272.

52. Berg, Christina et al. "Eating patterns and portion size associated with obesity in a Swedish population." *Appetite* 52, no. 1 (2009): 21–26. Accessed August 12, 2017.

53. Lee, Changhan, and Valter Longo. "Dietary restriction with and without caloric restriction for healthy aging." *F1000Research*, 2016. doi:10.12688/f1000research.7136.1.

54. Niederhoffer, Kate G., and James W. Pennebaker. "Linguistic Style Matching in Social Interaction." *Journal of Language and Social Psychology* 21, no. 4 (2002): 337–60. Accessed August 13, 2017.

55. Dallosso, H. M., P. R. Murgatroyd, and W. P. James. "Feeding frequency and energy balance in adult males." *Human Nutrition Clinical Nutrition* 36C, no. 1 (January 1982): 25–39.

56. Bellisle, France, Regina Mcdevitt, and Andrew M. Prentice. "Meal frequency and energy balance." *British Journal of Nutrition* 77, no. S1 (1997). doi:10.1079/bjn19970104.

57. Taylor, M. A., and J. S. Garrow. "Compared with nibbling, neither gorging nor a morning fast affect short-term energy balance in obese patients in a chamber calorimeter." *International Journal of Obesity* 25, no. 4 (2001): 519–28. doi:10.1038/sj.ijo.0801572.

58. Zauner, C. et al. "Resting energy expenditure in short-term starvation is increased as a result of an increase in serum norepinephrine." *American Journal of Clinical Nutrition* 71, no. 6 (2000): 1511–5. Accessed June 2000.

59. Heilbronn, Leonie K. et al "Effect of 6-Month Calorie Restriction on Biomarkers of Longevity, Metabolic Adaptation, and Oxidative Stress in Overweight Individuals." *Journal of the American Medical Association* 295, no. 13 (2006): 1539.

60. Belko, Amy Z., and Teresa F. Barbieri. "Effect of meal size and frequency on the thermic effect of food." *Nutrition Research* 7, no. 3 (1987): 237–42. doi:10.1016/s0271-5317(87)80013-1.

61. Weinsier, R. L. et al. "Energy Expenditure and Free-living Physical Activity in Black and White Women: Comparison before and after Weight Loss." *American Journal of Clinical Nutrition* 71, no. 5 (2000): 1138–46.

62. Seyfried, Thomas N. and Purna Mukherjee. *Nutrition & Metabolism* 2, no. 1 (2005): 30. doi:10.1186/1743-7075-2-30.

63. Brown, A. W., M. M. Bohan Brown, and D. B. Allison. "Belief beyond the evidence: using the proposed effect of breakfast on obesity to show 2 practices that distort scientific evidence." *American Journal of Clinical Nutrition* 98, no. 5 (2013): 1298–308. doi:10.3945/ajcn.113.064410.

64. Geliebter, Allan et al. "Skipping Breakfast Leads to Weight Loss but Also Elevated Cholesterol Compared with Consuming Daily Breakfasts of Oat Porridge or Frosted Cornflakes in Overweight Individuals: A Randomised Controlled Trial." *Journal of Nutritional Science* 3 (2014): http://www.ncbi.nlm.nih.gov/pmc/articles/PMC4473164/

65. Betts, J. A. et al. "The Causal Role of Breakfast in Energy Balance and Health: A Randomized Controlled Trial in Lean Adults." *American Journal of Clinical Nutrition* 100.2 (2014): 539–47. http://ajcn.nutrition.org/content/100/2/539.full.

66. Levitsky, David A. and Carly R. Pacanowski. "Effect of skipping breakfast on subsequent energy intake." *Physiology & Behavior* 119 (2013): 9–16. doi:10.1016/j.physbeh.2013.05.006.

67. Kral, T. V., et al. "Effects of eating breakfast compared with skipping breakfast on rat-ings of appetite and intake at subsequent meals in 8- to 10-y-old children." *American Journal of Clinical Nutrition* 93, no. 2 (2010): 284–91. doi:10.3945/ajcn.110.000505.

68. Dhurandhar, E. J. et al. "The effectiveness of breakfast recommendations on weight loss: a randomized controlled trial." *American Journal of Clinical Nutrition* 100, no. 2 (2014): 507–13. doi:10.3945/ajcn.114.089573.

69. Martin, Ambroise et al. "Is advice for breakfast consumption justified? Results from a short-term dietary and metabolic experiment in young healthy men." *British Journal of Nutrition* 84, no. 03 (2000): 337–44. doi:10.1017/s0007114500001616.

70. Taylor, M. A., and J. S. Garrow. "Compared with nibbling, neither gorging nor a morning fast affect short-term energy balance in obese patients in a chamber calo-rimeter." *International Journal of Obesity* 25, no. 4 (2001): 519–28. doi:10.1038/sj.ijo.0801572.

71. Kinsey, Amber and Michael Ormsbee. "The Health Impact of Nighttime Eating: Old and New Perspectives." *Nutrients* 7, no. 4 (2015): 2648–662. doi:10.3390/nu7042648.

72. Kinsey, Amber W. et al. "Influence of night-time protein and carbohydrate intake on appetite and cardiometabolic risk in sedentary overweight and obese women." *British Journal of Nutrition* 112, no. 03 (2014): 320–27. doi:10.1017/s0007114514001068.

73. Sofer, Sigal et al. "Greater Weight Loss and Hormonal Changes After 6 Months Diet With Carbohydrates Eaten Mostly at Dinner." *Obesity* 19, no. 10 (2011): 2006–014. doi:10.1038/oby.2011.48.

74. Gonnissen, H. K. et al. "Overnight energy expenditure determined by whole-body indirect calorimetry does not differ during different sleep stages." *American Journal of Clinical Nutrition* 98, no. 4 (2013): 867–71. doi:10.3945/ajcn.113.067884.

75. Nedeltcheva, Arlet V. et al. "Insufficient Sleep Undermines Dietary Efforts to Reduce Adiposity." *Annals of Internal Medicine* 153, no. 7 (2010): 435. doi:10.7326/0003-4819-153-7-201010050-00006.

76. Harvie, Michelle et al. "The effect of intermittent energy and carbohydrate restriction v. daily energy restriction on weight loss and metabolic disease risk markers in over-weight women." *British Journal of Nutrition* 110, no. 08 (2013): 1534–547. doi:10.1017/s0007114513000792.

77. Chapelot, D. "The Role of Snacking in Energy Balance: a Biobehavioral Approach." *Journal of Nutrition* 141, no. 1 (2010): 158–62. doi:10.3945/jn.109.114330.

78. LeGrand, E. K. "Why Infection-induced Anorexia? The Case for Enhanced Apopto-sis of Infected Cells." *Medical Hypotheses* 54, no. 4 (April 2000): 597–602. Accessed August 15, 2017.

79. Murray, M. J., and A. B. Murray. "Anorexia of infection as a mechanism of host defense." *American Journal of Clinical Nutrition* 32, no. 3 (March 1979): 593–96.

80. Kanra, G. Y., H. Özen, and A. Kara. "Infection and anorexia." *Turkish Journal of Pedi-atrics* 48 (2006): 279–87.

81. Ibid.

82. LeGrand, E. K. "Why infection-induced anorexia? The case for enhanced apoptosis of

infected cells." *Medical Hypotheses* 54, no. 4 (April 2000): 597–602. Accessed August 16, 2017.

NOTES FOR "WINE?" SECTION, PAGES 143–168:

1. Yeomans, Martin R. "Alcohol, appetite and energy balance: Is alcohol intake a risk factor for obesity?" *Physiology & Behavior* 100, no. 1 (2010): 82–89. doi:10.1016/j .physbeh.2010.01.012.

2. Yeomans, M. R., S. Caton, and M. M. Hetherington. "Alcohol and food intake." *Current Opinion in Clinical Nutrition & Metabolic Care* 6, no. 6 (November 2003): 639–44. Accessed August 16, 2017.

3. Berridge, Kent C. "Food reward: Brain substrates of wanting and liking." *Neuroscience & Biobehavioral Reviews* 20, no. 1 (1996): 1–25. doi:10.1016/0149-7634(95)00033-b.

4. Liangpunsakul, Suthat. "Relationship between alcohol intake and dietary pattern: Findings from NHANES III." *World Journal of Gastroenterology* 16, no. 32 (2010): 4055. doi:10.3748/wjg.v16.i32.4055.

5. Arif, Ahmed A. and James E. Rohrer. "Patterns of alcohol drinking and its association with obesity: data from the third national health and nutrition examination survey, 1988–1994." *BMC Public Health* 5, no. 1 (2005). doi:10.1186/1471-2458-5-126.

6. Tobon, F. and E. Mezey. "Effect of ethanol administration on hepatic ethanol and drug-metabolizing enzymes and on rates of ethanol degradation." *Journal of Laboratory and Clinical Medicine* 77, no. 1 (January 1971): 110–21.

7. Milton, K. "Ferment in the Family Tree: Does a Frugivorous Dietary Heritage Influence Contemporary Patterns of Human Ethanol Use?" *Integrative and Comparative Biology* 44, no. 4 (2004): 304–14. doi:10.1093/icb/44.4.304.

8. Guthrie, G. D. et al. "Alcohol as a nutrient; interactions between ethanol and carbohydrate." *Alcoholism: Clinical and Experimental Research* 14, no. 1 (March 1990): 17–22.

9. Mccarty, M.F. "Does regular ethanol consumption promote insulin sensitivity and leanness by stimulating AMP-activated protein kinase?" *Medical Hypotheses* 57, no. 3 (2001): 405–07. doi:10.1054/mehy.2001.1404.

10. Oneta, C. M. et al. "First pass metabolism of ethanol is strikingly influenced by the speed of gastric emptying." *Gut* 43, no. 5 (1998): 612–19. doi:10.1136/gut.43.5.612.

11. Mojzer, Eva Brglez et al. "Polyphenols: Extraction Methods, Antioxidative Action, Bioavailability and Anticarcinogenic Effects." *Molecules* 21, no. 7 (2016): 901. doi:10.3390/ molecules21070901.

12. Chen, Wen-Pin, Tzong-Cherng Chi, Lee-Ming Chuang, and Ming-Jai Su. "Resveratrol enhances insulin secretion by blocking KATP and KV channels of beta cells." *European Journal of Pharmacology* 568, no. 1–3 (2007): 269–77. doi:10.1016/j .ejphar.2007.04.062.

13. Milne, J. C. et al. "Small molecule activators of SIRT1 as therapeutics for the treatment of type 2 diabetes." *Nature* 29, no. 450 (November 2007): 712–6. Accessed August 16, 2017.

Petroni, K., M. Trinei et al. "Dietary cyanidin 3-glucoside from purple corn ameliorates doxorubicin-induced cardiotoxicity in mice." *Nutrition, Metabolism and Cardiovascular Diseases* 27, no. 5 (2017): 462–69. doi:10.1016/j.numecd.2017.02.002.

14. Lila, Mary Ann. "Anthocyanins and Human Health: An In Vitro Investigative Approach." *Journal of Biomedicine and Biotechnology* 2004, no. 5 (2004): 306–13. doi:10.1155/s111072430440401x.

15. Okla, Meshail et al. "Ellagic acid modulates lipid accumulation in primary human adipocytes and human hepatoma Huh7 cells via discrete mechanisms." *The Journal of Nutritional Biochemistry* 26, no. 1 (2015): 82–90. doi:10.1016/j.jnutbio.2014.09.010.

16. Wang, S. et al. "Resveratrol induces brown-like adipocyte formation in white fat through activation of AMP-activated protein kinase (AMPK) α1." *International Journal of Obesity* 39, no. 6 (2015): 967–76. doi:10.1038/ijo.2015.23

17. Momken, I. et al. "Resveratrol prevents the wasting disorders of mechanical unloading by acting as a physical exercise mimetic in the rat." *The FASEB Journal* 25, no. 10 (2011): 3646–660. doi:10.1096/fj.10-177295.

18. Dolinsky, Vernon W. et al. "Improvements in skeletal muscle strength and cardiac function induced by resveratrol during exercise training contribute to enhanced exercise performance in rats." *The Journal of Physiology* 590, no. 11 (2012): 2783–799. doi:10.1113/jphysiol.2012.230490.

19. Balodis, Iris M., Marc N. Potenza, and Mary C. Olmstead. "Binge drinking in undergraduates: relationships with sex, drinking behaviors, impulsivity, and the perceived effects of alcohol." *Behavioural Pharmacology* 20, no. 5–6 (2009): 518–26. doi:10.1097/fbp.0b013e328330c7

20. Giacosa, Attilio et al. "Mediterranean Way of Drinking and Longevity." *Critical Reviews in Food Science and Nutrition* 56, no. 4 (2014): 635–40. doi:10.1080/10408398.2012.747484.

21. Marcadenti, Melissa Markoski, et al. "Molecular Properties of Red Wine Compounds and Cardiometabolic Benefits." *Nutrition and Metabolic Insights*, 2016, 51. doi:10.4137/nmi.s32909.

22. Gepner, Yftach et al. "Differential Effect of Initiating Moderate Red Wine Consumption on 24-h Blood Pressure by Alcohol Dehydrogenase Genotypes: Randomized Trial in Type 2 Diabetes." *American Journal of Hypertension* 29, no. 4 (2015): 476–83. doi:10.1093/ajh/hpv126.

23. Shai, I., et al. "Moderate alcohol intake and markers of inflammation and endothelial dysfunction among diabetic men." *Diabetologia* 47, no. 10 (October 2004): 1760–7. Accessed August 17, 2017.

24. Djousse, L., et al. "Alcohol Consumption and Risk of Cardiovascular Disease and Death in Women: Potential Mediating Mechanisms." *Circulation* 120, no. 3 (2009): 237–44. doi:10.1161/circulationaha.108.832360.

25. Agarwal, D. P. "Cardioprotective Effects Of Light-Moderate Consumption Of Alcohol: A Review Of Putative Mechanisms." *Alcohol and Alcoholism* 37, no. 5 (2002): 409–15. doi:10.1093/alcalc/37.5.409.

26. Jimenez, Monik et al. "Alcohol Consumption and Risk of Stroke in Women." *Stroke* 43, no. 4 (2012): 939–45. doi:10.1161/strokeaha.111.639435.

> Klatsky, A. L., et al. "Alcohol drinking and risk of hospitalization for ischemic stroke." *American Journal of Cardiology* 88, no. 6 (September 15, 2001): 703–6. Accessed August 17, 2017. https://www.ncbi.nlm.nih.gov/pubmed/11564405.

27. Kopp, P. "Resveratrol, a Phytoestrogen Found in Red Wine. A Possible Explanation for the Conundrum of the 'French Paradox'?" *European Journal of Endocrinology* 138, no. 6 (1998): pp. 619–20.

> Streppel, M. T., et al. "Long-term wine consumption is related to cardiovascular mortality and life expectancy independently of moderate alcohol intake: the Zutphen Study." *Journal of Epidemiology & Community Health* 63, no. 7 (2009): 534–40. doi:10.1136/jech.2008.082198.

> Corder, R. et al "Oenology: Red wine procyanidins and vascular health." *Nature* 444, no. 7119 (2006): 566. doi:10.1038/444566a.

28. Harman, D. "Free radical theory of aging: an update: increasing the functional life span." *Annals of the New York Academy of Sciences* 1067 (May 2006): 10–21. Accessed August 17, 2017. https://www.ncbi.nlm.nih.gov/pubmed/16803965.

29. Rizvi, S. I., and P. K. Maurya. "Alterations in antioxidant enzymes during aging in humans." *Molecular Biotechnology* 37, no. 1 (September 2007): 58–61. Accessed August 17, 2017. https://www.ncbi.nlm.nih.gov/pubmed/17914165.

30. Micallef, Michelle, Louise Lexis, and Paul Lewandowski. "Red wine consumption increases antioxidant status and decreases oxidative stress in the circulation of both young and old humans." *Nutrition Journal* 6, no. 1 (2007). doi:10.1186/1475-2891-6-27.

31. Parr, Adrian J. and G. Paul Bolwell. "Phenols in the plant and in man. The potential for possible nutritional enhancement of the diet by modifying the phenols content or profile." *Journal of the Science of Food and Agriculture* 80, no. 7 (May 15, 2000): 985–1012. Accessed August 17, 2017. https://www.researchgate.net/publication/227963605_Phenols_in_the_plant_and_in_man_The_potential_for_possible_nutritional_enhancement_of_the_diet_by_modifying_the_phenols_content_or_profile.

32. Beckman, Carl H. "Phenolic-storing cells: keys to programmed cell death and periderm formation in wilt disease resistance and in general defence responses in plants?" *Physiological and Molecular Plant Pathology* 57, no. 3 (2000): 101–10. doi:10.1006/pmpp.2000.0287.

33. Kris-Etherton, Penny M. et al. "Bioactive compounds in foods: their role in the prevention of cardiovascular disease and cancer." *The American Journal of Medicine* 113, no. 9 (2002): 71–88. doi:10.1016/s0002-9343(01)00995-0.

34. Chatterjee, Ananya and Sandip K. Bandyopadhyay. "Herbal Remedy: An Alternate Therapy of Nonsteroidal Anti-Inflammatory Drug Induced Gastric Ulcer Healing." *Ulcers* 2014 (2014): 1–13. doi:10.1155/2014/361586.

35. Velazquez, K. T. et al. "Quercetin Supplementation Attenuates the Progression of Cancer Cachexia in ApcMin/ Mice." *Journal of Nutrition* 144, no. 6 (2014): 868–75. doi:10.3945/jn.113.188367.

36. Chirumbolo, Salvatore. "Role of quercetin in vascular physiology." *Canadian Journal of Physiology and Pharmacology* 90, no. 12 (2012): 1652–657. doi:10.1139/y2012-137.

37. Boelsterli, Urs A., Matthew R. Redinbo, and Kyle S. Saitta. "Multiple NSAID-Induced Hits Injure the Small Intestine: Underlying Mechanisms and Novel Strategies." *Toxicological Sciences* 131, no. 2 (2012): 654–67. doi:10.1093/toxsci/kfs310.

38. Sandoval-Acuña, Cristian, et al. "Inhibition of mitochondrial complex I by various non-steroidal anti-inflammatory drugs and its protection by quercetin via a coenzyme Q-like action." *Chemico-Biological Interactions* 199, no. 1 (2012): 18–28. doi:10.1016/j.cbi.2012.05.006.

39. Tanigawa, Tomoko et al. "( )-Catechin protects dermal fibroblasts against oxidative stress-induced apoptosis." *BMC Complementary and Alternative Medicine* 14, no. 1 (2014): doi:10.1186/1472-6882-14-133

40. Pandey, Kanti Bhooshan and Syed Ibrahim Rizvi. "Plant Polyphenols as Dietary Antioxidants in Human Health and Disease." *Oxidative Medicine and Cellular Longevity* 2, no. 5 (2009): 270–78. doi:10.4161/oxim.2.5.9498.

41. Acquaviva, R. et al. "Cyanidin and cyanidin 3-O-β-D-glucoside as DNA cleavage protectors and antioxidants." *Cell Biology and Toxicology* 19, no. 4 (2003): 243–52. doi:10.1023/b:cbto.0000003974.27349.4e

42. Lila, Mary Ann. "Anthocyanins and Human Health: An In Vitro Investigative Approach." *Journal of Biomedicine and Biotechnology*, no. 5 (2004): 306–13. doi:10.1155/s111072430440401x

43. Hou, De-Xing. "Potential Mechanisms of Cancer Chemoprevention by Anthocyanins." *Current Molecular Medicine* 3, no. 2 (2003): 149–59. doi:10.2174/1566524033361555

44. Mccalley, Audrey, et al. "Resveratrol and Calcium Signaling: Molecular Mechanisms and Clinical Relevance." *Molecules* 19, no. 6 (2014): 7327–340. doi:10.3390/molecules19067327

45. Tillu, Dipti V. et al. "Resveratrol Engages AMPK to Attenuate ERK and mTOR Signaling in Sensory Neurons and Inhibits Incision-Induced Acute and Chronic Pain." *Molecular Pain* 8 (2012). doi:10.1186/1744-8069-8-5

46. Peltz, Lindsay et al. "Resveratrol Exerts Dosage and Duration Dependent Effect on Human Mesenchymal Stem Cell Development." *PLoS ONE* 7, no. 5 (2012). doi:10.1371/journal.pone.0037162

47. Markus, M. Andrea, and Brian J. Morris. "Resveratrol in prevention and treatment of common clinical conditions of aging." *Clinical Interventions in Aging* 3, no. 2 (June 2008): 331–39. https://www.ncbi.nlm.nih.gov/pmc/articles/PMC2546476/
    Barger, Jamie L. et al "A Low Dose of Dietary Resveratrol Partially Mimics Caloric Restriction and Retards Aging Parameters in Mice." *PLoS ONE* 3, no. 6 (2008). doi:10.1371/journal.pone.0002264

48. Kosuru, Ramoji, et al. "Promising therapeutic potential of pterostilbene and its mechanistic insight based on preclinical evidence." *European Journal of Pharmacology* 789 (2016): 229–43. doi:10.1016/j.ejphar.2016.07.046.

49. Prinz, J. F. and P. W. Lucas. "Saliva tannin interactions." *Journal of Oral Rehabilitation*

27, no. 11 (November 2000): 991–4. Accessed August 17, 2017. https://www.ncbi.nlm.nih.gov/pubmed/11106991.

50. Giacosa, Attilio et al. "Mediterranean Way of Drinking and Longevity." *Critical Reviews in Food Science and Nutrition* 56, no. 4 (2014): 635–40. doi:10.1080/10408398.2012.747484.

51. Stampfer, Meir J., et al. "Effects of Moderate Alcohol Consumption on Cognitive Function in Women." *New England Journal of Medicine* 352, no. 3 (2005): 245–53. doi:10.1056/nejmoa041152.

    Espeland, M. A. et al. "Association between alcohol intake and domain-specific cognitive function in older women." *Neuroepidemiology* 27, no. 1 (May 24, 2006): 1–12. Accessed August 17, 2017: https://www.ncbi.nlm.nih.gov/pubmed/16717476.

    Scholey, A. B., and K. A. Fowles. "Retrograde enhancement of kinesthetic memory by alcohol and by glucose." *Neurobiology of Learning and Memory* 78, no. 2 (September 2002): 477–83. Accessed August 17, 2017. https://www.ncbi.nlm.nih.gov/pubmed/12431432.

52. Aquilano, Katia, et al. "Role of Nitric Oxide Synthases in Parkinson's Disease: A Review on the Antioxidant and Anti-inflammatory Activity of Polyphenols." *Neurochemical Research* 33, no. 12 (2008): 2416–426. doi:10.1007/s11064-008-9697-6.

53. Weyerer, S. et al. "Current alcohol consumption and its relationship to incident dementia: results from a 3-year follow-up study among primary care attenders aged 75 years and older." *Age and Ageing* 40, no. 4 (2011): 456–63. doi:10.1093/ageing/afr007.

54. Zuccala, Giuseppe et al. "Dose-Related Impact of Alcohol Consumption on Cognitive Function in Advanced Age: Results of a Multicenter Survey." *Alcoholism: Clinical and Experimental Research* 25, no. 12 (2001): 1743–748. doi:10.1111/j.1530-0277.2001.tb02185.x.

55. Singh, Manjeet et al. "Challenges for Research on Polyphenols from Foods in Alzheimer's Disease: Bioavailability, Metabolism, and Cellular and Molecular Mechanisms." *Journal of Agricultural and Food Chemistry* 56, no. 13 (2008): 4855–873. doi:10.1021/jf0735073.

56. Lila, Mary Ann. "Anthocyanins and Human Health: An In Vitro Investigative Approach." *Journal of Biomedicine and Biotechnology* 2004, no. 5 (2004): 306–13. doi:10.1155/s111072430440401x.

57. Kennedy, D. O. et al. "Effects of resveratrol on cerebral blood flow variables and cognitive performance in humans: a double-blind, placebo-controlled, crossover investigation." *American Journal of Clinical Nutrition* 91, no. 6 (2010): 1590–597. doi:10.3945/ajcn.2009.28641.

58. Scholey, Andrew, et al. "Effects of resveratrol and alcohol on mood and cognitive function in older individuals." *Nutrition and Aging* 2, no. 2,3 (2014): 133–138. Accessed August 17, 2017.

59. Esteban-Fernández, A., C. et al. "Neuroprotective Effects of Selected Microbial-Derived Phenolic Metabolites and Aroma Compounds from Wine in Human SH-SY5Y Neuroblastoma Cells and Their Putative Mechanisms of Action." *Frontiers in Nutrition* 4 (2017). doi:10.3389/fnut.2017.00003.

60. Schrieks, Ilse C. et al. "The Biphasic Effects of Moderate Alcohol Consumption with a Meal on Ambiance-Induced Mood and Autonomic Nervous System Balance: A Randomized Crossover Trial." *PLoS ONE* 9, no. 1 (2014). doi:10.1371/journal.pone.0086199.

61. Gea, Alfredo et al. "Alcohol intake, wine consumption and the development of depression: the PREDIMED study." *BMC Medicine* 11, no. 1 (2013). doi:10.1186/1741-7015-11-192.

62. Marcadenti, Melissa Markoski, Juliano Garavaglia, Aline Oliveira, and Jessica Olivaes. "Molecular Properties of Red Wine Compounds and Cardiometabolic Benefits." *Nutrition and Metabolic Insights*, 2016, 51. doi:10.4137/nmi.s32909.

63. Saleem, T.S. Mohamed and S. Darbar Basha. "Red wine: A drink to your heart." *Journal of Cardiovascular Disease Research* 1, no. 4 (2010): 171–76. doi:10.4103/0975-3583.74259.

64. Gepner, Yftach et al. "Effects of Initiating Moderate Alcohol Intake on Cardiometabolic Risk in Adults With Type 2 Diabetes." *Annals of Internal Medicine* 163, no. 8 (2015): 569. doi:10.7326/m14-1650.

65. Carrigan, Matthew A. et al. "Hominids adapted to metabolize ethanol long before human-directed fermentation." *Proceedings of the National Academy of Sciences* 112, no. 2 (2014): 458–63. doi:10.1073/pnas.1404167111.

66. Dudley, R. "Ethanol, Fruit Ripening, and the Historical Origins of Human Alcoholism in Primate Frugivory." *Integrative and Comparative Biology* 44, no. 4 (2004): 315–23. doi:10.1093/icb/44.4.315.

67. Dani, C. et al. "Phenolic content and antioxidant activities of white and purple juices manufactured with organically- or conventionally-produced grapes." *Food and Chemical Toxicology* 45, no. 12 (2007): 2574–580. doi:10.1016/j.fct.2007.06.022.

68. Breslow, Rosalind A., Ph.D., M.P.H., R.D, and Kenneth J. Mukamal, M.D. "Measuring the Burden—Current and Future Research trends: Results From the nIAAA Expert Panel on Alcohol and Chronic disease Epidemiology." *NIH: National Institute on Alcohol Abuse and Alcoholism*. Accessed August 16, 2017. https://pubs.niaaa.nih.gov/publications/arcr352/250-259.pdf.

69. Thomasson, Holly R. "Gender Differences in Alcohol Metabolism." *Recent Developments in Alcoholism* (2002): 163–79. doi:10.1007/0-306-47138-8_9.

70. Kwo, Paul Y. et al "Gender differences in alcohol metabolism: Relationship to liver volume and effect of adjusting for body mass." *Gastroenterology* 115, no. 6 (1998): 1552–557. doi:10.1016/s0016-5085(98)70035-6.

71. Milton, K. "Ferment in the Family Tree: Does a Frugivorous Dietary Heritage Influence Contemporary Patterns of Human Ethanol Use?" *Integrative and Comparative Biology* 44, no. 4 (2004): 304–14. doi:10.1093/icb/44.4.304.

72. Toshikuni, Nobuyuki. "Clinical differences between alcoholic liver disease and nonalcoholic fatty liver disease." *World Journal of Gastroenterology* 20, no. 26 (2014): 8393. doi:10.3748/wjg.v20.i26.8393.

73. Webb, Amy et al. "The Investigation into CYP2E1 in Relation to the Level of

Response to Alcohol Through a Combination of Linkage and Association Analysis." *Alcoholism: Clinical and Experimental Research* 35, no. 1 (2010): 10–18. doi:10.1111/j.1530-0277.2010.01317.x.

74. Joslyn, G. et al. "Chromosome 15q25.1 genetic markers associated with level of response to alcohol in humans." *Proceedings of the National Academy of Sciences* 105, no. 51 (2008): 20368–0373. doi:10.1073/pnas.0810970105.

75. Romeo, Stefano et al. "Genetic variation in PNPLA3 confers susceptibility to nonalcoholic fatty liver disease." *Nature Genetics* 40, no. 12 (2008): 1461–465. doi:10.1038/ng.257.

76. Lewandowska, Hanna, et al. "The role of natural polyphenols in cell signaling and cytoprotection against cancer development." *The Journal of Nutritional Biochemistry* 32 (2016): 1–19. doi:10.1016/j.jnutbio.2015.11.006.

NOTES FOR "YOU!" SECTION, PAGES 169–226

1. Martin, Bronwen, et al. "Sex-Dependent Metabolic, Neuroendocrine, and Cognitive Responses to Dietary Energy Restriction and Excess." *Endocrinology* 148, no. 9 (2007): 4318–333. doi:10.1210/en.2007-0161.

2. Martin, Bronwen, et al. "Conserved and Differential Effects of Dietary Energy Intake on the Hippocampal Transcriptomes of Females and Males." *PLoS ONE* 3, no. 6 (2008). doi:10.1371/journal.pone.0002398.

3. Heilbronn, Leonie L., et al. "Alternate-day fasting in nonobese subjects: effects on body weight, body composition, and energy metabolism." *American Journal of Clinical Nutrition* 81, no. 1 (January 2005): 69–73.

4. Varady, K. A. "Alternate Day Fasting: Effects on Body Weight and Chronic Disease Risk in Humans and Animals." Comparative Physiology of Fasting, Starvation, and Food Limitation, (May 17, 2012): 395–408.

5. Soules, M. R., et al. "Short-term fasting in normal women: absence of effects on gonadotrophin secretion and the menstrual cycle." *Clinical Endocrinology* 40, no. 6 (1994): 725–31. doi:10.1111/j.1365-2265.1994.tb02505.x.

6. Eshghinia, Samira, and Fatemeh Mohammadzadeh. "The effects of modified alternate-day fasting diet on weight loss and CAD risk factors in overweight and obese women." *Journal of Diabetes & Metabolic Disorders* 12:4 (2013): doi: 10.1186/2251-6581-12-4.

7. Shahabi, Sima, et al. "Does Islamic Fasting Affect Gonadotropin around Female Ovulation?" *Royan Institute International Journal of Fertility and Sterility* 4, no. 3 (2010): 94–97.

8. Van Dam, Eveline W. C. M., et al. "Increase in daily LH secretion in response to short-term calorie restriction in obese women with PCOS." *American Journal of Physiology—Endocrinology And Metabolism* 282, no. 4 (2001). doi:10.1152/ajpendo.00458.2001

9. Nonino-Borges, Carla Barbosa, et al. "Influence of meal time on salivary circadian cortisol rhythms and weight loss in obese women." *Nutrition* 23, no. 5 (2007): 385–91. doi:10.1016/j.nut.2007.02.007.

10. Hayward, Sara, et al. "Effects of intermittent fasting on markers of body composition

and mood state." *Journal of the International Society of Sports Nutrition* 11, no. Suppl 1 (2014). doi:10.1186/1550-2783-11-s1-p25.

11. Dohm, G. L., et al. "Influence of fasting on glycogen depletion in rats during exercise." *Journal of Applied Physiology* 55, no. 3 (September 1983): 830–33.

12. Proeyen, Karen Van, et al. "Training in the fasted state improves glucose tolerance during fat-rich diet." *The Journal of Physiology* 588, no. 21 (2010): 4289–302. doi:10.1113/jphysiol.2010.196493.

13. Varady, K. A. "Intermittent versus daily calorie restriction: which diet regimen is more effective for weight loss?" *Obesity Reviews* 12, no. 7 (2011). doi:10.1111/j .1467-789x.2011.00873.x.

14. Harvie, Michelle, et al. "The effect of intermittent energy and carbohydrate restriction v. daily energy restriction on weight loss and metabolic disease risk markers in overweight women." *British Journal of Nutrition* 110, no. 08 (2013): 1534–547. doi:10.1017/ s0007114513000792.

15. Intermountain Medical Center. "Routine periodic fasting is good for your health, and your heart, study suggests." *ScienceDaily* (May 20, 2011). Accessed August 16, 2017. https://www.sciencedaily.com/releases/2011/04/110403090259.htm.

16. Arnal, Marie-Agnès, et al. "Protein Feeding Pattern Does Not Affect Protein Retention in Young Women." *Journal of Nutrition* 130, no. 7 (July 1, 2000): 1700–704.

17. Carlson, Olga, et al. "Impact of reduced meal frequency without caloric restriction on glucose regulation in healthy, normal-weight middle-aged men and women." Metabolism 56, no. 12 (2007): 1729–734. doi:10.1016/j.metabol.2007.07.018.

18. Bhutani, Surabhi, et al. "Effect of exercising while fasting on eating behaviors and food intake." *Journal of the International Society of Sports Nutrition* 10, no. 1 (2013): 50. doi:10.1186/1550-2783-10-50.

19. Proeyen, Karen Van, et al. "Training in the fasted state improves glucose tolerance during fat-rich diet." *The Journal of Physiology* 588, no. 21 (2010): 4289–302. doi:10.1113/jphysiol.2010.196493.

20. Desbrow, Ben, et al. "The effects of different doses of caffeine on endurance cycling time trial performance." *Journal of Sports Sciences* 30, no. 2 (2012): 115–20. doi:10.108 0/02640414.2011.632431.

21. Wan, Ruiqian, Simonetta Camandola, and Mark P. Mattson. "Intermittent Food Deprivation Improves Cardiovascular and Neuroendocrine Responses to Stress in Rats." *Journal of Nutrition* 133, no. 6 (June 1, 2003): 1921–29. Accessed August 16, 2017.

22. Zangeneh, Farideh, et al. "The Effect of Ramadan Fasting on Hypothalamic Pituitary Ovarian (HPO) Axis in Women with Polycystic Ovary Syndrome." *Women's Health Bulletin*, no. 1 (2014). doi:10.17795/intjsh-18962.

23. Ogden, Cynthia L., et al. "Trends in Obesity Prevalence Among Children and Adolescents in the United States, 1988–1994 Through 2013–2014." *Journal of American Medical Association* 315, no. 21 (2016): 2292. doi:10.1001/jama.2016.6361.

24. Reynolds, N. C., and R. Montgomery. "Using the Argonne diet in jet lag preven-

tion: deployment of troops across nine time zones." *Military Medicine* 167, no. 6 (June 2002): 451–3.

25. Quinn, Jeffrey M., et al. "Can't Control Yourself? Monitor Those Bad Habits." *Personality and Social Psychology Bulletin* 36, no. 4 (2010): 499–511. doi:10 .1177/0146167209360665.

26. Harvey, Kirsty, Eva Kemps, and Marika Tiggemann. "The nature of imagery processes underlying food cravings." *British Journal of Health Psychology* 10, no. 1 (2005): 49–56. doi:10.1348/135910704x14249.

NOTES FOR THE "HOW?" SECTION, PAGES 227–268

1. Yamaguchi, Takahiro, et al "Antibiotic Residue Monitoring Results for Pork, Chicken, and Beef Samples in Vietnam in 2012–2013." *Journal of Agricultural and Food Chemistry* 63, no. 21 (2015): 5141–145. doi:10.1021/jf505254

2. Mesnage, Robin, et al. "Major Pesticides Are More Toxic to Human Cells Than Their Declared Active Principles." *BioMed Research International* (2014): 1–8. doi:10.1155/2014/179691.

3. USDA. "United States Standards for Livestock and Meat Marketing Claims, Grass (Forage) Fed Claim for Ruminant Livestock and the Meat Products Derived From Such Livestock." AMS.USDA.gov. Accessed August 18, 2017. https://www. ams.usda.gov/sites/default/files/media/Grass%20Fed%20Standard%20%20 %28WITHDRAWN%29.pdf.

4. Yamaguchi, Tomoko, et al. "Radical-Scavenging Activity of Vegetables and the Effect of Cooking on Their Activity." F*ood Science and Technology Research* 7, no. 3 (2001): 250–57. doi:10.3136/fstr.7.250.

5. Li, Ling, et al. "Influence of Various Cooking Methods on the Concentrations of Volatile N-Nitrosamines and Biogenic Amines in Dry-Cured Sausages." *Journal of Food Science* 77, no. 5 (2012). doi:10.1111/j.1750-3841.2012.02667.x

   Jinap, S., et al. "Effects of varying degrees of doneness on the formation of Heterocyclic Aromatic Amines in chicken and beef satay." *Meat Science* 94, no. 2 (2013): 202–07. doi:10.1016/j.meatsci.2013.01.013

6. Jiménez-Monreal, A. M., et al. "Influence of Cooking Methods on Antioxidant Activity of Vegetables." *Journal of Food Science* 74, no. 3 (2009). doi:10 .1111/j.1750-3841.2009.01091.x

Index

vegetarian diet, 70–72, 272. *see also* in recipes
vinegar, 56
vitamin D, 16, 74

W

water, 75–76, 134–35, 245
weight
gain, 44–46, 86, 130–31, 135–36, 138, 146–47, 149, 197, 200–1, 206
water (*continued*)
loss, 66, 79–80, 84–86, 123–25, 127–29, 136, 138, 146–47, 176–77, 192–93, 194, 197, 210
maintaining, 137, 148
what to shop, 244–45
wheat allergy, 12
wheat germ agglutinin (WGA), 14
where to shop, 240–43
white potatoes, 60–61
white rice, 61
white wine, 168, 265
whole chickens, 244
whole grains, 10, 15, 16, 21

wholesale, 241
willpower, 46–47, 97–99
window approach, 110–11, 196
wine
and antioxidants, 151–57, 167–68
consumption, 165–66
and enhancement, 158–161
health benefits, 166–68
and longevity, 151–57
pairing guide, 263–68
and Paleo, 56–57, 162–64
pairing, 263–68
and polyphenols, 152–57
and toxins, 164–65
weight benefits, 148
white, 168, 265
women. *see* female fasters
workaholic faster, 187–89

Y

"yes!" list considerations, *49–50*, 51–57

Z

zonulin protein, 11–12